The K Factor

The *K* Factor

Reversing and Preventing High Blood Pressure without Drugs

Richard Moore, M.D., Ph.D.

George Webb, Ph.D.

MACMILLAN PUBLISHING COMPANY
New York

Copyright © 1986 by Richard D. Moore and George D. Webb

All rights reserved.
No part of this book may be reproduced or transmitted in any form or by any
means, electronic or mechanical, including photocopying, recording or by any
information storage and retrieval system, without permission in writing from
the Publisher.

MACMILLAN PUBLISHING COMPANY
866 Third Avenue, New York, N.Y. 10022
Collier Macmillan Canada, Inc.

Library of Congress Cataloging-in-Publication Data
Moore, Richard, M.D., Ph.D.
The K factor.

Includes bibliographies and index.
1. Hypertension—Nutritional aspects—Popular
works.   2. Hypertension—Diet therapy—Popular works.
3. Potassium in the body.   4. Potassium—Physiological
effect.   I. Webb, George.   II. Title.   [DNLM: 1. Diet,
Sodium-Restricted—popular works.   2. Hypertension—
prevention & control—popular works.   3. Potassium—
popular works.   WG 340 M823k]
RC685.H8M57   1986   616.1'320654   86-4
ISBN 0-02-586190-5
                                                    •

Macmillan books are available at special discounts for bulk purchases for
sales promotions, premiums, fund-raising, or educational use. For details,
contact:

Special Sales Director
Macmillan Publishing Company
866 Third Avenue
New York, N.Y. 10022

10   9   8   7   6   5   4   3   2   1

Printed in the United States of America

This book is not intended as a
substitute for medical advice of
physicians. The reader should
regularly consult a physician in
general and particularly for any
symptoms. Because of individual
variations and the need for personal
monitoring during any health or life-
style transition, the reader should
also consult a physician before
embarking on the program described.

Contents

Acknowledgments

We would like to express our appreciation to the following who reviewed substantial parts of the book. Because of the wide range of material covered, their constructive criticism in their respective areas of expertise was essential. Especially encouraging was the spirit of cooperation with which criticism was given.

Lavon Bartel, Ph.D., Department of Human Nutrition and Foods, University of Vermont, Burlington (Chapter 10)

John Crabbé, M.D., University of Catholic Louvain, School of Medicine, Bruxelles (Chapters 6 and 7)

Mark Cohen, Ph.D., Professor of Anthropology, SUNY and University of Cambridge (Chapter 3)

Robert Kochan, Ph.D., Biodynamics Laboratory, University of Wisconsin, Madison (Chapter 11)

Jarek Kolonowski, M.D., University of Catholic Louvain, School of Medicine, Bruxelles (Chapters 6 and 7)

Wayne A. Gavryck, M.D., Internal Medicine, Turners Falls, MA (Chapter 24)

Judith Hallfrisch, Ph.D., Gerontology Research Center, National Institutes of Health, Baltimore (Chapter 10)

David W. Maughan, Ph.D., Department of Physiology and Biophysics, University of Vermont, College of Medicine, Burlington (Chapter 21)

H. Lawrence McCrorey, Ph.D., Department of Physiology and Biophysics, University of Vermont, College of Medicine, Burlington (Chapter 22)

Lorin J. Mullins, Ph.D., Department of Biophysics, University of Maryland School of Medicine, Baltimore (several chapters)

Henry Overbeck, M.D., Cardiovascular Research and Training Center, University of Alabama School of Medicine, Birmingham (Chapters 6 and 7)

Ethan Sims, M.D., University of Vermont, College of Medicine, Burlington (Chapters 6, 7, 9, and 12)

Ray Sjodin, Ph.D., Department of Biophysics, University of Maryland, Baltimore (Chapter 6)

Richard Steinhardt, Ph.D., Department of Zoology, University of California, Berkeley (Chapters 6 and 7)

Stahl Waterhouse, Ph.D., Department of Biological Sciences, SUNY, Plattsburg (Chapter 23)

Rachael Yeater, Ph.D., Human Performance Laboratory, West Virginia University, Morgantown (Chapter 11)

H. Allan Walker, M.D., Internal Medicine, Plattsburgh (Chapter 24)

Special appreciation to author Douglas Terman and to Dr. Lorin Mullins for urging me to write this book. Both Doug and Lorin have helped me sharpen my thoughts on many subjects. Special appreciation to Barb, whose support enabled much of the research on insulin to come into this world, and to Charlie, whose participation extended far beyond anything he might have imagined.   —RM

Foremost, thanks to my wife and family who put up with my preoccupation with the writing of this book, my weekend absences from home while holed up at Dick's house writing, and my piles of reprints all over our house.   —GW

We are both grateful to Allan Edmands, for editing the manuscript to improve its readability for the lay person. Among those at Macmillan who have helped edit the book, Alexia Dorszynski and Jill Herbers have earned our special appreciation. Thanks also goes to Oscar Dalem, for keeping our computers going through thick and thin. We appreciate the excellent drawings by Gary Nelson, and Seddon Johnson for the pictures on the overleaf. We are grateful to John Pizzonia for his tireless efforts with a variety of detail work related to this work.

And finally, special thanks goes to George's wife Norma who developed the majority of the recipes and tested them on his family. Norma also spent countless hours helping develop the menu plans and other parts of Chapter 10.

How to Use This Book

The K Factor can be read several ways. The section called "Straight Talk" actually provides a summary of the whole book, so be sure to read it.

Parts I and II are introductory; they tell you what the problem is, and what the answer is. The program will be more effective if you become familiar with this information. There are three different ways you can do this, but however you do it, you must read Chapter 1 in its entirety. After that, you can read the material straight through, skip part or all of any given chapter and read its summary, or read only the summaries at the end of each chapter and the summary of Part II.

Part III is the program. You can read this material before, during, or after you become acquainted with the material in Parts I and II. If you are going to embark on the program, it is essential that you read the introduction to Part III, as well as Chapter 9 in its entirety, first. Be certain to read pages 143 to 146 in Chapter 10 before starting the menu plan. Also, read Chapter 16 ("Keep Track of Your Blood Pressure") and consult the tally sheet and progress chart in Part IV before you start the program.

In Part V, we discuss why it has taken so long to realize that drugs are not the best answer for high blood pressure; we also talk about what constitutes scientific proof. Part VI provides information about salt, about the role of the kidneys and hormones in high blood pressure, and about what drugs do and how they do it. While reading these chapters will deepen your understanding of the program we advocate and give additional basis for our claims, they are not "required reading." You'll be able to follow and succeed at the program perfectly well without reading them.

Part VIII is written to assist your physician in working with you.

Straight Talk

There are striking examples of facts that have been ignored because the cultural climate was not ready to incorporate them into a consistent theme.

—Ilya Prigogine and Isabelle Stengers

There is now overpowering evidence that high blood pressure, one of the major health problems in the United States today, is usually an unnecessary disease that can easily be avoided and even cured—without drugs. Most cases of high blood pressure result from mistakes we make in preparing our food. Because only a few within the medical establishment have recognized this, we Americans are taking several *billion* dollars worth of drugs each year to treat the *symptoms* of this disease.

These drugs almost always make you feel bad: Lack of energy and decreased sex drive are only two of *many* side effects. Worse, except for the more severe cases of hypertension, aggressive use of drugs has either left unchanged or actually *increased* the rate of death in people with hypertension.

The most common type of high blood pressure—essential (or

primary) hypertension—is mainly the result of nutritional problems, with lack of exercise also playing an important role. The answer, therefore, is not to use drugs to treat a problem of nutrition, but rather to correct the nutritional deficiency itself. People eat their way into high blood pressure, and in this book we're going to tell you how you can *eat your way out of it*. Once you make the necessary changes, you're not only going to have more peace of mind about your blood pressure and greatly diminish your chance of being bedridden or dying of a stroke, but you're going to feel better *each day*.

You've probably already heard about sodium, commonly called salt. Well, part of the problem *is* sodium in the diet. The evidence is very strong that excess sodium, especially sodium chloride (table salt), helps cause essential hypertension.

But cutting down on sodium chloride isn't enough. Until recently, the roles of other important minerals have been generally overlooked; the mineral *potassium* is just as important as sodium, and what really counts is the balance between these two minerals. We call the balance between potassium and sodium the *K Factor* (K is the chemical symbol for potassium). We'll also show you that there is a probable connection between the *K Factor* and the commonly recognized contributors to high blood pressure: obesity and lack of exercise.

This new understanding of the cause of essential hypertension makes it possible to prevent or to get rid of this problem. By using the simple guides in this book, you're not going to have to sacrifice much. You will need to give up eating only *a very few things*. Mostly, what you will need to do is learn a few simple principles about preparing food so it retains its natural amount of the *K Factor*.

New Insight into Hypertension

How do we know that the *K Factor* works? We first came to realize that it is the *balance* between sodium and potassium that is important for hypertension through our research on the mechanism that regulates exchange of potassium for sodium in the body. This mechanism, called the sodium-potassium pump, is present in every body cell. By moving potassium into the cell in exchange for sodium, the pump keeps the amount of potassium high inside body cells and the amount of sodium low. In Part II, we discuss why the sodium-potassium pump is so important to life processes and to the state of your health.

As we did our research, we became aware of recent evidence that indicates that the sodium-potassium pump plays an important role in regulating cells that control blood pressure. Since this pump moves sodium and potassium in opposite directions, it seemed likely to us that potassium in the diet should produce an effect on the body opposite to dietary sodium. If diets low in sodium are good, diets high in potassium should also be good. In other words, since the normal function of the cell requires exchange of potassium for sodium, *exchange* of dietary potassium for sodium is the key.

Several other basic scientists have come to the same realization that an imbalance of these minerals can lead to high blood pressure. So too little potassium in the diet is as bad, and has essentially the same effect, as too much sodium. Too much sodium is bad. Too little potassium is bad. Too much sodium *and* too little potassium can be deadly. As we will see, when these factors are coupled with a lack of magnesium and calcium in the diet, the effect is even worse. But the real key is a proper balance between sodium and potassium. The *K Factor* is a measure of this balance.

Because the sodium-potassium pump keeps our body cells full of potassium, our bodies contain more potassium than sodium. In our bodies the balance (or ratio) between potassium and sodium (the *K Factor*) is high, with a value over 2. The *K Factor* is also naturally high in animals, and even higher in plants. So it is not surprising that we should be eating food with a high *K Factor*. Unfortunately, the diet of most Americans is often too high in the problem ingredient (sodium chloride) and too low in the good ingredients (potassium, calcium, and magnesium). In other words, the standard diet is too low in the *K Factor*.

Although most of the food we eat has a high *K Factor* in its natural form, by the time the commercial food processors are through with it and we cook it at home, the *K Factor* is reduced almost *tenfold*. In the preparation of the typical American meal, we tend to exchange the naturally abundant amounts of potassium in food for sodium. As you'll see in Chapter 3, this is especially true in the commercial preparation of canned foods, some frozen foods, and most fast foods (which are also fat foods).

So it's not so much what we eat, but the way it's prepared in the factory and in the home that causes problems. We have gotten into habits of food preparation that flip-flop the natural balance of potassium to sodium—actually reversing it! So the *K Factor* is greatly decreased. That's where the trouble starts, and that's where high blood pressure starts.

Lack of exercise and obesity compound the nutritional imbalance. As we will show later, the reason both weight reduction and exercise help return blood pressure to normal may well be that they assist the body's mechanisms that maintain a proper balance between potassium and sodium in each cell. In the 30 percent of people who inherit a genetic tendency toward hypertension, this man-made imbalance in our food overpowers the mechanisms in body cells that normally maintain a healthy balance between sodium and potassium. The imbalance leads to high blood pressure.

So it's not surprising that in those hypertensive patients who merely go on a low sodium diet, blood pressure is reduced in only about half. What is called for instead is a balancing of sodium and potassium, which can cure most cases of hypertension.

People Who Prepare Their Food Right Don't Have Hypertension

If a deficiency in the *K Factor* really is the main cause of high blood pressure, this condition should be uncommon in people who eat natural, unprocessed food (with its normally high potassium and low sodium or high *K Factor*). Sure enough, studies had already been made of populations in nonindustrialized areas all over the world where, we now realize, the people eat food with a naturally high *K Factor*. In none of these groups does *more than one percent* of the people have high blood pressure. Contrast this with industrialized countries such as the United States, where *about a third of the adults* have high blood pressure. When people from these native groups start eating food processed and cooked the way the typical American diet is, they develop just as much high blood pressure as we do. So these results are totally consistent with our conclusion.

Treating Hypertension with K Factor Already Tried—It Works

When it became clear to us that potassium and the *K Factor* have been the **missing connection** in the treatment of hypertension, we began wondering if anyone had ever used the *K Factor* to actually treat high blood pressure. This isn't mentioned in medical textbooks or taught in medical schools but we thought we would check further just to make sure. Since increasing dietary potassium in exchange for sodium (increasing the *K Factor*) is such a simple thing to do, and yet has not been a standard part of the treatment of hypertension, we had not expected to find medical reports that such a simple step could help restore blood pressure to normal.

It took us a while to find the references, but to our surprise, we discovered that this procedure had *already been shown to work* in people with hypertension. In fact, it has been demonstrated over and over again—in at least a dozen different scientific reports, beginning as early as 1928—that essential hypertension can be cured by increasing the amount of *K Factor* that people eat. Every time it was tried, it worked in at least two-thirds of the people!

In Part II we discuss some of these medical studies where the *K Factor* was increased toward what we consider the "normal" range. In most patients the blood pressure fell back to normal levels! In one carefully designed study from Australia in 1982, patients with essential hypertension were changed from a "normal" diet, which had a *K Factor* of less than 1, to a diet with a *K Factor* of about 6.6. 80 percent had very significant improvement in their hypertension and were able either to decrease the dose of drugs they had been taking or to stop taking them altogether.

In the meantime, George used the *K Factor* to bring his high blood pressure—160/100—down to 125/75 (well within the "normal" range) without any drugs at all! ("Doctor, heal thyself.")

Although he didn't realize he was doing it, Nathan Pritikin introduced one of the best known applications of the *K Factor* with his program which primarily involves diet and exercise to promote health. Pritikin long ago noticed that one of the things his program accomplished was the lowering of blood pressure in those with hypertension. This program has begun to get support from the medical establishment, although they don't yet recognize that, as far as blood pressure is concerned, the *K Factor* is much the most important thing. And other pioneers, such as Dr. Walter Kempner, using a diet with a good *K Factor* did not know *why* their programs worked.

The advantage of understanding why these programs work is that you can better tailor the program to your own life-style. Several of the programs that work, including Nathan Pritikin's Program and Dr. Cleaves Bennett's approach, require major changes in life-style. Maybe you won't have the inclination or time for a major change in life-style. Well, don't throw up your hands: although such things as meditation, relaxation techniques, or biofeedback are good, they aren't as important for your blood pressure as how you eat—*especially how your food is prepared*—and whether or not you exercise. You may not have time to do everything that would help, but you **can** find time to eat food prepared so that it retains the *K Factor.*

Once you understand the simple principles, it isn't necessary to limit yourself to foods such as rice and fruit juice, as in Kempner's diet. You can eat *almost anything*, providing it is prepared right. And you can do it so your food will have pretty much the same taste as you're already used to.

As chance would have it, some groups of people living in industrialized countries, such as Israel and Japan, have *unwit-*

tingly tried this approach—with success. The stories of these, and other groups of people who avoid hypertension by eating properly, are told in Chapter 3.

Why Not Known Before Now?

If this really works so well, why hasn't the establishment gotten on the band wagon? Why haven't you already heard about it? We'll discuss this more in Part V, but for now consider these facts. Whereas universities and medical schools used to provide the salary for most of their faculty, now most of the faculty in a medical school have to get grants in order to get part or all of their salaries. Without a grant, at best they'll lose some of their salaries or, at worst, their jobs. And to get a grant, it helps to not be controversial, to stick to safe and accepted ways of doing things—and to accepted ideas. Since each grant is reviewed by about a dozen people and it's possible that even one can sink it, it pays to not make waves—or enemies.

On top of that, some of the grants for high blood pressure research come from drug companies. The sales on just *one* of the drugs sold to people with high blood pressure netted over one-half **billion** dollars in the United States in just this past year. By comparison, how much money do you think can be made by telling people how to keep from getting sick in the first place? Sure, we hope this book makes us some money so we can conduct our research more independently of this system, but even extravagant sales would be *peanuts* compared to what could be made selling drugs for hypertension.

We're confident there isn't any deliberate intention to avoid doing the right thing. In fact, people in the system are under such pressure to specialize and concentrate on details that very few can be expected to have the time to look at the whole picture—to consider the really important issues. And a system like this doesn't exactly encourage going around saying that drugs really aren't the answer after all.

Besides, doctors are taught that it is good medicine to give medicine. The importance of nutrition and exercise has been largely ignored in their training. Not only that, until recently medicine has been almost entirely an art rather than a science. Things had to be done because they seemed to work—and we usually didn't understand why. Doctors have inherited certain ideas about what they should pay attention to.

Like anyone, they can only pay attention to those things they know about and can measure—like blood pressure. Well, it turns out that blood pressure being high is a *symptom* (technically, a "sign") and not the fundamental problem in hypertension. The main problem is that the *K Factor* in the body's cells is too low. Some evidence suggests this may lead to weakened blood vessels, which could blow out more easily even with normal blood pressure. So when drugs are used to get the blood pressure down without increasing the *K Factor*, experience shows you can still have serious problems and even die. On the other hand, animal experiments indicate that the *K Factor* can restore normal health and longevity even if the blood pressure *doesn't* come down. So high blood pressure is a symptom. Treating the symptom with drugs misses the point. Fortunately, the fundamental problem *can* be fixed—by paying attention not only to blood pressure, but especially to the *K Factor* in your diet, and to getting a little regular exercise.

Realizing the Importance of the K Factor

How did we both get from an unquestioning acceptance of the drug approach to our realization that hypertension is a disease of life-style? Our interest in high blood pressure grew out of our own research. But for each of us, it was a long, slow, and sometimes difficult path to come to the realization that in most cases, the answer to hypertension is not drugs, but proper nutrition and exercise.

When everyone around you is doing something a particular way, like treating blood pressure with drugs, it's hard to imagine doing otherwise—especially when doing otherwise might make you liable in a law suit. So during his internship, Dick too prescribed drugs to people with hypertension. Even after returning to full-time research, if he had been asked how to treat high blood pressure, Dick would have recommended drugs, probably diuretics. When George discovered he had high blood pressure, his first reaction was "Uh oh, now I'll have to take drugs"— especially after he found that reducing his dietary sodium wasn't enough to get his blood pressure down to normal. And for years, in his lectures to nursing students, George sometimes talked about hypertension and, of course, discussed the standard textbook treatment—drugs.

So at first, although we realized that extra potassium in the diet should help some cases of high blood pressure, we still couldn't accept the evidence that essential hypertension is a nutritional and life-style problem, even when it was staring us in the face. This was against everything we had been taught.

As we looked further into the matter, evidence kept accumulating that clearly indicated that restoring the *K Factor* in the diet would prevent and cure many cases of hypertension (see Part II). Slowly the evidence kept pushing us both toward the realization that most cases of hypertension are the consequence of modern life-style, primarily due to a nutritional deficiency and, to some extent, lack of exercise. This has been hard for us to accept. It means that one of us participated in treating a nutritional deficiency with drugs! So it's not surprising to us that, until recently, not many physicians have realized that drugs are not the primary answer to hypertension.

Once we realized that eating food with the proper *K Factor* will prevent and even cure many cases of essential hypertension, we decided this should be presented to the public. This decision involved ethical considerations. We knew we would be criticized for breaking the unwritten rule that doctors should not give information to the public that hasn't been widely accepted and agreed upon by all the authorities.

Although we think the evidence for the important role of the *K Factor* is overpowering, many authorities will not accept any new idea until a very large "controlled" clinical trial, involving hundreds or thousands of people, provides statistics to demonstrate its success. This is true even though hundreds of people have already had their high blood pressure reduced by various programs, all of which involve the *K Factor*. But a large clinical trial such as that described above will take several years to accomplish and may not be possible to do at all (see Chapter 19). Not only that, relying only on statistical studies is an oversimplified way of doing science. In the meantime, should this information be withheld from the public?

We think not. This conclusion was not arrived at lightly. It is based not only on considerable thought, but also on consultation with colleagues and people in other professions. If the program we recommend were a dangerous procedure, a good argument for withholding the information and our conclusions could be made. But how can keeping a natural balance in your food and getting moderate exercise be considered dangerous?

The only danger that we can foresee is if people were to decide to treat their high blood pressure without medical supervision or decide to stop drugs without consulting a physician. This can be very dangerous because, as we discuss in Chapter 9, there *are* cases of high blood pressure which have nothing to do with the *K Factor*. Also, even if drugs should be discontinued in a given patient, this *must* be done with caution, under professional care, since—as we point out later—serious, even lethal, problems can occur if due precautions are not taken.

No doubt in a few years we will have more detailed insight into how the *K Factor* helps hypertension. Many details remain to be worked out. But in the meantime, while the specialists are arguing over the details, dotting i's and crossing t's, a good deal of suffering can be prevented by the safe and simple steps we recommend in this book, so there is no reason to keep the information from the public.

A Bonus to This Approach

One advantage of this program is that it will not only help or cure your high blood pressure, it will greatly decrease your chance of having a heart attack and, according to a recent government study, probably even decrease your chance of getting certain types of cancer. It takes very little time and effort to get these benefits and it won't cost you anything.

The Full Story

In Part I, we state the problem: what high blood pressure is, its dangers, and the less than satisfactory results of using drugs to cure it.

In Part II, we describe the abundant evidence that shows that a high *K Factor* diet is an effective way to cure (and prevent) essential hypertension (for reasons we'll explain, and to avoid the confusion of "essential" with "necessary," we'll call it by its other name—primary hypertension). We also discuss other factors that can influence blood pressure. Parts I and II are provided mainly for background and don't have to be read in detail. The rest of the book gives the more specific hands-on information you'll need for actually following the program.

In Part III, we describe, step by step, how you and your doctor can cure your hypertension—not just treat the symptom.

In Part IV, we show you how to keep track of your progress while following our program.

In Part V, we discuss why the authorities have been so slow to realize the importance of the *K Factor* in primary hypertension.

In Part VI, we provide background information on salt and how the kidneys, hormones, nervous system, and drugs interact in controlling blood pressure.

In Part VII, we provide background information and recommendations for your doctor.

You can begin your journey to normal blood pressure and good health *today*. Just reduce the salt you add to your food, after consulting with your doctor. As you will see, it is important to be off all table salt, both at the table, and in your cooking, for one week before starting the menu plan in Chapter 10. During this time, you can read the book through Part III, stock your kitchen with appropriate foods and condiments (as listed on pages 130 through 134), and *see your doctor to discuss this program* before beginning.

A Final Thought

If you have high blood pressure, you're going to *have* to change your life-style. If you don't do it the way we describe here, you will have to take pills regularly each day and probably put up with consequences such as weakness or loss of sex drive. So taking drugs for high blood pressure is also going to have an effect on your life-style. The choice is up to you and your doctor.

The K Factor

PART ONE
The Problem

The Stepped-Care program suggests initiating therapy with a small dosage of an antihypertensive drug, increasing the dose of that drug, and then adding or substituting one drug after another in gradually increasing doses as needed until goal blood pressure is achieved, side effects become intolerable, or the maximum dose of each drug has been reached.

—Joint National Committee on Detection, Evaluation, and Treatment of High Blood Pressure: 1984 Special Report[1]

If you have high blood pressure, you've got lots of company. It has been estimated that 55 million adult Americans—almost 1 out of every 3—suffer from high blood pressure, or hypertension.[2] This condition is the most common threat to health in the United States.

Hypertension is considered life threatening because people who have high blood pressure run a high risk of dying or becoming crippled for life by a paralyzing stroke, heart failure, or kidney disease. What makes hypertension doubly dangerous is that you can have it and still feel absolutely normal, or even feel

1

great—until you are stricken with one of the grisly consequences of this "silent killer."

If the 55 million Americans afflicted by this condition could feel their blood pressure go up, the news media would be talking about the largest epidemic we have yet seen. Indeed, hypertension has now reached epidemic proportions. And this epidemic is costing many billion dollars a year to treat, to help people avoid the consequences. That figure does not take into account the cost incurred when the consequences strike: the cost of premature deaths or of such incapacitating handicaps as deafness or being bedridden for life with kidney disease, for example.

Twenty-five years ago, it looked as though drugs were the answer for hypertension. Almost everyone thought that.

Within the medical establishment, however, there were a few lone voices of dissent. Dr. Walter Kempner, of Duke University Medical School, kept pointing out that his rice-fruit diet was a proved success for lowering elevated blood pressure.[3] Also, Dr. Lewis Dahl of the Brookhaven National Laboratory[4] and Dr. Lot Page of Tufts University School of Medicine[5] could point to evidence that too much sodium was part of the problem.

But in view of the potency of the new drugs, thiazide diuretics, in decreasing blood pressure, not many people wanted to be bothered with changing their eating habits. As a result, the production of drugs to treat hypertension grew into a multibillion-dollar-a-year industry. That's a lot of dollars! But preventing the terrible consequences of hypertension—the death, the paralysis—seemed worth it. So over the past quarter-century, the use of drugs has become the accepted means of treating everyone with hypertension.

A lot of doctors have grown skeptical of drugs. Because of the frequent unpleasant side effects, many patients on drugs complain that they just don't feel good. But because of legal risks and lack of a good alternative, doctors continue to prescribe drugs for almost everyone with hypertension.

Then, in 1982, came the bombshell that cracked the very foundations of the dogma that drugs are the answer to hypertension. This bombshell was an article in the *Journal of the American*

Medical Association citing evidence that aggressive use of drugs failed to help about half of all the people suffering from hypertension.[6] In some cases, drug treatment actually increased the rate of death.

So far, no one has been able to explain away this evidence, and the significance is beginning to sink in. A major rethinking of the whole problem is underway, with an increased open-mindedness to other approaches, including nutrition. Already some in the medical establishment are beginning to back off from the blanket recommendation that everybody with hypertension be treated with drugs. For example, in late summer of 1985, the Vermont affiliate of the American Heart Association stated: "Changing one's lifestyle is the recommended method of controlling high blood pressure, but . . . may not be enough to control hypertension in everyone."[7]

Before going into specifics about the nondrug approach we're describing, let's look at the types of hypertension that exist and the drugs commonly used to treat them. That's what Part I is about. It's important that you know these facts before deciding how to use the rest of the book.

CHAPTER 1

What Is High Blood Pressure?

What It Isn't

High blood pressure, or *hypertension*, is not the same thing as heart disease, but it can make heart disease worse. By making the heart work too hard, hypertension can help trigger (or be a "risk factor" for) heart attacks.

Both heart disease and hypertension can kill you. Heart disease can cause you to spend the rest of your life with chest pain or shortness of breath. But hypertension can cause you to "stroke out" so that—even if you survive—you spend the rest of your life partially paralyzed, unable to hear, or unable to speak.

There are some similarities in the causes of hypertension and coronary artery heart disease. For a long time, we have understood that coronary artery heart disease is due to mistakes in life-style, especially nutrition (particularly an overindulgence in dietary fat). In this book, we present the evidence that most cases of hypertension are also due to mistakes in life-style—primarily nutrition, but also lack of exercise.

But there are also critical differences in their causes. An important cause of coronary artery heart disease is cholesterol. The most important contributor to hypertension, however, is a low *K Factor* in the food people eat.

Also, high blood pressure is not the same thing as, nor is it due to, "hardening of the arteries"—a layman's term that refers to the cumulative effects of age, poor nutrition, and hypertension upon the arteries.

Finally, hypertension is not a type of nervous tension.

What It Is

Whether or not your doctor decides that you have hypertension depends on how high your blood pressure is. That's all there is to it.

Blood pressure is the pressure the blood exerts against the walls of all your arteries (the large blood vessels that carry blood from your heart to your body's tissues). Your heart creates this blood pressure by pumping blood into the arteries. How can you tell if your blood pressure is too high? You can't—unless it's measured. In fact, almost half of the people with high blood pressure don't realize they have it.[1]

How It's Measured

Your doctor measures your blood pressure by inflating a cuff placed around your arm with enough pressure to squeeze shut the artery inside your arm. By releasing the pressure of the cuff and listening to the sounds of the pulsating blood as the artery reopens, your doctor can determine your blood pressure.

(We'll describe how you can measure your own blood pressure in Part V.)

What the Numbers Mean

There are two different numbers that make up your "blood pressure," and each represents a pressure, the maximum and minimum during a complete pulse cycle. Every blood pressure reading is expressed by these two numbers.

As an example, let's consider a blood pressure reading of 120/80 ("120 over 80"). This is not a fraction, even though it looks like one. The first number is always greater than the second.

The first number is the *systolic blood pressure*—the maximum pressure reached in the arteries while the heart is contracting and thus pumping blood into them. In our example, systolic blood pressure is 120, which is considered normal for a young adult. It's actually 120 *mm Hg*, which means the pressure is sufficient to push a column of mercury up a distance of 120 millimeters (mm), or about 5 inches. *Hg* is the chemical symbol for mercury, whose Latin (scientific) name is *hydrargyrum*, or "water silver."

The second number is the *diastolic blood pressure*—the minimum pressure of the blood, which occurs while the heart is relaxing between beats. In our example, diastolic blood pressure is 80, which is considered normal for a young adult.

The graph in Figure 1 shows how the blood pressure in your arteries changes as the heart beats. The horizontal lines show the "normal" values we used in our example.

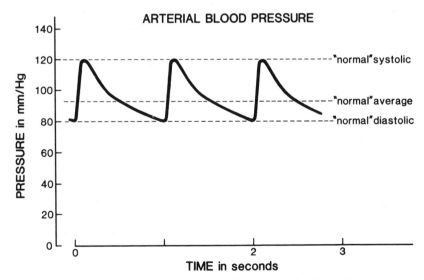

FIGURE 1. *How blood pressure changes as the heart beats.*

Because the heart generally relaxes for longer than it contracts, the diastolic blood pressure is closer to the average blood pressure than the systolic blood pressure is. Partly for this reason, high blood pressure, or hypertension, is usually defined on the basis of diastolic blood pressure.

When Is It High?

You are said to have hypertension if your diastolic blood pressure is 90 or higher or your systolic pressure is 140 or higher.[2] In the United States, a diastolic pressure between 85 and 89 was called normal until recently but is now considered high normal, partly because in 1979, new life insurance company statistics[3] showed that the death rate of people with diastolic pressures of 89 is greater than people with pressures of 80 (see Figure 2, page 10).

Types of Hypertension

There are two types of high blood pressure—*primary* (also called essential) and *secondary*. Of the 55 million hypertensives in this country, only about 5 percent have secondary hypertension. (It is called secondary because it is actually caused by another condition, such as kidney disease or an adrenal gland tumor.) The remaining 95 percent suffer from primary hypertension, a condition that has no "parent" disease.

We can now go a step further: Of the people with hypertension, there are borderline, mild, moderate, and severe cases, depending on the individual's diastolic blood pressure.

Table 1 at the top of the following page shows the breakdown.

And so if, after running tests, your doctor tells you you have primary hypertension and your reading is 130/92, you have a borderline case.

The Danger of Elevated Blood Pressure

But don't let the words *borderline* or *mild* deceive you. Figure 2 illustrates the consequences of having blood pressure above the normal range.

TABLE 1. *Classification of Blood Pressure**

Classification	Diastolic Blood Pressure (mm Hg)
Normal	less than 85
High normal	85–89
Borderline high blood pressure	90–94
Mild high blood pressure	95–104
Moderate high blood pressure	105–114
Severe high blood pressure	115 and over

*In the 1984 Report of the Joint National Committee of Detection, Evaluation, and Treatment of High Blood Pressure[4], this category is combined with "mild" hypertension. Since this is the group in which drugs evidently *increase* mortality, we and others use it to facilitate discussion. All the other categories in this table agree with those of the Joint National Committee.

Notice that your chances of death decrease as your diastolic blood pressure drops below the so-called "normal" value of 80 mm Hg. And with 70, you're even better off than with 75! On the other hand, as your diastolic pressure rises above 90, your chances of death increase dramatically. By the time your diastolic pressure reaches 100, your chance of dying in a given year is doubled! And that is not all: your chances of developing such severe handicaps as loss of hearing, kidney disease, a crippling heart condition, or paralysis due to stroke are greatly increased as your blood pressure gets higher.

Studies have shown that if you have hypertension and bring your blood pressure back to normal, you can reduce the chances of the occurrence of these harmful consequences of hypertension. Knowing these facts, how do you proceed if you have hypertension? The next chapter takes a look at the use of pills to treat high blood pressure.

Summary

Almost one in three American adults eventually develops hypertension. You are said to have hypertension if your diastolic blood

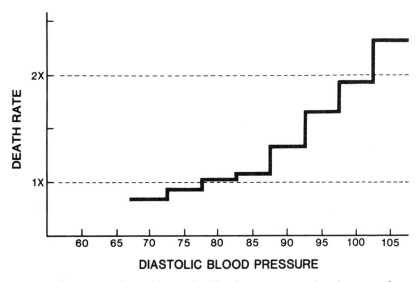

FIGURE 2. *The effect of diastolic blood pressure on the chances of death.* Death rate (read *vertically*): *1*× refers to the "normal" death rate for men and women (averaged together) with diastolic blood pressures 78 to 82 mm Hg; *2*× indicates a death rate twice as high. (Based on data from a large-scale life insurance study released in 1979).[5]

pressure is 90 or above. Although a diastolic pressure of 80 has been considered healthy, life insurance statistics indicate that as the diastolic pressure rises above about 74 mm Hg, the chances of death begin to increase.

High blood pressure kills or cripples people because it greatly increases the chance of a stroke, heart failure, or kidney disease. Because the chance of death increases dramatically as the diastolic pressure goes above 90—almost doubling at 100 mm Hg—you cannot afford to ignore high blood pressure even if you can't feel it. Reducing high blood pressure reduces the chance of death or crippling consequences.

CHAPTER 2

Drugs—The Usual Treatment

High blood pressure kills thousands of people every year and condemns additional thousands to a life of invalidism with paralysis, inability to speak or hear, heart failure, or kidney disease. So it's understandable that over the years, doctors have tried almost every imaginable approach to lowering elevated blood pressure. In the 1950s, the worst cases were sometimes treated by an operation called a *sympathectomy*, which removed some of the nerves that normally maintain blood pressure. Also, many severe cases of hypertension were cured by a special rice-fruit diet developed by Dr. Walter Kempner[1] of Duke University, but this diet was very restricted and tasteless. Dr. Kempner didn't know exactly why it worked, and the 1950s was not a time when the medical establishment was inclined to believe that diseases could be cured by what we do or don't eat.

After the astonishing success of penicillin and other "miracle" drugs during World War II, both doctors and the public were prepared to believe that a drug could be developed for almost anything. So most doctors breathed a sigh of relief at the appearance, in 1957, of the first drugs that could effectively lower elevated blood pressure. They were called *diuretics*.

11

It was very reasonable. Almost no one disagreed: drugs were the answer! After all, drugs got the blood pressure down, and that should put less stress on the arteries and the heart. And drugs were easy: easier than surgery and easier than anything as flaky as nutrition—which nobody believed in anyway. Just take your pills and things will be all right.

Of course, there were some unpleasant side effects, such as weakness, diarrhea, nausea, and loss of sex drive—but everything has its price. And, of course, you had to be prepared to take the pills for life. But they *did* get the blood pressure down, at least most of the time. More to the point, they seemed to be saving lives, since there were fewer deaths in people with hypertension who were treated with drugs.

To produce ever newer drugs designed to lower blood pressure, a whole industry was spawned. Today this industry takes in several *billion* dollars a year[2] in the United States alone. The use of drugs for treating primary hypertension has become the marching order of the day. Until recently, even the Joint National Committee on Detection, Evaluation, and Treatment of High Blood Pressure, a group appointed by the National Institutes of Health (NIH), recommended that doctors use drugs to treat everyone with hypertension.[3] So for the past twenty-five years, doctors treating patients with high blood pressure have typically prescribed drugs as the first line of defense.

But in the last couple of years, our assumptions about the use of drugs have been challenged. As bad as high blood pressure is, there is now reason to believe that drugs may actually *shorten* the life of many people with borderline hypertension.

Before we discuss this new development, let's briefly review the types of drugs that are used, how they're used, what they do, and their side effects.

Types of Drugs

Today the drugs doctors prescribe most often still are *diuretics*, such as chlorothiazide. (See Chapter 23 if you want to understand more about how these and other antihypertensive drugs work.) Their job is to stimulate the elimination of sodium and water through the kidneys. Other drugs include:

○ Inhibitors of sympathetic nerve function, such as propranolol and reserpine.

○ Dilators of blood vessels, such as hydralazine and minoxidil.

How Drugs Are Used

The government-supported Joint National Committee has recommended that when using drugs to treat primary hypertension, doctors follow the "stepped care" procedure, illustrated in Figure 3. As stated in the committee's 1984 report,[4] this approach consists of "initiating therapy with a small dosage of an antihypertensive drug, increasing the dose of that drug, and then adding or substituting *one drug after another* in gradually increasing doses as needed until goal blood pressure is achieved,

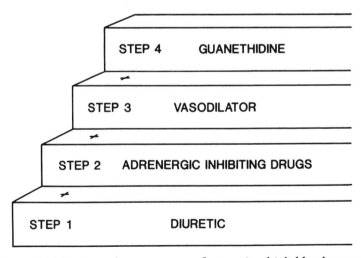

FIGURE 3. *The stepped-care program for treating high blood pressure with drugs.* After trying a "step" without success, the next step is added on top of the drug(s) already being used.

side effects become intolerable, or the maximum dose of each drug has been reached." (Italics ours.)

Until May 1984, the Joint National Committee recommended that doctors almost always use a thiazide diuretic as the first step. For reasons we will mention here and discuss in Chapter 23, it is now recommended that a "beta blocker" (one of the step-2 drugs), which works on nerves that control blood pressure, sometimes be used instead of thiazide diuretics to begin the first step.[5]

In addition to drugs, doctors have sometimes suggested one or more "natural" steps for treating high blood pressure, such as cutting down on salt or losing weight. But the big emphasis has been on drugs.

Side Effects of These Drugs

Besides lowering blood pressure, all these antihypertensive drugs can produce undesirable side effects. This is not surprising, since they alter basic body functions not only in the blood vessels but in the nervous system and kidneys as well.

Typical side effects of some of the more commonly used antihypertensive drugs include urinary loss of potassium, fatigue, gastric irritation, nausea, vomiting, abdominal cramps, diarrhea, dizziness, headache, rash, weakness, nasal congestion, impotence (loss of sex drive), congestive heart failure, mental depression, and loss of short-term memory.[6]

Sometimes other drugs are used to treat these side effects.

How common are these side effects? In a government-sponsored study of over five thousand patients being treated with drugs for high blood pressure, the number of patients who discontinued drug treatment because of side effects during a five-year period ranged from a low of 23 percent for black women to 41 percent for white men.[7] Some side effects are almost always produced by certain drugs but go unnoticed by the patient because laboratory tests are required to see them. For example, thiazide diuretics cause increased loss of potassium through the urine and often increase blood cholesterol, and propranolol (a beta blocker) causes an increase in blood triglycerides (a type of fat that is a risk factor for heart attacks).[8]

The most frequent side effects for each of the commonly used drugs are listed in the table on page 346 in Chapter 23, Antihypertensive Drugs.

Warning: If you are currently taking a drug for high blood pressure, do not suddenly stop taking it on your own, as this could trigger a heart attack, a stroke, or sudden death. *Any* change in your current medication should only be made in consultation with your physician.

The Justification for Using Drugs

The Joint National Committee has recommended the use of drugs with understandable reason: in spite of the many side effects, drugs can be successful in reducing both the damage from and the number of deaths due to hypertension. By the mid 1960s, it had been demonstrated that when they were used for very severe cases of hypertension, drugs could reduce both the complications and the higher death rate.[9] In 1970, a study conducted by the Veterans Administration[10] showed that drugs were effective in reducing fatal and nonfatal complications in those patients with diastolic pressure of 105 mm Hg or higher. The complications that were reduced included stroke, heart failure, kidney failure, and worsening of the hypertension. Recent studies, including one of 10,940 men and women in the United States (Hypertension Detection and Follow-up Program),[11] and another study of 3,427 men and women in Australia (the Australian Therapeutic Trial),[12] have demonstrated that treatment with antihypertensive drugs, designed to lower the blood pressure toward normal, results in an overall decrease in both fatalities and serious complications among patients with mild hypertension.

So in spite of the fact that some physicians had begun to worry about the "increasing number of totally unexpected adverse effects,"[13] for the last twenty-five years, almost all people with primary hypertension have faced the prospect of a lifetime of treatment with drugs.

The "Boomerang" of Drug Treatment

But in 1984, the picture began to change. In 1984, the Joint National Committee issued a Special Report,[14] in which it was recommended—for the first time—that people with borderline hypertension be started on treatment programs that do *not* use drugs.

What happened to trigger the Special Report? The trigger was the completion by the National Institutes of Health of a seven-year study called the Multiple Risk Factor Intervention Trial[15] (or MRFIT, pronounced "Mister Fit"), involving 12,866 men who were judged to be at high risk for heart attacks because they smoked, had elevated serum cholesterol, and had high blood pressure. This study, which cost U.S. taxpayers $100 million, produced a totally unexpected and shocking result. Together with scientific developments discussed in the next few chapters, this finding, along with other scientific advances, is causing a complete rethinking of the treatment and prevention of primary hypertension.

To the surprise of many scientists and doctors, in people with diastolic blood pressure between 94 and 99 mm Hg, the MRFIT study found that even though drugs did lower the blood pressure, there was no evidence that they affected the rate of death. Even more shocking was the finding that for people with borderline hypertension—90 to 94 mm Hg—aggressive use of drugs according to the stepped-care program apparently increased the rate of death. Only for people with diastolic blood pressure greater than 100 mm Hg—moderate or severe hypertension—was the death rate clearly decreased through the use of drugs.

Another study in Australia came up with similar findings. This study reported that in people with mild hypertension, those treated with thiazide diuretics had a higher than expected rate of death and a higher than expected incidence of heart attacks.[16] Moreover, the use of drugs to reduce blood pressure also increased the death rate of those subjects in the MRFIT study who had abnormal electrocardiograms (a record of the electrical activity of the heart). Indeed, this latter finding of the

MRFIT study prompted an editorial in the *Journal of the American Medical Association* which commented that the implications of these surprising findings are so major as to demand caution and would cause considerable debate and prompt follow-up studies *"since the results fly in the face of current medical dogma and practice"*[17] (italics ours).

New Recommendations

The Joint National Committee's Special Report[18] now recommends that drugs not be used, at least initially, if "risk factors" are absent and the diastolic blood pressure is between 90 and 94 mm Hg. Risk factors include elevated blood cholesterol, family history of heart disease, having a smoking habit, and experiencing emotional stress. These factors are conditions known to increase greatly the chances of having a heart attack or a stroke.

The Special Report recommended seven "natural" steps to good health, as alternatives to drugs for people with borderline cases of primary hypertension. Reduce weight if you're obese, reduce your dietary sodium to less than 2 grams per day, reduce your alcohol consumption, reduce your consumption of saturated fats, stop smoking, exercise, and get involved in some kind of relaxation therapy to minimize stress. The alarming results of the MRFIT and other studies have led Dr. W. McFate Smith,[19] of the U.S. Public Health Service, and Dr. Norman M. Kaplan,[20] of the University of Texas, to make recommendations that go further than those of the Joint National Committee. They have suggested that patients with diastolic blood pressures between 90 and 100 mm Hg not be treated with drugs unless they have risk factors.

Why Were We on the Wrong Path?

Any form of treatment that costs the country billions, makes almost everyone feel bad, and appears to help only the more severe cases while hurting the borderline cases can hardly be considered a success. How could an entire society, professionals and laymen alike, go so far down a path that has so much missed the most important destination: good health and long life?

Our near-total reliance upon drugs is an ultimate result of some fundamental assumptions of Western, especially American, culture. As Pogo used to say, "The problem is not them [the medical establishment and the pharmaceutical companies]. The problem is us." All of us.

We will explore some of these assumptions in detail in Part V, but the following are the main points:

○ Historically, our culture has regarded science primarily as a means to dominate nature, rather than to understand it.

○ Technology, which is really the application of science, is often confused with science itself. Our culture idolizes technology. This idolatry inspires a blind faith that the presumed benefits of technology will ultimately outweigh any undesirable side effects.

○ Drugs, such as the "miracle drug" diuretic pill that apparently reduced blood pressure, are decidedly high tech. Nutritional solutions, such as Kempner's rice-fruit diet, are low tech.

○ A lot of money is behind drugs. Pharmaceutical companies naturally want to see a good return on their sizable investment, and they therefore bombard doctors with intensive marketing efforts.

○ Patients themselves demand drugs. The American public by and large wants a pill to cure anything that ails them.

○ Doctors are wary of malpractice suits and are therefore wary of prescribing outside the accepted, conventional treatments—that is, drugs—lest they be liable if something goes wrong.

○ In general, doctors know very little about nondrug programs. For example, in medical schools, there is little if any training in either nutrition or exercise physiology.

○ It is difficult to accept a nondrug solution if there is no overall understanding of the problem—a master concept, or paradigm—within which we can see how a nondrug treatment, such as nutrition, can work.

In Part II, we will show you the evidence that proper nutrition and moderate exercise will lead to reduction of elevated blood pressure in most people with primary hypertension. We will also discuss recent evidence indicating that a dietary approach can improve your health and increase your life span even when blood pressure doesn't come down.

Summary

Because of the deadly consequences of hypertension, doctors have made a large effort to lower elevated blood pressure. Since the late 1950s the approach has focused almost exclusively on using drugs. This condition currently costs people in the United States several billion dollars each year—just for the drugs used to treat it. On top of this are the costs due to premature death, prolonged hospitalization, permanent invalidism due to stroke or kidney disease, or decreased productivity due to drug side effects. Nor is it possible to put a price tag on the damage in human terms.

Because they do reduce the deadly consequences of hypertension overall, the high cost of drugs has been considered justified. However, because of the cost of drug treatment, and lack of knowledge of alternative approaches, many elderly citizens on fixed income simply give up on treatment for their high blood pressure. More importantly, a growing body of evidence has led many physicians to question the wisdom of using drugs, with their frequent side effects, to treat this condition. Of particular concern is a body of evidence which suggests that in cases of borderline hypertension, drug treatment may actually be worse than no treatment at all. If drugs are used, pills must be taken *for life*—every day without fail (with some drugs, skipping even a day or two can cause problems). And some doctors worry about the fact that nobody really knows what effects these drugs may have over a 20- to 30-year period.

PART TWO
The Answer

If too much salt is used in food the pulse hardens. . . . The corresponding illness makes the tongue curl up and the patient unable to speak.

—Su Wen, 2600 B.C.[1]

It's been over four thousand years since the Emperor Su Wen recognized that salt leads to hypertension—"the pulse hardens"—and to strokes—"makes . . . the patient unable to speak." Yet in A.D. 1984, high blood pressure is still a problem and the importance of table salt is still being debated. Some specialists say the amount of sodium in your diet doesn't matter. Others continue to claim that hypertension is relieved by decreasing dietary sodium. Still others say that people with hypertension should eat foods with more calcium and magnesium, as well as potassium—but need not decrease dietary sodium.

It might seem that all is in a state of confusion. But sometimes confusion is the beginning of wisdom. We are now in the middle of a major shift in our understanding of hypertension. This shift is leading to a complete rethinking of methods of prevention and treatment. We now realize that there were unproved assumptions underlying the dogma that drugs were the answer to primary hypertension.

New Scientific Insights

Fortunately, at the same time that we are realizing that drugs are not the answer for most people with high blood pressure, our new view of primary hypertension offers a better alternative. This new view, which comes from scientific studies of how living cells work as well as from studies of people with hypertension, extends the old idea that both the problem and the answer involve salt.

This new view of primary hypertension is supported by the convergence of five main lines of evidence, all of which indicate that the real key to primary hypertension is not just sodium, or even just potassium, but the *balance* between potassium and sodium. And with this new understanding, we begin to see how such apparently unrelated factors as obesity, lack of exercise, too much dietary fat, too little dietary magnesium and calcium, and improper balance of dietary potassium and sodium can all produce the same result. All these factors lead to an imbalance between potassium and sodium in the body's cells. (This imbalance can also lead to a calcium imbalance inside cells; we'll explain how this imbalance can cause high blood pressure.)

What follows is a brief outline of the five lines of evidence. Each of these lines of evidence will then be described in greater detail later in this part of the book. Chapter 8 will also explore some other factors of lesser importance.

The five lines of evidence include:

1. *Cultural evidence.* The diet most of us eat is "abnormal" if we compare it to what our ancestors ate. These "primitive" diets all had a *K Factor* that was at least ten times higher than in our modern diets. There are several groups of native people in the world today that still eat this "primitive" diet. High blood pressure is very rare among these people.

2. *The K Factor cure: human studies.* We will show you results of
   several medical studies on people, which have demonstrated
   time and again that most cases of primary hypertension can
   be helped—and in many cases cured—by a combined reduction in dietary sodium *and* an increase in dietary potassium.
3. *The K Factor cure: animal studies.* We will discuss experiments with laboratory animals with high blood pressure that
   show that increasing the *K Factor* in the diet restores a normal span of life *even if it doesn't reduce blood pressure.* The
   importance of this finding can't be emphasized enough. It
   means that something other than just elevated blood pressure
   needs to be corrected, and that increasing the *K Factor* can do
   it.
4. *The K Factor and the living cell.* It was our own involvement in
   basic research into how the living cell regulates its levels of
   sodium, potassium, and calcium that led us individually to
   recognize the importance of the ratio of potassium (K) to
   sodium (Na)—the *K Factor*—in the diet and to become interested in its application to hypertension. We will give a simplified explanation of how sodium and potassium play a role
   in the regulation of the living cell and discuss the importance
   of this in hypertension.
5. *The K Factor, weight, and exercise.* You've probably heard that
   if you have hypertension, the loss of excess weight reduces
   elevated blood pressure. And recent studies show that regular
   aerobic exercise can help reduce elevated blood pressure even
   when there is no loss of weight.
   We will discuss recent scientific research that indicates
   that both obesity and lack of exercise cause abnormal levels
   of hormones that normally help the body regulate its balance
   between potassium and sodium.

*All lines of evidence taken together point to the conclusion that
most people get high blood pressure because they eat too little potassium (and, in some people, too little magnesium or calcium) and
too much sodium. Lack of exercise and especially being overweight
are the other major factors in causing high blood pressure.*

CHAPTER 3
High Blood Pressure Is Not Inevitable: Cultural Evidence

We used to think high blood pressure just happened. Later we realized that primary hypertension occurs only in those with an inherited, or genetic, tendency. Since it wasn't clear that the genetic weakness affected the body's ability to handle salt, nor could we at that time change a person's genes, it seemed inevitable that some people would get high blood pressure. Therefore, it was natural to focus on anything, such as drugs, that could lower the blood pressure.

You've just learned that the drug approach currently used has lots of drawbacks: It's expensive, it often saps your energy and sex drive, you're stuck with taking pills for the rest of your life, and your life may actually be shortened. If hypertension were inevitable (and assuming drugs were the only solution), a lot of us could look forward to a pretty dismal future.

But studies of population groups living today in different places around the world indicate that high blood pressure is not a necessary part of the human condition. Anthropologists have now studied blood pressure in over thirty groups of natives, including African hunter-gatherers and tribes in Australia and in South America. *None* of these groups has been afflicted with high blood pressure until they adopt a "civilized" life-style. Hospital records in Africa illustrate that in the early part of this century high blood pressure just wasn't observed in such primitive areas. But after adopting a civilized life-style, including the use of salt and processed foods, these same records show that hypertension began to occur in these people.[1] So the lack of high blood pressure in these native groups before eating such processed and salted foods is not due to an inherited resistance to high blood pressure. Because no exceptions to this have been found, anthropologists who have looked into the matter are agreed that *hypertension is a cultural disease*—a disease of lifestyle. In other words, hypertension is *not* inevitable.

But what aspect of our modern culture leads to high blood pressure? The evidence indicates that most cases of high blood pressure are produced by "modern" methods of food preparation and by insufficient exercise.

The Stone Age Diet

The first "diet" for low blood pressure was eaten thousands of years ago. Studies of the tools the Stone Age people used to obtain their food and the location of their living sites suggest that about one-third of their diet was meat from wild animals and the other two-thirds was from plants. This indicates that they ate foods that were very low in sodium and very high in potassium. As we will be demonstrating in the chapters to come, such a diet would have prevented hypertension. Of course, we don't know what their blood pressure actually was. But examination of their bones gives us reason to believe that if they escaped childhood diseases and didn't meet an unhappy fate with a tiger or other wild beast, many of our ancient ancestors lived at least into their fifties, a point where bones no longer reliably indicate age.[2]

The Stone Age Diet Today
It turns out that in spite of "civilization," there are a few places left in the world where primitive people are still eating

the diet of our ancient ancestors. In every such group that has been studied, no more than 1 percent of the people have high blood pressure. Even though 5 to 10 percent commonly live to their sixties or seventies, those individuals don't develop hypertension.[3] Contrast this to the United States, where about 30 percent of the adults have high blood pressure. The percentage is even higher in U.S. black adults. Also, in the United States, incidence of high blood pressure increases with age. This is not true of those groups still eating the diet of our ancestors.

Following is a list of some of the low-blood-pressure groups that have been studied. All have diets high in potassium and low in sodium.

Aita people, Solomon Islands[4]

Australian aborigines[5]

Botswana natives[6]

Carajas Indians, Brazil[7]

Cuna Indians, Panama[8]

Eskimos, Greenland[9]

Kenya natives[10]

Melanesians, northern Cook Islands[11]

New Guinea natives[12]

South African natives[13]

Tarahumara Indians, northern Mexico[14]

Ugandan natives[15]

West China natives[16]

Yanomamo Indians, Brazil[17]

Not only do these groups of people have almost no hypertension, they also seldom have heart attacks or diabetes.

Nathan Pritikin, founder of the Pritikin Program for health, was among the first to realize the importance of these observations. Pritikin was especially impressed by the fifty thousand Tarahumara Indians who live in the Sierra Madre mountains of northern Mexico, near the southern border of the United States.

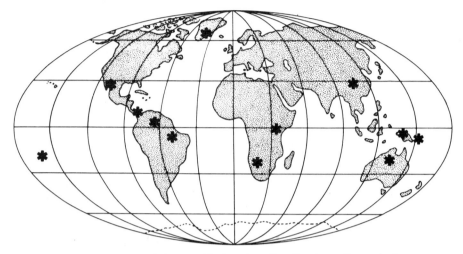

FIGURE 4. *Map of the world showing distribution of populations with diets high in potassium, low in sodium.*

Pritikin noticed their unusual health and stamina (they run up to 200 miles in their games of kickball, which last several days). He had also noticed that scientists have been unable to find any evidence that these people ever die from heart disease.[18] These Indians eat primarily corn and beans, supplemented with squash and chili peppers. Pritikin focused upon the fact that their diet has a very low fat content (about a fourth of that of the average person in the United States), is low in cholesterol, and is also high in fiber. We would add the important fact that their diet is high in potassium and low in sodium.[19]

When people from such "primitive" groups move to "modern" cities and begin eating processed foods, which are lower in potassium and higher in sodium than were the natural foods they had been eating, they then develop high blood pressure with the same frequency as do modern folk.[20]

Many attempts have been made to explain away these observations. Because primary hypertension occurs only in those with a genetic weakness, it's understandable that some have suggested these groups don't have high blood pressure because they all inherit a resistance to it. But these people are so diverse geographically and racially[21] (see Figure 4) that it is almost inconceivable that they all have a genetic resistance to high blood pressure whereas Europeans, Americans, and Japanese do not.[22] Besides, when these people *have* adopted a modern life-style, if anything, they have *more* hypertension than Europeans and Americans. If anything, one could argue that there has been some genetic adaptation of Europeans and Americans which makes them slightly less prone to the harmful effects of a Western life-style than the "primitive" people who are probably more genetically similar to our ancient ancestors.[23] It has also been argued that these "primitive" people have low blood pressure because they are comparatively thin. But many of the Cuna Indians of Panama are moderately fat; they do, however, eat a high–*K Factor* diet, and less than 1 percent of the adults have high blood pressure.[24] In addition, the "primitive" Qash'qai tribe of nomads in southern Iran are thin, but they eat a low–*K Factor* diet and have as much high blood pressure as do people in the United States.[25]

It has even been argued that high blood pressure is caused by stress. The very word *hypertension* suggests tension or stress. So some might wonder if these primitive people escape hypertension because of the simple, idyllic life they supposedly live. But neighboring villages of Brazil's Yanomamo Indians and other tribes in the Amazon rain forest are constantly at war, with between 30 and 42 percent of adults males dying in battle.[26] Although stress is difficult, if not impossible, to measure, it seems reasonable to assume these people have more than their share. Yet in spite of living with daily fear, they have no high blood pressure.[27]

The K Factor

As we have seen, "primitive" people in widely separated parts of the world have an extremely low incidence of hypertension when compared with modern Western societies. The only consistent explanation seems to be the "Stone Age diet" they all have in common—a diet very low in sodium and high in potassium.

It is the central premise of our book that such a diet is the key for you, too, to prevent or reverse your own hypertension.

We refer to the ratio of potassium to sodium as the *K Factor*. K is the chemical symbol for potassium, whose Latin (scientific) name is *kalium*. (The chemical symbol for sodium, by the way, is Na, from its Latin name *natrium*.)

If a food has the same amount (by weight) of potassium as sodium, its *K Factor* is 1. If it has more potassium than sodium, its *K Factor* is greater than 1. If there's twice as much potassium as sodium, the *K Factor* is 2; if there's three times as much, the *K Factor* is 3, and so on. On the other hand, if the food has more sodium than potassium, the *K Factor* is less than 1. If there's twice as much sodium as potassium, the *K Factor* is 0.5; if there's three times as much, the *K Factor* is 0.33, and so on. The *K Factor* of the diet of our ancient ancestors was probably in the range of 16![28]

We will be showing you how a diet with a high *K Factor*—the kind of diet eaten by our "primitive" cousins and our Stone Age ancestors—can help you get rid of any hypertension problem you have.

Comparing the K Factor in Different Ethnic Diets

By looking at several different populations living in the world today, we can see the relation between the frequency of hypertension and the level of the *K Factor* in their food.

Modern Americans and Japanese are eating diets with less than 3 percent of the *K Factor* of the diet of our ancient ancestors and the Yanomamo Indians.

Although this table alone is not conclusive, notice that once the *K Factor* drops below about 2 (or 1.6 in the table), the frequency of hypertension goes way up. It appears that about two-thirds of us inherit a resistance to hypertension regardless of what we eat. The other third will end up with hypertension if we eat foods with a lower *K Factor*—especially if we don't get any

TABLE 2. *Frequency of Hypertension in Various Populations*

K Factor*	Percentage with Hypertension	Population
20	less than 1	Yanomamo Indians, Brazil[29]
4.9	less than 1	!Kung people, northern Botswana[30]
1.6	2	Vegetarians in Tel Aviv[31]
1.1	26	Nonvegetarians in Tel Aviv[31]
0.39	27	Blacks and whites in Evans County, Georgia[32]
0.36	33	Residents of northern Japan[33]

*The dietary *K Factor* was estimated by measuring the amount of sodium and potassium in the urine of these people. Since most of the dietary sodium and potassium is excreted in the urine under normal conditions, the ratio of urinary potassium to sodium is a good approximation of the dietary *K Factor*.

regular exercise. In some people, magnesium and calcium are also very important, but the simplest single measure that correlates with high blood pressure appears to be the *K Factor*.

It is well known that in the United States, high blood pressure is even more common in blacks than in whites. Some specialists have suggested that this difference is genetic, and others have suggested that it is because blacks eat more salt than whites. But in one study, black men actually had about a quarter less sodium in their diet than whites even though they had more high blood pressure.[34] However, because of deficient potassium, the food they ate *did* have a very much lower *K Factor* than the food eaten by the whites. At least three other studies have also found that a lower dietary *K Factor* is associated with the higher blood pressure in U.S. blacks.[35]

Dr. Louis Tobian of the University of Minnesota School of Medicine has pointed out that whereas primitive hunter-gatherers eat about 8 grams of potassium in their daily diets, in the United States, white males eat less than 3 grams and black males eat only about 1.5 grams of potassium each day.[36] Based upon studies we will describe in Chapter 5, he suggests this is responsible for the fact that blacks are 18 times more likely to have hypertensive kidney failure than are whites.

Low Incidence of Hypertension in Some Modern Populations

You don't have to wear a loincloth or live away from modern civilization to avoid hypertension. Everything points to the way you eat and to exercise as being the critical factors.

In Japan, high blood pressure is even more common than in the United States. In 1959, researchers compared two northern Japanese villages.[37] Both villages had similar sodium intake but different blood pressures. The group with the lower blood pressure was found to consume much more potassium in their diet.

As a test of this explanation, the researchers had the hypertensive persons eat about six apples, which are high in potassium, each day. This resulted in a significant drop in their blood pressure. (Perhaps we should change the old adage to Six apples a day keeps the doctor away.) However, as we describe in Part VI, eating even two or three apples each day has a definite tendency to decrease blood pressure.

A 1985 study of eight thousand Japanese men living in Hawaii found that those who ate more potassium and calcium had significantly lower blood pressure than those who didn't.[38]

Vegetarian groups consistently have lower average blood pressures than matched control groups.[39] For example, hypertension hits over a quarter of the people living in Tel Aviv. Yet only 2 percent of the vegetarians living in that city have hypertension.[40] Other than the way they eat, these vegetarians have an almost identical life-style to the nonvegetarians. We must emphasize that one of the principal distinctions of a vegetarian diet is its high *K Factor*, relative to most nonvegetarian fare.

What Is an Acceptable K Factor?

Four lines of evidence indicate that to prevent hypertension, the *K Factor* should be at least three.

The first line of evidence comes from Table 1, which suggests that hypertension is uncommon (about 1 percent) when the *K Factor* is above 2. In Chapter 4, we discuss medical studies in which the *K Factor* approach was consistently successful in lowering blood pressure when the value was 3 or above. In Chapter 5, we will discuss data from animal studies, which indicate that 2 is sometimes not high enough. Finally, the *K Factor* of human milk might also provide a guideline, since that recipe evolved over millions of years to provide optimal nutrition for human infants. That value, about 3.5,[41] reinforces a tentative choice of a *K Factor* of at least 3.

However, keep in mind that our ancestors ate a diet with a much higher *K Factor*.

Therefore, until more complete data are obtained, we recommend you shoot for a *K Factor* of well above 3 in your diet. A *K Factor* of 3 requires eating three times as much potassium as sodium, which is about the proportion occurring naturally in your body. Remember, the ratio between the amount of potassium and the amount of sodium you eat is more important than the absolute amounts. Chapter 10 contains specific recommendations for obtaining the proper level of *K Factor*.

Summary

Hypertension is not an inevitable part of the human condition. Rather it is clear that even in those with the genetic tendency, high blood pressure is due to the way they live—that is to lifestyle. The psychological stress of modern civilization is not the main culprit.

There is evidence from studies of various population groups which suggests that proper nutrition and exercise can keep blood pressure from getting too high. The food our ancient ancestors ate and, for the most part, the food eaten by "primitive" populations today has a much higher ratio of potassium to sodium (that is, a higher *K Factor*) than we get today. The primitive groups eating this diet today have a very low incidence of hypertension, and we can assume the same was true of our ancestors.

This isn't surprising, since our ancestors had adapted to the diet over millions of years. We have inherited that adaptation. Our bodies are designed for the Stone Age diet and for exercise. Since our bodies are used to—and tuned for—the type of balance in that "primitive" (Stone Age) diet, it's not surprising that when we use technology to upset the balance in our food, we run into trouble. Eating food with an artificially low *K Factor* puts stresses on our body that not only can lead to hypertension but may lead to other problems as well. (We'll talk about that later.)

We will discuss other evidence supporting a high–*K Factor* diet in the next few chapters.

CHAPTER 4

The K Cure:
Human Studies

Every profession creates channels that become ruts in which ambitious people in the field have to stay; otherwise, they're not respectable.

—Daniel Boorstin, noted historian and
Pulitzer Prize winner, quoted in
U.S. News & World Report, March 5, 1985

Now you've seen some of the evidence that eating food with a high *K Factor*—a high ratio of potassium to sodium—can prevent hypertension. But what if you already have high blood pressure? Can increasing the *K Factor* bring it back to normal?

Let's take a look at some of the medical studies of the effects of raising the *K Factor* to reduce high blood pressure. The subjects of these experiments were modern people who had been eating food with a low *K Factor* and had developed high blood pressure; the experiments had them change to a diet with a high *K Factor*. If you already have high blood pressure, these studies should be of great interest to you. Of course, it's too late now to change what you ate in your youth. But these studies show that you can change what you eat *now* and begin to benefit from the change *right away.*

So far there have been at least twelve reports of treating hypertension by increasing the *K Factor.* All told, a few thousand patients have been treated this way, with success rates varying from 67 to 100 percent.

The Background: Before the 1980s

Treating hypertension by reducing sodium intake and increasing potassium intake is hardly a new idea. At the beginning of Part II, we quoted Su Wen (2600 B.C.), who described in gruesome detail the consequences of too much sodium in the diet. Another ancient medical text—a physician's prescription book from Sumeria (c. 2000 B.C.)—mentions that potassium should be included in the diet.[1] But the most complete evidence about the *K Factor* began to accumulate at the very beginning of this century. And now there is lots of it.

The Ambard-Beaujard Report (1904)

One of the earliest modern medical studies of a high–*K Factor* diet for treating hypertension was conducted and summarized in a report way back in 1904 by two French physicians, Ambard and Beaujard.[2] These two doctors increased the *K Factor* by decreasing the amount of table salt (sodium chloride) and raising the amount of potassium-rich foods in the diet of their patients. They succeeded in lowering the blood pressure in five out of eight of these patients.

The Addison Study (1928)

The first study in which the *K Factor* was increased by giving potassium salts was conducted in the 1920s by a Toronto physician, W.L.T. Addison. The results of this study were reported in the *Journal of the Canadian Medical Association* in 1928.[3] Addison got his inspiration from a paper written in Paris by a researcher named Blume, who had discovered that potassium displaces sodium in the body to cause a diuresis—that is, an increased excretion of water and sodium through the kidneys. In 1924, Addison had reported that giving calcium reduced the blood pressure in many of his hypertensive patients.[4] We will explain the possible reason for this in Chapter 6. (Very recently Dr. Lawrence Resnick,[5] of Cornell University Medical College in New York City, and his co-workers,[6] have confirmed the ability of calcium to lower blood pressure in certain patients with hypertension.) In those patients whom calcium didn't help, Addison found that giving them potassium salts often brought their blood pressure down, frequently back to normal. In 1928, he reported the results of treating five hypertensive patients with potassium chloride or potassium citrate.[7] To increase potassium intake, he also put all five patients on a low-salt, meatless diet that emphasized fish once daily, vegetables, fruits, cereals and milk. In each case, giving extra potassium lowered the blood pressure.

The most dramatic case was a sixty-four-year-old man whose blood pressure was initially 182/128. After taking large amounts of calcium chloride each day, his blood pressure decreased to 165/117 and stayed there for several months. When this man was then given 7.8 grams of potassium citrate (840 mg potassium) each day instead of the calcium chloride, his blood pressure decreased to 140/88. In each of the five patients, substitution of sodium chloride for the potassium salt resulted in return of the blood pressures to the previously elevated levels, which were then lowered again by returning to the potassium salt.

Addison's success is illustrated in Figure 5, a graph of the blood pressure of one of his patients. On day 1, this patient had a blood pressure of 162/98 and was given potassium chloride (KCl). By day 5, his blood pressure was down to 150/82. He was then given table salt—sodium chloride (NaCl)—and by day 9, his blood pressure was up to 186/118. Then he was given potassium bromide (KBr); in two days, his blood pressure was down to 144/104. Then he was given sodium bromide (NaBr), which, in another two days, brought his blood pressure back up to 172/116. Finally, he was given potassium citrate; in three days, his blood pressure was down to 134/78.

Addison clearly demonstrated the fact that sodium makes

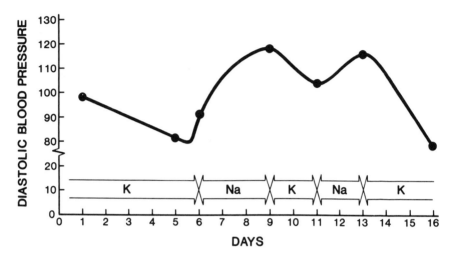

FIGURE 5. *Patients' blood pressure in response to potassium (K) or sodium (Na).*

blood pressure go up and calcium or potassium can make it go down. By giving either calcium or potassium, he was able to lower the blood pressure in 70 percent of his hypertension patients.[8]

In this landmark paper, Dr. Addison concluded: "One has forced on one the concept that the prevalence of arterial hypertension on this continent is in large part due to a potash [potassium] poor diet, and an excessive use of salt [sodium chloride] as a condiment, and as a preservative of meat." This was printed in 1928!

Priddle and McQuarrie (the 1930s)

Studies by Dr. W. Priddle in 1931[9] and by Dr. McQuarrie and associates in 1936[10] also indicated that a high potassium intake lowers blood pressure in people with hypertension. Dr. Priddle achieved 100 percent success in reducing the blood pressure of forty-five hypertensive patients by giving them potassium citrate combined with a low-sodium diet.

The Kempner Diet (1940s)

In the 1940s, Dr. Walter Kempner popularized a rice-fruit diet that succeeded in lowering the blood pressure by at least 20 mm Hg in two out of three of his hypertensive patients, with most of the rest having at least a partial reduction of blood pressure toward normal.[11] This diet emphasized fruits and vegetables.

Although it was not stressed at the time, the Kempner rice-fruit diet is in reality a low-sodium (about 160 mm per day)/high-potassium diet. In fact, the *K Factor* in this diet can be as high as 20.[12] Unfortunately, most Americans found the recipes used in this diet too tasteless. (But don't you worry. We'll show you a very tasty way to achieve a high *K Factor*.)

The Dahl Report (1972)

By 1972, a scientist who provided the basis for much of our present understanding about sodium, potassium, and hypertension, Dr. Lewis Dahl, had recognized what he considered the indisputable effectiveness of Kempner's rice-fruit diet. Dr. Dahl concluded that the rice-fruit diet was often useful in treating even severe cases of hypertension.[13] This conclusion was based not only upon Dr. Kempner's reports but also upon Dr. Dahl's own observations of several physicians who were themselves incapacitated by progressive hypertensive heart disease and were able to return to practice after several months on the Kempner diet.

The Pritikin Experience (1960s–1985)

In the previous chapter, we discussed Nathan Pritikin's observations of the Tarahumara Indians of northern Mexico, who eat corn, beans, squash, and chili peppers (a remarkably high–*K Factor* diet), and who are capable of running up to two hundred miles in a game of kickball that lasts several days. For the past twenty years, Pritikin and his followers have been placing people on a program that includes a similar diet, along with moderate exercise (not 200 miles). By now, Pritikin's Longevity Centers have experience with over ten thousand people. Of those who had hypertension, 85 percent were off drugs and had normal blood pressure within four weeks on this diet-exercise program.[14]

Recent Controlled Medical Studies

Although the results of the early medical studies of increasing the *K Factor* in the diet were dramatic, they were not designed so that they could be analyzed with statistics. However, more recently medical studies have been conducted in which people given high–*K Factor* diets were compared with control groups of hypertensives eating their usual diet. The results could then be statistically analyzed.

These studies have demonstrated that lowering sodium chloride does lower blood pressure and that raising dietary potassium lowers it still further. These scientifically controlled studies are described in detail in Chapter 20.

The Australian Experiment (1982)

If you are taking pills for high blood pressure and would rather not, a scientifically controlled study conducted by Dr. Trevor Beard and others will be of special interest.[15] In Australia, ninety volunteers were all taking medicine that had brought their blood pressure into the normal range. The volunteers were randomly assigned to each of two groups. One group followed a special high-potassium, low-sodium diet; the other didn't. Everything else was the same in both groups, and the doctors and nurses didn't know who was in which group.

Before the study, most of the volunteers were eating food with a *K Factor* of less than 1; that is, they were eating more sodium than potassium. The forty-five volunteers who changed their diet (under the advice of a nutritionist) ended up eating over six times as much potassium as sodium, or a diet with a *K Factor* greater than 6.

In the high–*K Factor* diet group, four out of five of the volunteers were able to reduce their dose of blood pressure medicine, and one out of three was completely able to stop taking any drugs by the end of the twelve-week study! In the control group, less than one out of ten was able to stop taking medicine. The reason the control group showed any improvement at all is that the extra blood pressure measurements and attention to health associated with participating in the study had a beneficial effect. This is why a control group is necessary.

Notice that this was done under their doctors' supervision. **Warning:** *Don't try to do this without your doctor. Suddenly stopping some kinds of medicines can be lethal!*

The London Experiments (1982)

How are we to know if the people on the high–*K Factor* diet were cured because of their faith in the diet? Two studies, by Dr. Graham MacGregor and his co-workers in London, took care of this problem, since the volunteers did not even know which group they were in.[16]

Everybody ate a similar diet, supplemented with pills. In the first experiment, both groups ate a low-sodium diet that dropped their blood pressure.[17] To test that this drop was not
. due to something else in the diet, one group was then given sodium chloride pills, while the other group received lookalike blank (placebo) pills. In the second experiment, one group received potassium pills, while the control group received placebos.[18] Until the studies were over, nobody (except the drug company that provided the pills) knew which was which. Statistical analysis of the results showed beyond any reasonable doubt that reducing sodium or increasing potassium in the diet each produce a partial reduction of blood pressure of people with hypertension.

Dr. MacGregor and his co-workers pointed out that the increase in potassium intake could be achieved with a potassium-based salt substitute (such as is commonly found in grocery stores in the U.S.) and an increase in vegetable and fruit consumption. They stated: "Moderate dietary sodium restriction with dietary potassium supplementation may obviate or reduce the need for drug treatment in some patients with mild to moderate hypertension."

A Japanese Study (1981)

A Japanese group reached almost the same conclusion as the MacGregor studies: "A high-potassium diet has a beneficial effect on blood pressure in patients with mild or moderate essential hypertension, particularly in patients on a high sodium diet."[19] This Japanese group also pointed out that an increase in potassium intake of about 2.34 grams (2340 milligrams) each day could be achieved with a potassium-based salt substitute and a moderate increase in fresh fruit and vegetable consumption. They ended their report with the statement:

Dietary alteration of sodium and potassium intake may obviate the need for drug treatment in many patients with essential hypertension and it might also improve the efficacy of drugs in those patients in whom dietary measures alone are insufficient. Education of the population at risk of hypertension to conform with a more suitable ratio of sodium to potassium in their diet may reduce the prevalence of hypertension and the high cost of drug treatment. The cooperation of the food industry in labeling the approximate sodium content of their foods and in using potassium rather than sodium based additives would help people comply with such an alteration in diet.

Our Personal Experience

The conclusions we have provided evidence for in this chapter are further validated by the personal experiences of each of the authors of this book. As we mentioned in the introduction, Straight Talk, George brought his own blood pressure down from higher than 160/100 to about 125/75 by switching to food with a high *K Factor* (about 4).

Actually this occurred in two stages: First he went on a low-sodium diet without changing the amount of potassium; he succeeded in getting his pressure down to about 140/90. For the next six months, it didn't go lower than this. Then, while staying on the same sodium intake, George started increasing his potassium consumption. Within a couple of weeks, his pressure was down to about 135/80, and since then it has usually been as low as 125/75. During the year and a half he has been on this high–*K Factor* diet (the one we recommend in this book), his pressure has stayed down and he has never felt better.

Lowering sodium is very beneficial, but raising potassium is equally important. You've got to do both.

Dick must have genetic resistance to high blood pressure, because his blood pressure has remained the "classic" 120/80 all his life in spite of the fact he used to eat a fair amount of foods that contain extra salt (fast foods, potato chips). After realizing the importance of ingesting normal levels of the *K Factor* for body cells to function properly, however, he considered the possibility that a low *K Factor* might not only lead to hypertension but to other problems (we'll mention these in Chapter 6). So Dick switched his methods of food preparation to the way we describe in Part III, and for the past year, his blood pressure has been 115/70. This is about the same as those native populations who eat the diet of our ancient ancestors!

But What about Negative Reports?

The McCarron Report

In the summer of 1984, the widely publicized report by Dr. David McCarron and co-workers claimed that there is no relationship between blood pressure and sodium in the U.S. population.[20] This report was generated by examining computer tapes that contained information about a large, government-sponsored survey of diet and blood pressure. Because people with hypertension usually receive treatment to lower blood pressure, all those *known* to have hypertension were removed from the data (before the statistical examination). However, as we mentioned at the beginning of Chapter 3, these are precisely the people who probably have a genetic weakness in their ability to handle salt. This could explain the report's unusual conclusion that sodium actually appeared to cause a slight reduction in blood pressure. This report appears to contradict all the evidence on sodium we've been presenting.

Another possible explanation for the unusual results of this study was that the subjects included in it were those eating more than 3 grams of sodium each day. People on low-salt diets were not included. Therefore, the study fails to take into account people on the "threshold" level of sodium intake—about 2 grams a day. That is, if your diet includes the relatively low level of potassium typical of Americans, and if you are already eating more than about 2 grams of sodium a day (the threshold amount), it doesn't make much difference whether you eat 3 grams or 5 grams of sodium a day. If you have an inherited tendency to get high blood pressure, you'll be sure to get it. On the other hand, if you eat less than 2 grams of sodium per day, and you get enough potassium, magnesium, and calcium, and keep your weight in control with enough exercise, you probably won't develop high blood pressure, no matter what your inherited tendency is.

Incidentally, the study did show that people who ate more potassium—fresh fruits and vegetables—had lower blood pressure.

As reported in the March 15, 1985, issue of the *Journal of the American Medical Association*, Dr. Harvey Gruchow and co-workers[21] reanalyzed the computer tapes studied by Dr. McCarron. This new analysis utilized a powerful ("multi-variant") statistical technique to analyze the same data and found that people in the United States who eat more sodium do indeed have higher blood pressure, while those who eat more potassium have lower blood pressure.

For a discussion of the limitations of statistical studies, see Chapter 19.

The Richards Report

In 1984, a very careful study of "Blood-pressure response to moderate sodium restriction and to potassium supplementation in mild essential hypertension" was published by Dr. Mark Richards of New Zealand.[22] The results showed that moderate restriction of sodium *or* addition of dietary potassium had "variable effects" on diastolic pressure in people with mild primary (essential) hypertension. They concluded that the changes in blood pressure were very small and not statistically significant. This study was meticulous, and the analysis of the data was very rigorous. As a result, several specialists have quoted this study as indicating that potassium is ineffective in treating primary hypertension.

However, when the total picture is considered, an entirely different conclusion emerges. Analyzing the data to take into account *both* potassium and sodium shows that when potassium was added, the *K Factor* still was only 1.9—less than the minimum value of about 3—because the amount of sodium was so high (over 4 grams per day). When sodium was restricted, potassium was also decreased, and the *K Factor* was only 1.3—even further from the value required for an effect upon blood pressure. So when the whole picture is considered, this study provides evidence that is totally consistent with the conclusion of the previous chapter—that the *K Factor* must be above 3 to lower blood pressure—and also illustrates the critical importance of considering both potassium *and* sodium.

The Bottom Line

It's all well and good to say that a high *K Factor* can restore your blood pressure to normal levels. But the real question in any treatment of hypertension is: Will it protect you from death and crippling consequences, such as paralyzing strokes? There is very good reason to believe that the *K Factor* approach *will* protect you from death and crippling consequences, whether or not it lowers your blood pressure.

Dr. Priddle first commented on this back in 1962, when he reported his experience of treating people with hypertension using a high–*K Factor* nutritional program over a period of thirty years: "Although admittedly, in a considerable percentage of cases, there appeared to be little influence on the blood pressure levels, we were impressed with the low incidence of complications and the improved survival rate. From these clinical observations, we felt that in many cases perhaps the tempo of the disease was decreased in spite of the stationary or slowly increasing blood pressure readings."[23]

In the next chapter, we will briefly outline the results from animal experiments that confirm Dr. Priddle's impression. These results clearly indicate that increasing the *K Factor* can restore life span and health to normal, even in cases in which the blood pressure doesn't return to normal. And that's the bottom line.

Summary

On at least ten different occasions, beginning first in 1904, and then in 1928, doctors have repeatedly observed that increasing the dietary *K Factor* reduced high blood pressure. In 1981 and 1982, three "controlled" studies conducted according to accepted medical standards confirmed that increasing dietary potassium, and therefore the *K Factor*, can help lower the blood pressure.

In all studies where the *K Factor* was increased to 3 or higher, a sizable decrease in blood pressure occurred in 60 percent to 100 percent of the patients.

CHAPTER 5
The K Cure: Animal Studies

Experiments on laboratory animals have taught us many important things about hypertension. Of course, the biological systems of humans have unique features, and it would be folly to overgeneralize from the conclusions of animal studies in every respect. Nonetheless, the systems of most mammals are remarkably similar to those of humans, and this fact has made animal studies relevant to human medical research for some time. Moreover, researchers have far wider experimental latitude with laboratory animals than they do with humans.

Animal studies have clearly demonstrated that increasing the dietary *K Factor* can bring blood pressure down, increase the life span of the animals, and provide some protection from kidney disease. Of all the things we have learned from experiments on laboratory animals, one thing stands out in importance above all others:

Increasing the K Factor with potassium protects against crippling strokes and premature death, even when it doesn't decrease blood pressure.

The Gordon-Drury and Meneely-Ball Studies (1950s)

In the previous chapter, we quoted Dr. W. Priddle, who concluded from his experience in treating people who had hypertension that increasing the *K Factor* in their diets resulted in fewer complications and in improved rates of survival, even when it didn't lower blood pressure. Dr. Priddle's observations of the protective effect of potassium on his patients has also been borne out in animal experiments.

In 1956, Dr. David Gordon and Dr. Douglas Drury reported that giving extra potassium to hypertensive rabbits prevented internal bleeding due to ruptures in the small arteries in their intestines.[1] Two years later, in Nashville, Tennessee, Dr. George Meneely and his colleague Con Ball were experimenting with laboratory rats, making them hypertensive with a diet high in sodium chloride (salt).[2] Scientific papers are usually pretty dry, but these two pioneers managed to slip a little "tongue-in-cheek" past the editor. After the usual technical summary, they concluded, "Salt is rough on rats"—which should hardly be surprising to you by now.

But their study also came up with some results that are astonishing indeed: When the dietary *K Factor* was increased by the addition of potassium chloride while keeping sodium chloride in the food constant, the average life span of the hypertensive rats was increased by 50 percent, even when the elevated blood pressure didn't go down! These two researchers pointed out that the extra life span conferred on these rats by potassium was equivalent to twenty to twenty-four years for a human!

Incidentally, it was probably these two scientists who, in 1958, first suggested the use of the dietary *K Factor* as an indicator of the likelihood that a person will develop hypertension.

The Dahl Study (1972)

In 1972, Dr. Lewis Dahl and co-workers confirmed the conclusions of the Meneely-Ball study: Blood pressure was lowered by increasing the *K Factor* in the food of a group of rats that had become hypertensive on a high-sodium diet. And, more significant, the rats on a high–*K Factor* diet lived much longer than the others.[3]

This study also showed that not only is the *K Factor*, or ratio of potassium to sodium, important, but the absolute amounts of sodium and potassium also affect blood pressure. When the *K Factor* was kept constant, increasing the amount of both sodium and potassium threefold resulted in a significant rise in blood pressure. *This result highlights the fact that you must not only increase the potassium in your diet but also decrease the amount of sodium.* (At the other extreme, the effect of too little potassium cannot be totally countered just by decreasing sodium. Over the range of potassium and sodium most of us get, the balance is the important thing.)

The Tobian Study (1983)

The special protective effect of increasing the *K Factor* by giving potassium has also been demonstrated by Dr. Louis Tobian, chief of the Hypertension Section of the University of Minnesota Medical School. At the 1983 meeting of the American Association for the Advancement of Science, Dr. Tobian reported on experiments that confirm that even when blood pressure is not lowered, increasing dietary potassium decreases death and restores a normal life span to hypertensive rats.[4] Dr. Tobian's work went further and also showed that the increased dietary potassium also protects the rats against kidney damage. In particular, he showed that potassium prevented the ruptures of the small arteries in the kidneys that occurred in the rats not receiving potassium.[5]

In Dr. Tobian's more recent studies, which he described in 1984 at the Medical Grand Rounds at the University of Vermont Medical College, he found that increased potassium not only increases the life span of hypertensive rats but protects them against stroke by preventing rupture of the blood vessels in the brain. Again, this is true even when the rats' blood pressure has not been lowered.

Lowering Hypertension in Pets—A Personal Anecdote

As we have seen, animal studies have relevance to human medicine. Personal experience demonstrates that what we discover about humans can also be relevant to the health of pets. As we mentioned in the previous chapter, each of the authors of this book has discovered the benefits of a high–*K Factor* diet. George was also able to apply his experience to a canine senior citizen: Queenie, his fourteen-year-old Chesapeake Bay retriever. Queenie had begun to tire on their morning jog. The vet discovered high blood pressure, lung congestion, and an enlarged heart. A glance at dog food labels confirmed that almost all dog food has added salt. George had unwittingly been giving his dog high blood pressure in her food bowl every night.

George found a health food store that sold unsalted, high-potassium dog food. Queenie liked the food, and her energy began to pick up within three weeks. Within two months, she was running with George again.

An Understanding of Hypertension Begins to Emerge

In the 1960s and 1970s two independent lines of research began to crack the enigma of primary hypertension, while a third, apparently unrelated at the time, began to clarify a connection between the "sugar hormone," insulin, and potassium.

POTASSIUM-SODIUM EXCHANGE PROVIDES A KEY. The first line of research was underway by 1959, when Drs. Emanuel, Scott, and Haddy showed that elevation of potassium in the blood directly causes arteries to relax, thus making it easier for the blood to flow through them.[6]

In 1972, Dr. Chen and co-workers[7] showed that this relaxing effect of potassium is due to stimulation of a mechanism which exchanges potassium for sodium across the surface membrane of cells. The mechanism is called the sodium-potassium pump and turns out to play a central role in primary hypertension. That same year, Dr. Henry Overbeck,[8] presently of the University of Alabama School of Medicine, began to tie things together when he demonstrated that the development of hypertension in animals was associated with a decreased effectiveness in the ability of potassium to relax and dilate their arteries. In that study, Dr. Overbeck hypothesized that the depressed response to potassium might be due to slowed activity of the sodium-potassium pump.

DAHL'S PREDICTION SETS THE STAGE. A second line of research began in 1969 when Dr. Lewis Dahl, together with doctors Knudsen and Iwai, showed that in the salt-sensitive hypertensive rat, the sustained rise in blood pressure is due to a substance circulating in the blood.[9] A master of the use of deductive logic and intuition in research, Dahl and his co-workers suggested that in normal animals and people, this substance, probably a hormone, is released into the blood when the kidneys need to excrete excess sodium from the body. But in salt-sensitive hypertensive rats, or humans with an inherited tendency to hypertension, a high salt intake "will invoke the release" of this "sodium-excreting hormone," which in these animals will also cause high blood pressure. How this "hormone" might act on blood vessels, let alone on the kidneys, was at that time a mystery.

INSULIN COMES INTO THE PICTURE. The third line of investigation involved basic research into the biophysical effects of insulin. At that time, the researchers never dreamed that the "sugar hormone" insulin has anything to do with primary hypertension. But you never know where basic research will lead—until you get there. In 1973 and in 1975, Dick and his students provided convincing evidence that insulin stimulates the sodium-potassium pump.[10] This conclusion was supported by experiments reported in 1977 by Drs. Torben Clausen and Peter Kohn in Denmark,[11] and in 1980 by Drs. Kitasato and co-workers in Japan.[12]

THE PICTURE BEGINS TO COME TOGETHER. The first two lines of research came together in 1976 when Drs. Francis J. Haddy, presently of the Uniformed Services University of Health Science in Bethesda, and Henry W. Overbeck proposed that Dahl's "sodium-excreting hormone" might act by depressing activity of the sodium-potassium pump.[13] Since 1976, an ever-increasing body of evidence has accumulated to confirm that some hypertensive animals or people with primary hypertension,[14] or hypertension associated with pregnancy,[15] have elevated blood levels of Dahl's "sodium-excreting" and pressure elevating hormone. This substance, now called a "natriuretic" hormone, also inhibits the exchange of potassium for sodium in the cells of the body.[16]

This substance is released from the brain[17] and normally plays a useful role. With moderate salt intake, or in people without the genetic weakness associated with primary hypertension, the mild inhibition of sodium-potassium exchange by this substance causes the kidneys to excrete extra sodium.[18] But in people with a genetic tendency to hypertension, the elevation of the blood level of this substance by excess salt appears to inhibit the exchange of potassium for sodium in the cells of the small arteries which control blood pressure.[19] Modern concepts about the role of the cell surface membrane led Drs. Haddy and Overbeck, and also Dr. Mordecai Blaustein of the University of Maryland, to point out that this inhibition should cause the small arteries to squeeze down and thus increase blood pressure.[20]

The third line of evidence, involving insulin, began to relate to high blood pressure only in the early 1980s, as we'll explain in Chapter 7.

The Take-home Lesson

There is every reason to believe that the protective effect of potassium will work not only in laboratory animals but also in human beings. Based on his experience with his own patients, Dr. Priddle had concluded that potassium was improving their health and protecting them from premature death even when blood pressure remained elevated. *The importance of this can't be overemphasized.* After all, preventing strokes and premature death is the really important thing, not just lowering the numbers on the blood pressure machine.

The *K Factor* approach gets at the primary problem, whereas drugs do not, since they are developed and chosen only on the basis of their ability to lower blood pressure, without thought to whether or not they help the primary problem. With the exception of Dr. Tobian and a few others, medical doctors have tended to overlook this ability of a high *K Factor* to get at the primary problem, perhaps because the role of potassium, sodium, and calcium in the regulation of the living cell is not discussed in most medical textbooks. But to cell biophysicists, the effect of potassium is not surprising, since, as we outline in the next chapter, a deficiency of body potassium might be expected to retard the normal protein synthesis that would be required to keep the walls of arteries strong.

To emphasize the primary role of potassium and sodium in hypertension, Dr. Tobian has stated, "An alteration of the amounts of sodium and potassium in the diet of populations susceptible to hypertension may be the most practical way to decrease the incidence of the disease."
We agree!

Summary

Animal studies confirm that increasing the dietary *K Factor* can reduce elevated blood pressure. Of great significance is the fact that even when the blood pressure doesn't come down, adding potassium to the diet of hypertensive animals helps prevent the damage to blood vessels in intestine, kidneys, and the brain, thus preventing kidney disease, strokes and prolonging life. Besides the changes that cause the blood pressure to go up, there must also be some weakness in the walls of the arteries in order to account for all the damage done by hypertension. And increasing the *K Factor* by eating food containing more potassium appears to correct this weakness.

The animal studies show that the problem of hypertension goes deeper than just an elevation of blood pressure. In the 1970s, evidence began to appear that hypertension involves changes in the living cell's ability to exchange potassium for sodium—a change which produces other problems within the cell. The first indication of this was the discovery that in some animals with hypertension and in people with primary hypertension, there are increased levels of a "natriuretic" hormone which appears to inhibit exchange of potassium for sodium in the cell. Then it was discovered that reduced effectiveness of insulin, such as seen in diabetes—another condition which leads to high blood pressure—also reduces the ability of body cells to exchange potassium for sodium.

The *K Factor* approach gets at the primary problem—an imbalance between potassium and sodium in the living cell. Restoring this balance is the only reasonable way to expect to lower blood pressure, plus restore normal strength and flexibility to arteries and so prevent strokes and other consequences of hypertension.

CHAPTER 6
The Action at the Cell Membrane

The cell membrane is like the surface of the earth, that's where the action is.

Suppose you could place a tiny remote camera inside a body cell of someone with high blood pressure. Amid the complex, swirling patterns of membranes and proteins, amid the dancing molecules and atoms, amid the carefully regulated voltages between different regions of the cell, amid the kaleidoscopic, synchronized movements orchestrated in those special rhythms peculiar to life—what would you see that was different about the cell in a person with primary hypertension? And which body cells would be most involved?

In the answer to these questions lies the key to understanding, and therefore to curing and preventing, high blood pressure. For like all diseases, *hypertension represents a disturbance in the organization and function of body cells.*

In this chapter, we will trace how our explorations into the ordering of the cell led each of us into hypertension research and our realization of the importance of the *K Factor*. We present the

55

biophysical evidence in simple form. We hope that in following our story you will appreciate the evidence on the microscopic, cellular level that supports this book's recommendations.

The Order of the Cell

Our involvement in this story actually began a quarter-century ago, when we each became active in basic scientific research without any goal other than to understand the fascinating phenomenon called the living cell. At the time, it never entered our minds that our research would lead us into studying hypertension. We were motivated by curiosity and by wonder, without much thought to practical applications.

Amid the dynamic, constantly changing patterns of the cell, there are hints of an underlying order. In fact, the living cell consists of matter that is highly organized, organized to a degree not observed in nonliving things. A big question nagging biophysicists is: How do living cells build up so much order?

Since the cell is part of the physical universe, we know that none of the laws of physics is violated in this cellular order. There really can be no "magic." In particular, we know that this order does not violate the famous Second Law of Thermodynamics, or the "Entropy Law": The entropy—disorder, or chaos—of any closed system must increase as time goes on. (Those of you who are parents are probably familiar with the effects of this law every time you look at your child's room.)

So to rephrase the burning question: How do living cells keep their entropy so low?

We now understand the basic concepts. The entropy decreasing in our body cells is connected to the increasing entropy in another part of the universe: the sun. Of course, the connection is the available energy (some physicists would say negative entropy) in sunlight, which plants can capture and use to make food, which provides the fuel that our cells can use to order themselves. We are literally tied to our star. But we do not yet really deeply understand the answer to our question. There's still a lot to learn.

Nonetheless, we do have partial answers and we have glimpses. In science, as in any activity, one does what one can. So we, the authors of this book, looked at part of the problem; we studied what we could study. Back in the late 1950s, it was known that one mechanism at the cell surface functions to keep sodium outside and potassium inside the cell and thus helps keep the cell organized.

This was something we could study.

Pumps and Batteries

Drawing analogies to familiar, everyday objects when discussing the functions of actions at the cellular level is often useful. A good number of the functions in the cell that are important to our discussion closely resemble the functions of ordinary pumps and batteries.

The Sodium-Potassium Pump

The mechanism we each began to study back in the fifties is called thè *sodium-potassium pump*, which moves sodium out of the cell in exchange for potassium moving in (see Figure 6).

This ordering—potassium to the inside, sodium to the outside—is similar to the ordering you might use when you put your plates in one cabinet and your glasses in another.

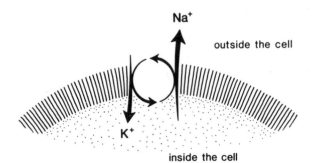

FIGURE 6. *The sodium-potassium pump: Na is sodium, K potassium.*

By moving sodium out of the cell and potassium into the cell, the sodium-potassium pump keeps the *K Factor* of the cell high. In fact, this is why almost all natural foods have a high *K Factor*. Their own cells have a lot more potassium than sodium. The sodium-potassium pump in relation to the cell as a whole is illustrated in Figure 7.

We call this mechanism a pump because it takes energy to run it, since both the sodium and the potassium are being moved "uphill"—that is, from areas of low concentration to areas of high concentration. It's the same general idea with any pump: It takes energy to move water out of a well, and the mechanism we use is a water pump.

The sodium-potassium pump gets its energy from food burned by the cell. According to some estimates, about one-third of the calories we eat are used to run the sodium-potassium pumps located on the surface membrane surrounding every single body cell.[1]

If by now you've guessed that by eating high–*K Factor* foods,

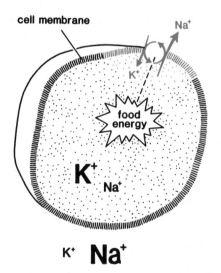

FIGURE 7. *The sodium-potassium pump in the cell.* Large letters indicate a high concentration, small letters a low one.

you prevent high blood pressure by stimulating the activity of the sodium-potassium pump, which maintains the balance between potassium and sodium in the cell, you're right. The connection is a little bit complicated (we go into more detail in Part V), and some details are still a bit fuzzy, but we'll oversimplify a bit in this chapter to give you the general picture.

THE ROLE OF INSULIN IN STIMULATING THE PUMP—DICK'S INVOLVEMENT IN HYPERTENSION RESEARCH. In the 1960s, one of us (Dick) discovered—and in the early 1970s, his and other research groups confirmed—that insulin stimulates the activity of the sodium-potassium pump.[2] From this fact, Dick's group predicted that the defective insulin action seen in diabetes should affect the activity of the sodium-potassium pump. They found evidence to support this hypothesis with tests on diabetic animals.[3]

In fact, Dick, together with Dr. John Munford, now at Wabash College, and others, showed that the level of sodium inside muscle cells is increased in animals when they become diabetic.[4] In the next chapter, we explain how the effect of insulin on the sodium-potassium pump may play a part in causing hypertension in overweight people.

One day Dick received a phone call from Dr. Henry Overbeck, who was mentioned in the last chapter. He was interested in what Dick knew about ways to increase the activity of the sodium-potassium pump. Henry mentioned evidence that primary hypertension is probably due to a decrease in the activity of the sodium-potassium pumps in the tiny muscle cells surrounding blood vessels. (We will explain how this works later in the chapter.)

Dick replied that if the evidence was correct, his own work indicated that diabetics would tend to have hypertension. "Well, they do!" replied Henry. From that moment, Dick became interested in hypertension.

The Sodium Battery

In the process of its work of keeping potassium in the cell and sodium out, the sodium-potassium pump helps produce an electrical voltage between the inside and the outside of the cell. This voltage is shown by the plus and minus signs in Figure 8.

In a single, tiny muscle cell, the cell membrane voltage is almost a tenth of a volt. The exact causes of this voltage are beyond the scope of this chapter, but it is partly due to the fact that the sodium-potassium pump pushes more sodium out than potassium in, and partly due to the fact that the cell membrane is leakier to potassium than to sodium. If the sodium-potassium pump is slowed, the concentration of sodium and potassium inside the cell after a while will come closer to the concentration outside, and the membrane voltage will become much smaller.

Because the sodium-potassium pump keeps potassium inside the cell and sodium outside, sodium is much less concentrated inside the cell than outside. This results in a tendency for sodium to move into the cell (a "chemical potential"). In addition, sodium is positively charged, whereas the inside of the cell is negatively charged. Because opposite charges attract each other, the positive charge of the sodium gives it a tendency to move into the negatively charged cell interior. This tendency may be

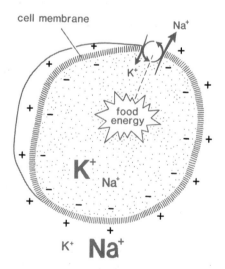

FIGURE 8. *The cell membrane voltage.*

called the electrical potential for sodium. The combined effect of the difference in the chemical concentrations of sodium on the two sides of the membrane and the electrical potential is called the electrochemical potential.

Because of this electrochemical potential, the cell membrane itself acts like a battery—that is, a device that produces a voltage that can drive electric current. We shall call this potential energy of sodium in relation to the cell the *sodium battery* (see Figure 9).

In a flashlight battery or car battery, the electric current is carried by negatively charged particles called electrons. In the cell membrane sodium battery, though, the electric current is carried by positively charged sodium atoms (or sodium ions).

The potential in the sodium battery is capable of work, just as the potential available in a car battery is. The "electric generator" that charges the sodium battery and makes all that work potential is the sodium-potassium pump.

Since the Nobel Prize–winning work of Alan Hodgkin and Andrew Huxley in 1952, it has been known that the potential

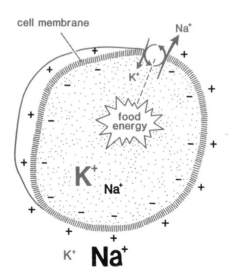

FIGURE 9. *The sodium battery.*

produced by the sodium-potassium pump and stored in the sodium battery plays a key role in the transmission of signals along nerves.

FUNCTIONS OF THE SODIUM BATTERY—GEORGE'S INVOLVEMENT IN HYPERTENSION RESEARCH. The electrochemical potential also plays many other roles. Take the electric eel. Do you know how it generates all that electricity? You guessed it: The sodium-potassium pump and the sodium battery have something to do with it.

In fact, one of us (George) did some research on how this works. In the electric eel, thousands of special cells are lined up so their sodium batteries all point in one direction. All these batteries together act like one big battery. And with each cell able to produce about a tenth of a volt, it can really add up—to 600 volts! (Incidentally, the Italian physicist Count Alessandro Volta got his idea for inventing batteries after studying how the cells in electric fish are stacked up to produce their electricity. Today your car battery has six cells stacked together to make a total of 12 volts, 2 volts from each cell.)

After his work on the electric eel, George studied the sodium-potassium pumps in red blood cells. George's library research uncovered studies indicating that the amount of sodium inside the cells of animals and humans with hypertension may be higher than normal due to an alteration in the movements of sodium and potassium through the surface membrane of these cells. George then decided to devote all his efforts to hypertension research. He did some preliminary work that showed that the sodium concentration is higher inside red blood cells from hypertensive men than cells from men with normal blood pressure.[5]

We will now explain how a higher-than-normal concentration of sodium inside our body's cells could cause high blood pressure.

The Calcium Pump

We have seen how the sodium battery is charged by the action of the sodium-potassium pump, which derives its energy from food. But the sodium battery itself drives another pump, one that is very important to hypertension: the calcium pump.

How can one pump drive another? The connection is the sodium battery. Remember, the electrochemical potential of the sodium battery comes from the stored energy of all that sodium pushed out of the cell by the sodium-potassium pump but "wanting" to come back in because of its natural electrical tendency. One type of calcium pump acts by letting some of the sodium back into the cell; the energy that is released thereby drives calcium out of the cell (see Fig. 10).

This calcium pump operates by a very simple trick. Imagine a wheel with nets to hold rocks; three small rocks are placed on one side and one large rock (weighing a bit less than the total of the three small rocks) is placed in a net on the other. The effect of gravity on the three small rocks is greater than on the one large one, so the wheel uses the energy of the three small rocks going down to lift the one large one. Similarly, as illustrated in Figure 10, this type of calcium pump picks up three sodium atoms (each

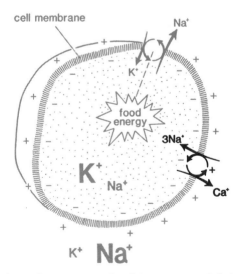

FIGURE 10. *The sodium-powered calcium pump.* Calcium is represented by its chemical symbol Ca. K⁺ = potassium, Na⁺ = sodium.

carrying one positive charge) at a time. The effect of the sodium battery on these three sodium ions (atoms with excess charge are called ions) into the cell is greater than on the one calcium ion (which carries two positive charges), so the energy of three sodium ions going into the cell drives the one calcium out. There is now good evidence that this type of calcium pump exists in the surface membrane of smooth muscle from arteries.[6]

Let's look at this calcium situation more closely.

The dissolved calcium inside a healthy living cell should be kept more than ten thousand times lower than outside. Keeping the calcium low is especially important in a muscle cell, because even a small rise in the calcium inside will cause the muscle to contract. The muscles that allow us to move and to maintain our posture can relax completely (due to a very low internal calcium level) or they can contract (shorten) when the internal calcium is raised due to the action of nerve signals sent to the muscle cells from our brain.

The tiny muscle cells that surround blood vessels and help control blood pressure work the same way, except that they generally don't relax completely: they maintain some degree of tension, which in turn depends on the internal level of calcium. The big difference in the levels of calcium inside and outside muscle cells, plus the negative charge inside these cells, causes a strong tendency for the positive calcium to leak into the cell. Therefore, it takes energy to keep the level of calcium inside the cell from rising too high.

This situation is sort of like being in a leaky boat. How do you keep the water (calcium) inside the boat (cell) from rising? Well, there are two things you can do: You can bail, or pump, the water back out, or you can plug up the leaks. A smart seaman would do both.

And the cell is smart. It does both. It has tiny pumps (the calcium pump we're discussing here) in the surface membrane, which bail or pump the calcium back out. And it keeps the membrane itself from getting too leaky to calcium so the calcium doesn't get back in.

The fully charged sodium battery is required for both tasks. We have already discussed how it provides energy to the calcium pump. But it also helps keep the membrane from becoming leaky to calcium. It turns out that there are atom-size "holes" in the cell membrane, through which calcium can leak. But these holes close when the membrane voltage is high enough—that is, when the sodium battery is fully charged.

When the membrane voltage is slightly discharged, these holes open, letting in calcium, which causes the muscle cells in blood vessels to contract and narrow the blood vessel. The blood vessel muscle cells are slightly discharged most of the time, so that calcium is constantly leaking in to provide a continuous muscle tone.

Let's review this process so far by tracing the causation sequence backward: In order for the muscles to be relatively relaxed (low muscle tension), there must be a far lower concentration of calcium inside the cell than outside. This means that the calcium must be pumped out and must be prevented from leaking back in. For this to happen, the sodium battery must be charged: There must be a high concentration of sodium outside the cell and a low concentration inside, and the membrane voltage must be charged. That means that the sodium-potassium pump must be active. And that means that your body must have a proper balance of potassium to sodium—in other words, a high *K Factor* (see Figure 11).

A high *K Factor* literally keeps your cells charged and prevents the muscles in your arteries from contracting more than they should. The higher calcium level in the cell on the right causes greater muscle contraction or tone. In the next section, we will discuss how hypertension is brought about by excessive muscular contraction of the muscles in the blood vessel walls.

A Low K Factor May Contribute to Other Problems

Before going on, let's just stop to think about possible consequences of the sodium batteries running down. We've shown that this would lead to more calcium inside body cells. In a short while, we will show that this will tend to cause the cell to accumulate more acid also. Neither of these is good.

There is some evidence that if the sodium battery runs down, particularly if the voltage across the cell membrane drops, cells

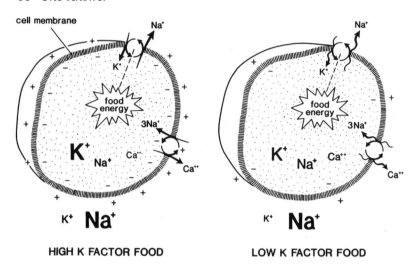

FIGURE 11. *How the* K Factor *affects the calcium level inside cells.*

can divide faster. A biophysicist, Clarence D. Cone, former head of NASA's Langley Research Center in Hampton, Virginia, has reported that division and growth of both "malignant (and normal) cells in cultures can be effectively 'turned-off' by suitably lowering the intracellular sodium concentration while elevating the potassium concentration, and the blocked cells soon die: the key factor . . . is the lowering of the intracellular sodium level."[7] In other words, Dr. Cone's work as well as other considerations suggest that cells cannot divide uncontrollably if their sodium battery is fully charged. This makes one worry about the possibility of uncontrolled cell division, or cancer. In fact, one study has suggested that too much sodium in the diet (remember, this tends to cause the sodium battery to run down) may contribute to causing cancer of the digestive system.[8]

In the early part of the century, a German physician, Dr. Max Gerson, used a nutritional regimen to treat a variety of diseases, including high blood pressure. This treatment included foods containing large amounts of vitamin A and potassium and low amounts of sodium. Albert Schweitzer's wife, who had apparently terminal tuberculosis, recovered after Gerson treated her.

When he was in his seventies, Schweitzer tried Gerson's nutritional therapy and was able to stop taking insulin. In 1928, a woman wih inoperable cancer of the bile duct prevailed upon Gerson to try this diet therapy on her. Both she and two others with inoperable, metastasized cancer were apparently cured by Gerson's approach. Over the years, he claimed that about 30 percent of his cancer patients recovered, but after coming to America and obtaining his New York medical license in 1938, he wrote, "the knife of the AMA was at my throat . . ." and had difficulty being accepted. Some physicians, including Dr. George Miley, executive director of New York's Gotham Hospital, were impressed by Gerson's treatment. Nevertheless, because it has been believed that cancer cannot be cured by diet, apparently no investigation into any possible validity of Gerson's approach has ever been conducted.[9]

We also know that proper healing of wounds requires electricity in the body. As just one example, broken bones won't heal unless a voltage develops between the two pieces. Although the role of electricity in the regulation of living cells is hardly discussed in medical textbooks, this role is not at all surprising to those who have considered the physics, in addition to the biochemistry, of the living cell.

Because of the possible consequences (however remote: such as slow wound healing or perhaps even cancer) of not having the sodium battery fully charged, Dick (who is genetically resistant to high blood pressure) has switched his eating habits to those outlined in this book—as well as resumed regular exercise.

Artery Muscle Tension and Blood Pressure

So how do all these pumps and batteries relate to high blood pressure?

Before we go further with the new scientific insights connecting potassium, sodium, and calcium to hypertension, let's review what produces blood pressure in the first place and how it is controlled.

As we said in Chapter 1, your blood pressure is created by

your heart pumping blood into your large arteries. If the blood could easily flow through these large arteries, nourish the cells, and return through large veins, not very much pressure would be created. But the large arteries branch out into more than 100,000 very tiny "resistance arteries," or arterioles, as they're called. Because of their very small size (less than one-hundredth of an inch in diameter), these arterioles produce a resistance to the flow of blood out of the large arteries. Thus, blood pressure is due to the heart pushing blood against the resistance of the arterioles.

The situation is very much like yet another water pump (the heart), this one pushing water (blood) into a garden hose (arteries). Either increasing the pumping or narrowing the nozzle (arterioles) on the end of the hose (arteries) will increase the water pressure (blood pressure) in the hose (arteries). (See Figure 12.)

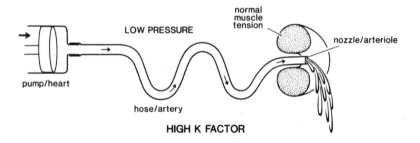

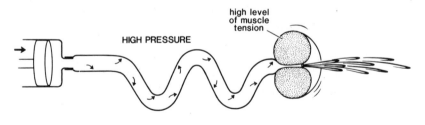

FIGURE 12. *The pump, hose, and nozzle system.*

Because the arterioles are located at the end, or "periphery," of the arterial system, the resistance they produce is called peripheral resistance. Since the arterioles can either constrict or relax, they can either increase or decrease the peripheral resistance to blood flow.

The signals that tell the muscles in the walls of the arterioles whether to constrict or to relax are carried by hormones in the blood or by nerves. But it is ultimately the level of calcium inside the muscle cells that determines the degree of contraction or tension and, therefore, the diameter of the arterioles (nozzle).

Several studies have shown that in primary hypertension, the elevated blood pressure is due to an increase in peripheral resistance rather than to an increase in the volume of blood pumped by the heart. In the early stages of primary hypertension, the increased peripheral resistance is due to increased contraction of the tiny muscle cells surrounding the arterioles—that is, increased muscle tension. Therefore, to decrease blood pressure, we have to allow these tiny muscle cells to relax their grip on the arterioles. Figure 13 shows cross sections of a relaxed and a contracted arteriole.

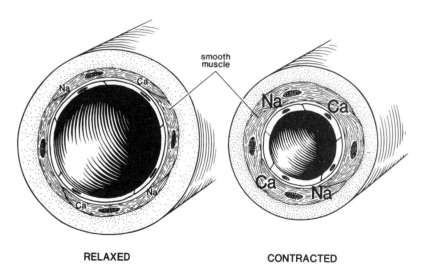

RELAXED   CONTRACTED

FIGURE 13. *Cross sections of arterioles.*

If the hypertension is severe and has been present for several years, scar-type tissue may form in the arterioles, which can make it impossible for them to relax. That's one reason it's important to detect and treat hypertension *before* too much damage is done.

From K Factor to Blood Pressure: The Causal Chain

As we have seen, the high blood pressure in patients with primary hypertension is brought about by excessive peripheral resistance in the arterioles. The peripheral resistance, in turn, is the result of excessive tension, or contraction, of the muscle cells encircling the arteriole walls. And we know that muscular contractions are caused by an increase of calcium inside the cell.

An overabundance of calcium inside the cell, in turn, can be caused by either a slow calcium pump (pushing less calcium out of the cell) or by holes in the cellular membrane allowing calcium to leak back inside the cell. Either of these can result from a sodium battery that is run down. And either slow sodium-potassium pumps or too few sodium-potassium pumps will allow the sodium battery to run down. This causal chain is diagramed in Figure 14, which is a repeat of Figure 11.

We have hinted that a low–*K Factor* diet will slow the sodium-potassium pump. But just how does this work?

Recall from the last chapter the evidence that when too much sodium is retained in the body, the brain releases a hormone (a natriuretic factor) that slows the exchange of potassium for sodium by the sodium-potassium pumps in the small arteries. (We describe this further in Chapter 22.) Since potassium tends to decrease the amount of sodium in the body, a low ratio of potassium to sodium in the diet, or a low *K Factor*, will tend to elevate this substance, thus leading to slowing of the sodium-potassium pumps in the body. Several studies indicate that this natriuretic hormone is elevated in many people with primary hypertension.

But there is another way that a low–*K Factor* diet may slow the sodium-potassium pumps. Because potassium is pumped into cells, there has to be enough potassium on the outside of the cell in order for the sodium-potassium pump to work well, moving the potassium from the outside to the inside. If the po-

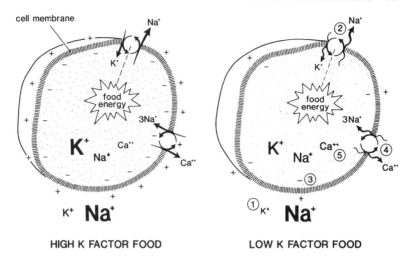

HIGH K FACTOR FOOD   LOW K FACTOR FOOD

FIGURE 14. *The* K Factor *and cellular calcium: 2 = sodium-po-tassium pump, 4 = calcium pump*. These and other numbers show the causal chain, as described in the text, of events leading from a low–*K Factor* diet to a higher level of calcium inside the cell and, thus, high blood pressure.

tassium ions in the blood (and outside the cells, number 1 in Figure 14) are few and far between, they won't bump into the sodium-potassium pumps as often. This means that the pumps will slow down (number 2 in Figure 14). In fact, the speed of the sodium-potassium pump depends on the level of blood (serum) potassium. There is evidence that in the normal range of plasma potassium, the level of potassium has a significant effect upon the sodium-potassium pump's speed.[10]

One way to test the idea that increasing levels of serum potassium, within the "normal" range, relax the small arteries and do so by speeding up the sodium-potassium pump, is to add potassium to arteries and see what happens—especially if we block the sodium-potassium pump. When this experiment is done, increasing the level of potassium from 3.6 to 6.0 meq/L causes the small arteries to relax so they let blood flow through more easily.[11] Not only that, but when a drug called ouabain, which specifically inhibits the sodium-potassium pump, is added to the small arteries first, potassium no longer makes them dilate. So the evidence seems pretty good that part of the blood pressure effect of potassium is due to its direct stimulation of the sodium-potassium pump so the sodium battery can remain charged and the muscle cells in the small arteries can stay relaxed.

So you can see that either adding too much sodium to your body (by eating too much of it) or taking away potassium (by eating too little) could slow the sodium-potassium pumps' charging of the sodium batteries (number 3 in Figure 14), which then slows down the calcium pumps (number 4) and increases membrane leakiness to calcium, which increases calcium inside the cells (number 5), which increases muscle tension, peripheral resistance, and finally blood pressure (recall figures 12 and 13). The importance of the connection between slowing of the sodium-potassium pump and the resulting slowing of the calcium pumps in developing high blood pressure was first emphasized in 1977 by Dr. Mordecai Blaustein, chairman of the department of Biophysics and Physiology at the University of Maryland School of Medicine.[12]

Dr. Blaustein calculates that even a 5 percent elevation of sodium inside the arterioles should result in a 15 percent elevation of free intracellular calcium, which in turn could cause as much as a 50 percent increase in resting tension of the arterioles.[12]

Superimposed on all this are inherited differences in other hormone systems that regulate the sodium-potassium pumps and the leakiness of our cell membranes (which makes the pumps work faster just to keep up). Thus, because of our inheritance, some of us are more likely to develop high blood pressure when we eat a low–*K Factor* diet than are others of us. But remember from Chapter 3 that if you eat foods with a high *K Factor*, it's unlikely that you'll get hypertension regardless of your inheritance.

In the final analysis, to keep the calcium low inside the tiny muscle cells so your arterioles can relax, your body must have a normal balance between potassium and sodium: the sodium batteries must be charged.

IS CALCIUM BAD? From what we have said in this chapter up until now, you might expect that extra dietary calcium would be bad for hypertension. If calcium builds up in the cell, we get too much muscle tension, too much peripheral resistance, and too much blood pressure.

But we saw in Chapter 4 how Addison demonstrated that a high-calcium diet helped control blood pressure. How can this be?

When we look at the cell a little closer, this isn't so surprising. A charged sodium battery is not the only thing that prevents leakiness in the cell wall. Paradoxically, the very presence of lots of calcium outside the cell membrane (remember, 10,000 times more calcium outside than inside), pressuring to get in, helps keep the membrane tight and thus slows the leak of calcium into the cell. If the amount of calcium in the blood drops very much, the membrane becomes leaky. As a result, the calcium level inside the cell actually goes up. To keep the calcium low inside, you've got to keep it high outside! Surprising at first sight, but true.

So either a low *K Factor* or a low amount of dietary calcium can cause hypertension.

HOW ABOUT MAGNESIUM? How does magnesium help? Magnesium in the blood outside the cell, like calcium, helps stabilize the cell membrane by helping to keep it tight and to prevent leaks. Not only that, magnesium is necessary for the sodium-potassium pump to operate properly. So it should not be surprising that sufficient magnesium must be present to enable the sodium battery to be kept charged.

In Chapter 8, we will present evidence that too little magnesium in the diet can also help cause high blood pressure.

The Acid and the "Building Block" Pumps: Maintaining Protein Strength

The sodium battery is important not only for keeping your blood pressure from getting too high. It is also important in maintaining protein structure itself—in particular, to keep the walls of the arteries strong.

Protein makes up the substance of cell tissue. For any cell to maintain itself, it must have sufficient protein. But complete proteins cannot pass from the blood into the cell; they are too large to get through the cell's surface membrane. Therefore, the cell must make its own protein inside by zipping together smaller protein building blocks, which scientists call amino acids. (These amino acids do not make the cell more acid but are called acids for technical reasons.) These building blocks, or amino acids, are small enough that they can be transported through the cell's surface membrane.

Inside the cell, there is enzyme machinery bound together in what is called *ribosomes*, which act like little factories to make protein. The raw material, amino acids, goes into these little factories, or ribosomes, where it is put together on an assembly line that is directed by a template material called RNA (ribonucleic acid). There are twenty different types of natural amino acids, each a different type of building block. The ribosome zips these together into a chain, which then folds up into different forms, depending upon the exact sequence of amino acids. The sequence is like a message, or language, in which there are twenty different letters. As in any language, the meaning of the message is determined by the exact sequence of the letters, building blocks, or amino acids in this case. The RNA carries the instructions for sequence of assembly from the genetic material, DNA, in our genes and forms the template that determines the exact sequence of amino acids and thus the identity of each protein.

Since protein can't be made without them, the amino acids need to be brought into the cell. On the other hand, acid (hydrogen ions: H^+) has to be moved out of the cell. For example, the cell's enzyme machinery in the ribosomes that zips the amino acid building blocks together can be inhibited by acid (H^+).[14] In order for your cells to have enough protein structure to be strong, amino acids must be moved in and acid must be moved out.

The sodium battery does not merely empower the calcium

pump; it also drives an amino acid pump and an acid (H⁺) pump (see Figure 15).

Notice that the acid (H⁺) pump works by letting sodium move in while moving H⁺ out. The amino acid pump works differently: Sodium and an amino acid move in together. But the principle is the same: The energy for moving some amino acids into the cell ("uphill," or against its natural tendency) comes from the sodium battery, just as the energy for moving the acid uphill (out of the cell) comes from the sodium battery.

So if the sodium-potassium pump slows (from a low–*K Factor* diet) and therefore the sodium battery runs down, the delivery of amino acid building blocks will slow, and acid will accumulate in the cell. There are a number of ways an increase in acid *or* an increase in calcium inside the cell could decrease the rate at which proteins are made or could have dramatic effects on the type of proteins that are made or the way they are assembled into larger structures.[15] Thus it is entirely possible that less protein, or the wrong kind of protein, will be manufactured in the cells of people with primary hypertension. The cells themselves would be weaker.

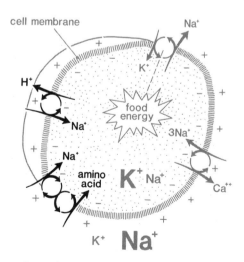

FIGURE 15. *The sodium-powered amino acid and H⁺ pumps.*

Increasing the *K Factor* (which will help the sodium-potassium pumps and so charges the sodium battery) decreases
the chances of strokes (blowout of arteries) even when the blood
pressure doesn't come down as we described in the previous
chapter. In addition, in 1985 a research group in Australia[16] reported that even in people with normal blood pressure, people
who eat high levels of sodium, or a low *K Factor*, develop increased stiffness of their arteries. This indicates that a high
K Factor is necessary for strong, pliable arteries, built from sufficient protein. Conversely, it's not surprising that a deficiency of
the *K Factor* seems to lead to weak arteries from insufficient or
improper protein (see Figure 16).

Testing the Model

What we have presented in this chapter is oversimplified.
Many details remain to be worked out and confirmed. Nevertheless, several predictions necessarily follow from the model presented here. Demonstrating that any one of these predictions is
wrong would invalidate, or disprove, the model or at least require it to be modified (see Chapter 19 for a discussion of scientific "proof"). Among the predictions that have been confirmed
by scientific studies are:

PREDICTION 1: The potassium in body cells (and therefore
total body potassium) will be decreased in people with primary hypertension.

Confirmation: In fact, Scandinavian scientists have shown
that in people with untreated primary hypertension, the total
amount of potassium in their bodies is significantly decreased.[17]

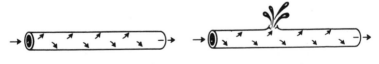

HIGH K FACTOR FOOD   **LOW K FACTOR FOOD**

FIGURE 16. *A strong and a weak artery.*

PREDICTION 2: The potassium level in the blood plasma of people with hypertension should tend to be decreased.

Confirmation: In Chapter 23, we present evidence that shows that people with hypertension generally have a slightly lower level of potassium in their blood plasma.

PREDICTION 3: The sodium inside the cells of the body should be increased in people with primary hypertension.

Confirmation: The white blood cell is an easily studied cell with many sodium-potassium pumps. Many studies have shown, apparently without exception, that there is an elevated level of sodium in white blood cells from people with hypertension compared to people with normal blood pressure.[18]

PREDICTION 4: Increasing the level of potassium in the blood should cause the small resistance arteries to relax.

Confirmation: Raising plasma potassium from 3.6 meq/L to 6 meq/L produces a significant relaxation of the small arteries, with a resulting drop in blood pressure.[19]

PREDICTION 5: Inhibiting the sodium-potassium pump in the small resistance arteries should block this relaxing effect of potassium.

Confirmation: Inhibiting the sodium-potassium pump with a specific inhibitor blocks this action of potassium on these small arteries.[20]

PREDICTION 6: Because the muscle cells of Type II diabetics are resistant to the effects of insulin, their sodium-potassium pumps should slow down, allowing increased levels of sodium inside the muscle cells. Therefore, Type II diabetics should be more likely to develop high blood pressure.

Confirmation: Having diabetes mellitus greatly increases a person's chances of developing high blood pressure.[21]

PREDICTION 7: Giving adequate potassium compared to sodium in the diet should help lower elevated blood pressure.

Confirmation: In Chapter 5, we documented studies that show that increasing the ratio of potassium to sodium, the *K Factor*, in the diet can restore blood pressure toward normal in people with hypertension.

All in all, the evidence for the following statement is very strong:

The real problem isn't just blood pressure; it's deeper than that. It involves an imbalance between potassium and sodium, and also calcium, deep within the living cell. Drugs don't get at that problem; the K Factor approach does.

Summary

When the diet is high in sodium chloride and/or low in potassium, the sodium-potassium pumps tend to slow, allowing the sodium battery to run down. Thus it should not be surprising to find that either an excess of sodium or a deficiency of potassium in the diet can contribute to high blood pressure.

On the other hand, extra potassium can stimulate the sodium-potassium pump and recharge the sodium battery! A fully charged sodium battery also helps keep cell calcium levels low, thus relaxing arterioles and keeping the blood pressure low. The battery also helps promote the manufacture of proteins by the cells. A discharged sodium battery might also explain a decreased strength of artery walls in people or animals with hypertension.

One might say that in the body, sodium and potassium balance each other. As an approximation, sodium and potassium may be seen as representing opposing forces. As such, they must be kept in a kind of balance if you are to function the way nature intended.

One "pushes" where the other "pulls." One is the yin and the other yang. To have a complete effect, both must be changed.

That's why we use the *K Factor*: It's a measure of the balance between potassium and sodium.

CHAPTER 7

Where Does Being Fit Fit In?

Being overweight greatly increases your chances of developing primary hypertension. And if you are overweight, it can be more difficult to get your blood pressure down than it would be for someone whose weight is normal. Losing even half of the excess pounds can reduce blood pressure significantly. In two studies,[1] dietary reduction of weight in obese people with hypertension lowered diastolic blood pressure to normal levels in three out of every four cases, even though no drugs were used!

When it is combined with exercise, weight loss can be especially effective. A large-scale study, the Chicago Prevention Evaluation Program, has demonstrated the effectiveness of increased physical activity, together with dietary restriction, in reducing blood pressure. The subjects were advised to engage in "modest" light exercise at least three times per week and to reduce caloric intake by 30 percent. This program produced an average weight loss of 11.7 pounds, which was sustained over five years. In the 67 middle-aged hypertensives who were not receiving antihypertensive drugs, systolic blood pressure was reduced by an average of 13.3 mm Hg and diastolic by an average of 9.7 mm Hg.[2]

Regardless of body weight, people who fail to get regular exercise tend to have more high blood pressure. Regular exercise programs have been shown to reduce blood pressure even when no weight loss occurs.[3] This works both in people with hypertension who are obese and also in those with normal body weight. When twenty-seven obese hypertensive women were given a six-month course of physical training, there was a significant decrease in blood pressure in all of them. This decrease in blood pressure toward normal was correlated not with change in body fat but with the degree of reduction of elevated serum insulin and also with the reduction of serum triglycerides.[4] Increased physical activity can also produce a substantial reduction of blood pressure in hypertensives of normal body weight.[5]

The dramatic ability of aerobic exercise to lower elevated blood pressure in many patients was recently demonstrated in a study conducted at the University of Florida by Dr. Robert Cade and his co-workers.[6] All of the 105 patients who completed the exercise program started with a diastolic blood pressure of over 90 mm Hg. Roughly half (47) were receiving antihypertensive drugs, and the other half were not. No attempt was made to alter the diet or to restrict dietary sodium.

The exercise program began with each patient walking one mile each day and progressed, at a rate tailored individually, until each patient was running two miles every day. Within three months after reaching two miles per day, 101 of the 105 patients had significant drops in blood pressure. Of the four whose blood pressure failed to respond, one had kidney disease and the others had reduced kidney function due to long-standing high blood pressure.

Of those receiving antihypertensive therapy, roughly half were able to discontinue all drugs and yet achieve lower blood pressure than when they started. Most of those who were still receiving drugs were able to decrease the amount. The decrease in blood pressure was not due to weight changes, since the decrease was as great in those patients who gained weight as in those who lost weight during the study.

Of seven patients who entered the study with severe hypertension (diastolic pressure greater than 115 mm Hg), two developed normal blood pressure and two others decreased to borderline hypertension. The most dramatic response was seen in a thirty-four-year-old woman who entered the study with primary hypertension and blood pressure of 160/120. After three months of running two miles per day, her blood pressure remained an excellent 110/74 without any drugs.

This study has been criticized because of lack of controls (see statistical analysis in Chapter 19) to eliminate other factors, such as time or other life-style factors. However, fifteen of the patients *themselves* served as "controls." These fifteen were persuaded to stop exercising after three months. After three more months of sedentary life, the average diastolic blood pressure of this group rose from the postexercise value of 82 mm to 100 mm Hg! Several other studies have also indicated that exercise can lower blood pressure without change in weight. Recently Drs. John Martin and Pat Dubbert at the Veterans Administration Hospital in Jackson, Mississippi, conducted a classic "controlled study" involving nineteen people with primary hypertension. This study showed that 10 weeks of aerobic exercise for 30 minutes three to four days a week produces a significant drop in blood pressure.[7] This drop in blood pressure was not accompanied by any significant change in body fat.

So there isn't much doubt that getting regular exercise is an important step (pun intended) in keeping your blood pressure normal and that if you are overweight, it is essential to get rid of some of those excess pounds of fat.

Weight Loss, Exercise, and Increasing the K Factor—Why Do All Three?

If you lose weight, increase your *K Factor*, and exercise regularly, you will not only get the maximum reduction in your blood pressure, but you will produce the best "tune-up," or balance, in your body's cells. In practice, the different elements of the *K Factor* program all tie together. The *K Factor* eating approach not only helps your blood pressure by increasing the

K Factor but, by cutting down the fat you eat, it also helps you lose pounds. The *K Factor*-and-exercise approach helps your blood pressure *and* helps you keep the weight off. So in practice, the steps are related. They work together. But is this just a coincidence?

Do Losing Excess Weight, Getting Exercise, and Eating Food with a High K Factor Have Something in Common?

At first sight, it must seem, even to most professionals, that obesity and lack of exercise are one thing and a deficient *K Factor* is another. That's easy to understand, because only in the last few years have scientific articles begun to appear that point toward possible connections tying together the *K Factor*, losing weight, and getting exercise. One connection appears to involve the "sugar" hormone, insulin.

When referring to insulin, we put quotes around the word *sugar* because we now know that insulin regulates not only the absorption of carbohydrates and other nutrients such as fat and protein, but insulin also helps regulate the activity of the sodium-potassium pump.[8] By helping to control the sodium-potassium pump, insulin helps maintain the balance of potassium to sodium in body cells and can also slow the excretion of sodium by the kidneys. So eating food with a high *K Factor*, exercising, and maintaining normal body weight to keep insulin levels normal all help maintain the normal balance in your body's cells.

It All Comes Together Here

One of the hidden problems of being overweight is that it causes your blood insulin levels to rise. Lack of exercise also tends to result in an elevation of blood insulin.[9] In fact, although we don't yet know the reasons, even people with high blood pressure who are not overweight seem to have an increase in blood insulin.[10]

Another group that tends to be hypertensive is people with Type II diabetes, the type that usually begins in adults who are overweight. Though Type II diabetics suffer from a resistance to the action of insulin on their muscle and fat cells, they actually have elevated blood levels of insulin.[11] It now appears that *all* groups with primary hypertension may have elevated insulin levels. We now know that an elevated level of insulin can stimulate the sodium-potassium pumps in the kidney and thus cause the kidney to retain sodium in the body.[12] The elevated insulin levels can also increase the activity of the sympathetic nerves that make your blood pressure go up.[13] Again, this may involve the sodium-potassium pump, helping to regulate the amount of "chemical transmitter" (noradrenaline) that carries signals from sympathetic nerves to small blood vessels (arterioles), telling them to contract.

Obesity

In obesity, the elevated blood insulin partly compensates for a decreased ability of fat cells to respond to insulin. But the kidney responds to these elevated insulin levels by speeding up its sodium-potassium pumps to pump sodium from the newly formed urine (kidney ultrafiltrate) back into the blood. So if you're overweight, your body tends to retain the sodium you eat instead of excreting it as it should. This can upset the balance between potassium and sodium in body cells, leading to a decrease in energy of the "sodium battery" and an increase in calcium inside the tiny muscle cells of the arterioles, causing your blood pressure to go up.

Fortunately, losing those excess pounds of fat tends to get the insulin level back to where it should be. (Losing muscle *doesn't* help—that's one reason very low calorie diets aren't recommended for weight loss.) And when that happens, one or both of two things follow: the lowered blood insulin allows the kidneys to excrete more sodium and water, and the sympathetic nerves to quiet down,[14] thus relaxing the arterioles. Both effects help produce a dramatic drop in blood pressure.

Again, we see that a balance between potassium, sodium, and calcium in the cell is the key to hypertension.

Exercise

Recent studies[15] have shown that regular exercise, even when it doesn't cause weight loss, decreases the blood level of insulin and changes the levels of other hormones related to potassium and sodium balance. This may explain why a long-term exercise program can decrease blood pressure.

So being fit tunes up not only your muscles but also the body's mechanisms that regulate the balance between potassium and sodium. So stay tuned up, and tune in to what you eat and how you prepare it. If you just give your body a chance, it'll keep your blood pressure—and blood vessels—in good shape.

Simple Sugars Can Raise Blood Pressure

Overfeeding sucrose to rats with hypertension stimulates their sympathetic nervous system,[16] elevating the blood pressure still further. Overfeeding the same amount of calories as fat had no effect on either sympathetic activity or on blood pressure. In rats with normal blood pressure, overfeeding sucrose produced the same effects, but less dramatically. This effect of sugar is probably due to the resulting increase in blood insulin levels, since experiments have shown that where blood glucose is kept unchanged, elevation of insulin levels increases sympathic activity and blood pressure.[17]

Fasting

A dramatic way to illustrate the connection between insulin and hypertension is fasting. In obese people on a "protein sparing," or partial, fast, elevated blood pressure will almost always decrease toward normal within less than a week. That's because fasting is one way to lower quickly but temporarily the levels of blood insulin and other hormones that regulate the body's ability to keep a proper balance between potassium and sodium. These changes, especially the lower insulin levels, allow the kidneys to get rid of excess body sodium and water. (Incidentally, that's why the first pounds lost on a very low calorie diet are mostly not fat but water.) Fasting also decreases the activity of the sympathetic nervous system,[18] presumably secondary to the decreased insulin levels.[19]

We strongly recommend against a total fast, since after the first day, your body begins to burn up your muscle and other protein. Don't try even a partial fast without your doctor's supervision.

Summary

There is evidence that increasing the *K Factor* in the diet (increasing potassium and decreasing sodium), losing excess pounds of fat, and getting regular exercise are in many ways *doing the same things* inside the body. They all work together to normalize the balance in your body's cells. Although some effects involve the sympathetic nervous system and others involve the kidneys, evidence keeps appearing that indicates that changes in the sodium-potassium pump are part of the mechanism whereby either exercise or weight loss can restore elevated blood pressure toward normal.

One interesting observation is that apparently all groups with primary hypertension seem to have elevated blood levels of insulin—which causes the kidneys to retain sodium in the body. Both weight loss and exercise help lower these insulin levels and this may be part of the mechanism that allows these activities to help reduce elevated blood pressure.

Although many details remain to be worked out, the common theme that appears is that to cure your high blood pressure without drugs, you need to keep up the *K Factor* in your food and to eliminate factors, such as obesity and lack of exercise, that prevent the body from maintaining a normal balance between potassium and sodium.

CHAPTER 8

Other Factors That Influence Blood Pressure

The Key Factors

In this book, we emphasize the three key factors to naturally prevent or cure primary hypertension:

- Diet, especially the *K Factor*.
- Weight control.
- Exercise.

The most effective way to lower your blood pressure is to combine these three factors. But the overall scientific evidence suggests that eating foods with a proper ratio of potassium to sodium, or *K Factor*, is *the* most important factor in determining whether a person with a hereditary tendency for hypertension develops high blood pressure.

Other factors, however, do have roles to play—some of them important roles. We have already mentioned that getting enough dietary calcium is important; in about a third of the people with primary hypertension, it is perhaps a key factor.

And dietary chloride may be almost as harmful as sodium (so table salt, which contains both sodium *and* chloride, is doubly bad).

We now discuss, in what we think is the order of importance, these other factors.

Magnesium and Calcium

In the cell, the movements of calcium and of magnesium are linked to sodium and, through the sodium-potassium pump, thus to potassium. Adequate blood levels of calcium and magnesium are necessary to stabilize and prevent leakiness of the membrane that surrounds each body cell and are essential for normal balance of the levels of sodium and potassium across this membrane. Thus it is not surprising that adequate amounts in the diet of calcium and magnesium are important in the prevention and treatment of some cases of hypertension.

MAGNESIUM. There are now several reasons to suspect that a dietary factor in primary hypertension is deficiency of magnesium. The incidence of hypertension is high in regions that have naturally soft water—that is, mineral-poor water—or magnesium-poor soil.[1] (Water softeners are doubly bad, since most of them add sodium in addition to removing magnesium and calcium.) Rats fed a diet deficient in magnesium develop significant hypertension within twelve weeks.[2]

Deficient dietary magnesium might be expected to result in lower levels of magnesium in the blood serum that bathes the body cells. This in turn could tend to make the cell membranes less stable and more leaky to sodium, potassium, and calcium. So an adequate level of magnesium in blood serum is probably important in stabilizing these membranes and allowing the small muscle cells that control blood pressure to remain relaxed. In fact, experiments on blood vessels in dogs have shown that increasing blood magnesium does dilate the arteries.[3] Lowering blood magnesium levels in animals and in humans is often associated with increases in peripheral resistance, with resulting increases in blood pressure.[4]

Some people with primary hypertension do indeed have low

levels of magnesium in their blood serum.[5] In these people,[6] lower serum magnesium levels have been found together with increased activity of a blood hormone, renin, that acts to increase blood pressure (see Chapter 22). A recent study has shown that the level of free magnesium inside blood cells is about 25 percent lower in those people with primary hypertension than it is in the rest of the population.[7]

There is another way magnesium deficiency could contribute to high blood pressure. Magnesium loss increases the tendency of the body to lose potassium, and administration of magnesium is sometimes required in order to enable the body to replenish its stores of potassium.[8] Not only that, but administration of magnesium has been reported to increase sodium excretion by the kidneys, and magnesium deficiency decreases urinary sodium, possibly due to a decrease in a sodium-retaining hormone, aldosterone.[9] So the fact that prolonged use of the sodium-excreting thiazide diuretics results in not only a decrease in body potassium but also a decrease in body magnesium content[10] reinforces the desirability of using nondrug approaches— especially for those with mild hypertension.

The idea of using magnesium isn't new; it was first recommended as the treatment of severe hypertension due to kidney disease as early as 1925.[11] In one specific type of hypertension, that associated with preeclampsia of pregnancy, the most effective way to decrease the blood pressure has been for years, and still is, to give magnesium. And it has been reported that giving supplemental magnesium to pregnant women prevents preeclampsia and hypertension.[12]

In one of the few recent clinical studies testing the effects of magnesium on primary hypertension, eighteen hypertensive patients who had been taking diuretics for some time were given magnesium aspartate hydrochloride tablets each day (365 mg of magnesium per day). This resulted in an average reduction in diastolic blood pressure of 8 mm Hg.[13] Unfortunately, there were no placebo controls in this study.

Especially since magnesium deficiency can contribute to a potassium deficiency, the evidence appears strong that adequate magnesium intake is necessary to prevent or to reverse primary hypertension. Unfortunately, many of us don't get enough of this previously overlooked mineral, perhaps because of widespread areas of magnesium-deficient soil in the United States. The average daily consumption has been claimed to be as low as 200 to 250 milligrams, compared to the National Academy of Sciences Recommended Dietary Allowance (RDA) of 300 milligrams daily for nonpregnant women, 450 milligrams daily for pregnant women, and 350 milligrams daily for men, except 400 milligrams per day for fifteen- to eighteen-year-old men. Good food sources of magnesium include bananas, black-eyed peas, buckwheat flour, whole wheat flour, kidney beans, lima beans, avocados, and our old standby, the potato.

CALCIUM. Evidence from animal studies, from correlation of dietary nutrients with hypertension in humans, and from a consideration of the interplay between calcium, magnesium, sodium, and potassium inside the living cell all suggests that sufficient calcium in the diet is important in preventing hypertension. As far back as 1924, Addison[14] had reported that not only supplemental potassium but also calcium chloride could lower the blood pressure of hypertensive patients.

In the last few years, interest in calcium has revived. In one controlled study, half of a group of volunteers with normal blood pressure were given a daily tablet containing 1 gram of calcium and the other half received a placebo tablet (one that appeared identical but contained no calcium).[15] The group receiving the calcium showed a significant reduction in blood pressure.

In a study by Dr. Lawrence Resnick and his colleagues at Cornell University Medical College in New York City, an increase in dietary calcium decreased diastolic blood pressure, sometimes by as much as 10 to 20 percent, in the 30 percent of patients with primary hypertension who had low blood levels of a substance, called renin, that can affect blood pressure.[16] Increasing dietary calcium was more effective in those with low initial levels of blood-serum calcium and in those hypertensives with high dietary levels of sodium.

A study in Guatemala of thirty-six pregnant women with normal blood pressure also showed that calcium supplementation can decrease blood pressure.[17] To eliminate possible psychological effects in this study, the women did not know whether they were taking placebo (fake) pills or the pills that actually contained calcium. This was a "double blind" study, because both those studied *and* those doing the studying were "blind"—that is, ignorant of who got the placebo pills and who got ᵗhe real thing. This information was released by the pill manufacturer only at the end of the study. Near the end of their pregnancies, the average diastolic blood pressures of the women taking placebo pills was 71.9 mm Hg; in the group taking 1 gram of calcium per day, it was 68.8 mm Hg; and in the group taking 2 grams of calcium per day, it was 64.5 mm Hg.

Some statistical analyses of the large HANES I Data Base of eating habits and blood pressure in the United States found that the higher the intake of calcium, the lower the blood pressure tended to be.[18] In this study, dietary calcium was estimated by asking each person to name the foods eaten the previous day. As we discuss in Chapter 19, other statistical evaluations of the HANES I Data Base suggest that dietary calcium may not be so important.

In addition, still other studies have suggested the reverse: that is, the higher the urinary calcium, the higher the blood pressure. These studies were undertaken in Italy,[19] Belgium,[20] and Korea.[21] The dietary calcium was estimated by measuring calcium excretion in the urine. But this method may not always reflect the amount of calcium in the diet. Several conditions can cause loss of body calcium: certain diseases, excess sodium chloride, too little exercise. Some suggest that too much dietary protein can also do it. Therefore, these conditions can increase calcium in the urine even when the diet is deficient in calcium.

When hypertensive rats were put on a low-calcium diet, they became even more hypertensive, whereas when they were on a high-calcium diet, the rats became much less hypertensive.[22] When normal rats are given extra sodium chloride in their diet (amounts comparable to that in the typical American diet), they begin to lose calcium from their bones into the urine. The effect of excess sodium chloride again demonstrates the counterbalance between sodium (bad for blood pressure) and potassium and calcium (good for blood pressure).

The effect of calcium on blood pressure is also consistent with our understanding of the cellular mechanisms that are involved in keeping the cell membrane "tight" so the proper balance between potassium, sodium, and calcium within the cell can be maintained, as we described in Chapter 6.

In summary, there are several clues that indicate that a drop in dietary calcium can contribute to high blood pressure.

Chloride

Although the hypertensive effect of table salt (NaCl) is commonly attributed to the positive sodium ion, Na^+, there is evidence that the negative chloride ion, Cl^-, may also contribute, along with sodium, to the development of hypertension.[23] When sodium is given to people with a family history of hypertension, it raises the blood pressure only when given as NaCl. Other sodium salts, such as sodium bicarbonate, produce relatively little elevation of blood pressure. Also, Dr. Addison noticed that potassium citrate appeared more effective than potassium chloride in his treatment of humans with hypertension.[24]

The fact that sodium appears to depend on chloride to do its dirty work may not be so surprising in light of the fact that for sodium to be reabsorbed in the kidney and thus retained by the body, most of it must be accompanied by chloride. If sodium is accompanied by another substance, such as bicarbonate or the organic ions present in natural food, then the sodium will tend to be lost in the urine. So table salt (NaCl) is double trouble.

Dietary Fat

Beyond the small amount (probably much less than 15 percent of our calories) our body needs, there really is nothing good to say for dietary fat. Besides contributing to obesity, increasing the chances of the occurrence of some types of cancer, and being the main factor causing coronary vascular disease leading to heart attacks, excess dietary fat may contribute directly to hypertension. There is now some evidence that decreasing total fat content together with some increase in linoleic acid can help control primary hypertension.

Scientific studies have reported that decreasing dietary fat to provide only 25 percent of energy intake *and* increasing the ratio of polyunsaturated fat to saturated fat (P/S ratio) to about 1.0 results in a significant reduction in blood pressure. This effect is independent of weight reduction and is observed in normal people as well as in those with mild hypertension, although the effect appears to be greater among the latter.[25]

In these two studies, the reduction in dietary fat was accomplished by dietary substitution of vegetables and fresh fruits for fatty foods. This would be expected to increase dietary potassium. Although the amount of sodium in low-fat, high P/S–ratio diets was not changed, in the one study in which it was measured, dietary potassium was found to be increased by up to an additional 90 percent when the changes in dietary fat were made. Thus the decrease in blood pressure in some of these studies might have been due in part to the increase in dietary potassium.

LINOLEIC ACID. The increase in polyunsaturated fat in these diets was accompanied by an increase in dietary linoleic acid, the only fatty acid "required" in the diet, since the human body does not manufacture it from other foods. Since this fatty acid is required for synthesis of the hormones called prostaglandins, it has been speculated that the effect of the dietary change in these studies may be due to an increase in prostaglandin hormones, which are known to increase sodium excretion by the kidneys. This led to a study in which the effect of dietary content of linoleic acid upon blood pressure in mildly hypertensive humans was tested.

Increasing dietary linoleic acid from an average of 4.0 (plus or minus 0.3) percent of total calories to 5.2 (plus or minus 0.4) percent resulted in a significant reduction in diastolic blood pressure.[26] When the dietary linoleic acid was increased, excretion of potassium by the kidney was decreased by 40 percent. In addition, this increase of dietary linoleic acid decreased serum cholesterol by 7 percent, a small but significant amount. The ability of increased dietary linoleic acid (in the form of safflower oil) to lower elevated blood pressure has also been demonstrated in hypertensive rats in several studies[27] and in humans in a study done in Finland.[28]

Although the role of dietary fat as a contributing factor to hypertension is not yet completely understood, it is clear that a decrease of total fat intake together with some increase in linoleic acid cannot hurt and will probably help in controlling primary hypertension. In view of the bad effects of dietary fat in terms of obesity, cancer, and especially heart disease, decreasing dietary fat to no more than 20 percent of calories is a high priority for health and longevity.

Alcohol

It is very clear that heavy drinkers have much higher blood pressure than those who drink less.[29] One study of 83,947 persons with highly different occupations and ethnic backgrounds showed that this correlation is not explained by overweight or use of coffee or cigarettes.[30]

The effect of excessive amounts of alcohol on blood pressure is not surprising, since intoxicating amounts of alcohol may increase the leakiness of the cell membrane to sodium.[31] Not only that, alcoholism has often been associated with decreased levels of magnesium.[32] As discussed in Chapter 6, an increased leakiness can lead indirectly to an increase in the level of calcium inside the smooth muscles surrounding the small arteries, leading to narrowing of these arteries.

Vitamins C and D

The original analysis of the HANES I study indicated that people eating larger amounts of vitamin C had lower blood pressure.[33] A more recent analysis of the same data reached the same conclusion and also reported that higher levels of vitamin D in the diet were correlated with lower blood pressure. A probable explanation for these observations is that vitamin C is found in foods rich in potassium (fruits and vegetables) and vitamin D is found in milk (rich in calcium and also in potassium).

Psychological Stress

A commonly held view is that psychological stress can cause hypertension. In our opinion, this is highly speculative. As we have already discussed, it is questionable whether the people in the low blood pressure, unacculturated societies that have been studied are under less stress than are people in industrialized societies. Moreover, tranquilizers and sedatives are ineffective in treating hypertension. Nevertheless, there is evidence that in people with hypertension, the blood pressure is more sensitive to stress.

Stress operates through the sympathetic nervous system, which uses adrenaline to transmit signals from nerves to stimulate contraction of the smooth muscles in the walls of the arterioles. The action of the sympathetic nervous system explains how some of the drugs used to treat hypertension work. For example, the beta and alpha "adrenergic" blockers help lower blood pressure by blocking sympathetic nerve activity, thus allowing the small arteries to relax. So it's not surprising that in people who already have primary hypertension, there is evidence that psychological stress can make their blood pressure go still higher.

Some recent evidence indicates that some people respond to stress by losing more magnesium in their urine. This could contribute to a magnesium deficiency, with consequent bad effects on blood pressure.

One thing is certain: stress often leads to behavior, such as overeating or overdrinking, that is bad not only for our blood pressure but our general health.

Even in hypertension in which stress may be a contributor, however, potassium should help. This is supported by the finding that humans with normal blood pressure who are placed on a high-potassium diet do not show as great a rise in blood pressure, when subjected to mental stress, as do people in a control group on a "normal" diet.[34]

Meditation

Although the role of psychological stress is not clear, meditation and relaxation have been reported to be effective in producing long-term reductions in blood pressure.[35] (Relaxation also produces an immediate reduction of blood pressure, so that it is very important for you to relax completely while your blood pressure is being taken, in order to avoid a falsely high reading. Just by gripping the arm of your chair firmly, you can increase your systolic and diastolic blood pressures over 20 mm Hg.[36] Even the act of talking calmly while your blood pressure is being taken can raise your pressure readings by about 5 mm Hg.

Biofeedback

There is little doubt that with proper training, biofeedback can lower blood pressure.[37] The power of the brain (some would say of the mind) to control basic body functions such as pulse and blood pressure has been known by yogis for centuries.

But this is just another means for regulating, or controlling, blood pressure. True, biofeedback doesn't have the side effects of drugs, but like them, biofeedback is a means of treating the symptom, not of curing the primary problem. There is no evidence that biofeedback can restore the imbalance within the cell that causes hypertension in the first place.

Workaholism

It has been suggested that workaholics have higher than average blood pressures, but this is hard to quantitate. In our opinion, good health is best maintained by a balance between work and play as well as between sodium and potassium. We need a yin and a yang. One needs to work in order to feel a sense of accomplishment, but it is also important to laugh and enjoy life.

Climate

Some have suggested that climate may have some effect on blood pressure. For example, in an extensive study of blood pressures of adults living in England, it was noted that blood pressures were significantly lower when measured in the summer than when measured in the winter.[38] Presumably this was due partly to the decreased resistance to blood flow resulting from the dilation of the blood vessels in the skin in the summertime. It may also have been partly due to the greater availability in the summer of fresh fruits and vegetables (which are rich in potassium).

To keep things in perspective, one of the low-sodium, high-potassium groups that was found to have consistently low blood pressures was the Greenland Eskimos, who live where the weather is cool even in the summer.

Summary

There are many roads to primary hypertension. The most traveled are deficient dietary *K Factor*, lack of exercise, and obesity. Other commonly traveled roads are deficient dietary magnesium or calcium. But excess dietary fat or excess alcohol can also help get you there.

Thus there are many things you can and should do to reduce or prevent high blood pressure. From the evidence we have presented, it should be obvious that a total, or holistic, approach is required. To be really successful, you need to control your weight, get regular exercise, and—most important—eat food with a *K Factor* above 3!

Summary: Part Two

We have presented five lines of evidence that all converge to indicate that a lack of proper action of the sodium-potassium pump is a common factor in producing primary hypertension. This lack of balance in the exchange of potassium for sodium is caused by changes in life-style typical of modern industrialized countries and encountered for the first time in the four million years of human evolution; namely, a low–*K Factor* diet, lack of exercise, and obesity. Those who inherit especially strong regulatory systems don't get obvious hypertension, but those who don't inherit the extra margin of error do. The lines of evidence showed:

1. The fact that primary hypertension does *not* exist in some societies depends not upon the genetic inheritance of that society—but upon their life-style.
2. Since 1904 and 1928, a few pioneering physicians have repeatedly demonstrated that increasing dietary *K Factor* can restore normal blood pressure—often in even severe hypertension.
3. Studies on experimental animals indicate that increasing the dietary *K Factor* not only can often lower the blood pressure,

but more important, can restore normal health and life-span *even if* blood pressure remains elevated.

Other animal studies demonstrated that elevated blood pressure is due in part to changes in blood levels of hormones, which affect the exchange of potassium for sodium in body cells.

4. In the surface membrane of each body cell, potassium is exchanged for sodium by a mechanism called the sodium-potassium pump. Among other things, this "pump" indirectly supplies the energy required to: Keep calcium out of the cell, keep acid out of the cell, and bring into the cell some of the "building blocks" required to make protein.

Accordingly, if the activity of the sodium-potassium pump slows down in those muscle cells which encircle small arteries, the resulting increase of calcium inside the cell will lead to increased narrowing of the arteries and thus raise blood pressure. The decreased tendency to bring in "protein building blocks," plus the increased calcium and acid inside the cell probably disturbs protein synthesis, damaging the structure of these cells.

5. The evidence indicates that not only a low dietary *K Factor*, but obesity and lack of exercise, by causing hormone changes, disturb normal activity of the sodium-potassium pump. These disturbances appear to cause changes within the small arteries which make them more prone to constrict, and to increase activity of the sympathetic (adrenaline-like) nervous system which signals these arteries to constrict.

Because of increased insulin levels, many of these people probably have increased activity of the sodium-potassium pumps in their kidney cells, and that would lead to increased conservation of sodium within their bodies.

Several factors can contribute to cause primary hypertension in those who have the genetic tendency. There are many ways to disturb the balance between potassium and sodium in the body: not only a deficient dietary *K Factor*, but obesity, lack of exercise, and other factors, such as dietary magnesium and probably calcium, also play a role. However, in view of the evidence now available, the *K Factor*, obesity, and lack of exercise appear to be the most important. From a practical point of view, the key point is to realize that all of these factors are under *your* control. Together with your physician, you can take charge of your life in a way that will allow your body to heal itself and reduce the dangers of high blood pressure.

We're not saying that this view is completely "proven." (Nothing in science is ever *totally* proven—see Chapter 19.) But while no one line of evidence is conclusive in and of itself, the fact that they all point to the same conclusion is impressive. There is consistency here. Everywhere you look, there is either solid evidence, or at the least suggestive evidence, that potassium/sodium exchange by the sodium-potassium pump is involved in hypertension. When you see a pattern emerging, time and again, it's a good sign that it reflects some approximation of the real situation.

Although much remains to be learned, we now have enough understanding of how these factors operate to realize that by changing life-style, we can reverse and prevent the imbalance within the body cells which leads to primary hypertension.

In the meantime, you have a choice: diet and exercise therapy or drug therapy. The clinical evidence is strong that both can decrease mortality. But in the case of nutrition, there is no evidence indicating that it does harm.

Drugs affect only some of the *consequences* of this imbalance, such as retention of sodium or increased activity of the sympathetic nervous system, without correcting the underlying imbalance itself. So it's not completely surprising that two studies suggest that for borderline hypertensives, aggressive drug treatment may actually *increase* mortality. Many want to explain this evidence away. But although these studies may not be entirely conclusive, the burden of proof is on those who maintain that drugs are the preferred treatment.

Although you can't change your genetic inheritance, if you consider the evidence presented in this section, you will realize that the changes in primary hypertension such as sodium and potassium levels, natriuretic factor, insulin levels, and body fat can be reversed by increasing the dietary *K Factor*, getting adequate exercise, and losing any excess weight. Therefore it is possible for people with primary hypertension to get their body systems back into a natural mode of operation. We discuss how to do this in the next section. *A Word of caution:* if you have high blood pressure for a sufficiently long period of time, other secondary changes can occur (mentioned in Part VI) which can make the elevated blood pressure irreversible. *This emphasizes the importance of early detection, diagnosis, and treatment of high blood pressure.*

PART THREE
The Program

The goal of treating patients with hypertension is to prevent the morbidity [damage to well-being] and mortality [death] attributed to high blood pressure.

—Joint National Committee on Detection,
Evaluation, and Treatment of High Blood
Pressure: 1984 Special Report

The fundamental goal of our four-step program, outlined in this part of the book, is not *just* to get your blood pressure down—not just to decrease the numbers read from the blood pressure machine—but to improve your health. It is not intended to treat only part of the problem—blood pressure—but, far more important, to allow your body to restore its normal function, which will decrease your chance of death and increase your sense of well-being. The program is designed to help you be healthy, feel healthy, and live your allotted span of years.

101

It's Easy

This is not a rigid program; it does not require you to give up a lot of things you like. It is simpler and easier to stick to than other successful nondrug programs.

However, without understanding the program, you could put a lot of time and effort into a nondrug, or "natural," approach and make some simple oversights that would result in your not treating your hypertension successfully.

Once you do understand the simple principles we explain here, you'll be able to follow the program with relatively little effort. Soon it will become second nature to you. In particular, we predict that within a few years, almost all Americans will be selecting and preparing their food this way and exercising more.

But It's Up to You

Although it is essential that you consult with your physician, you must realize that in the final analysis, *you* are the one responsible for your health. Neither the government, insurance companies, the medical profession, modern technology, employee programs, nor anything else can really keep you well. Only *you* can do that.

So get involved with your own health care. You're the one who is going to live (or maybe not) with the results.

The Four Steps

What follows is a brief outline of the four steps of our program. Each of these steps will be described in more detail in this part of the book. That is, Step One is described in Chapter 9, Step Two in Chapter 10, and so on.

The steps are related and work together. To take just one example: your weight will reach its proper level (Step Four) more easily if you are eating the right kinds of foods (Step Two) and exercising regularly (Step Three).

The first step is to see your doctor.

Step One: See Your Doctor

First see your doctor for a complete examination. In fact, you need to have your blood pressure measured on at least three separate occasions before deciding if you have high blood pressure. Even if your blood pressure is normal, you should have periodic blood pressure checks, at least once every year, especially if your parents or other close relatives have had high blood pressure.

If you have high blood pressure, you need tests for specific disease conditions that may cause high blood pressure and you need a test for kidney function. Before you embark on our program, you need to rule out the possibility that you have some secondary condition. Such a condition, afflicting about 5 percent of all those with high blood pressure, often requires very special treatment and probably means that this program is not for you.

However, once you are assured that you are in the 95-percent group, you can begin following the other steps of our program. You will need the cooperation of your doctor. For one thing, you need professional advice about if, when, and how to change or discontinue any drug treatment you are currently on. Also, your doctor may help you determine just what kind of exercise—and how much of it—is safe for you (Step Three). Finally, the two of you together should be monitoring your progress with our program as a whole.

Step Two: Eat Right

You need to eat food that is richer in potassium and lower in sodium—in other words, food that has a high *K Factor*.

To do this, you don't really have to sacrifice many things you like to eat now. The key is not so much in what you eat as in *how it's prepared.* You need to buy the right foods in the supermarket, and you need to avoid a couple of common mistakes in preparing your meals at home. *You can actually eat your way out of high blood pressure!*

You can increase your dietary *K Factor* naturally by eating more of such foods as whole grains, fresh vegetables and fruits, and nonfat dairy products, and eating less processed foods, fast foods, junk foods, and—generally—food with added salt. You need to cut out table salt, both on the table and in your cooking. Instead, you can use salt substitutes (preferably without chloride), such as those we describe in the Appendix.

You should also include in your diet adequate amounts of calcium and magnesium, which can be found in dairy products (preferably nonfat and unsalted), nuts, whole grains, beans, and green leafy vegetables.

Finally, you need to decrease the amount of fat in your diet to no more than 20 percent of your total calories. And that 20 percent should be mostly polyunsaturated fat, such as liquid vegetable oil.

Step Three: Exercise

In some people, exercise alone is enough to restore their blood pressure to normal. A combination of eating right and adequate exercise can not only give you normal blood pressure and help you avoid heart attacks but can improve the quality of your life as well.

Exercise—aerobic exercise in particular—produces changes in blood hormones, thereby affecting the potassium and sodium balance inside the body's cells, which in turn helps reduce high blood pressure.

Also, for most people, exercise is an important or necessary part of keeping weight down to normal. Exercising even three times a week can make a noticeable difference.

Step Four: Help Your Body Find Its Proper Weight

Quite simply, avoid being overweight. Losing excess weight is often enough to restore blood pressure to normal levels.

Obesity causes changes in the levels of the blood hormones that regulate the exchange of potassium and sodium within the body. This has been proposed as an explanation for the well-established fact that obesity increases your chances of developing high blood pressure.

One of the side advantages of Step Two, a diet with a lot of fruits, vegetables, and grains (a high–*K Factor* diet), is that it is also a low-fat diet. Since fat has more than twice as many calories as the same weight of carbohydrates or protein, a diet rich in fruits, vegetables, and grains also helps you keep your weight down. Fruits, vegetables, and grains are also rich in fiber, which is necessary for a healthy diet and may help prevent some kinds of cancer.

A side benefit of an aerobic exercise program (Step Three) is that it helps you lose excess weight. In fact, 98 percent of weight-loss programs fail *unless* regular aerobic exercise is included.

Losing excess weight and maintaining normal weight are primarily consequences of proper nutrition (Step Two) and exercise (Step Three). However, to be effective, the *balance* between nutrition and exercise must be adjusted properly. A modern concept, the "set point," borrowed from control system theory, gives insight into this balance and is discussed in Step Four.

Other Things You Can Do

Changing behavior that is bad for your general health can also help keep your blood pressure normal.

For example, you should avoid excessive use of alcohol. Heavy drinking clearly increases your chances of getting high blood pressure. Also, minimize or, better yet, eliminate smoking. Smoking may contribute to the development of high blood pressure (and we know it is a major factor in causing heart attacks).

Finally, minimize the effects of stress. Although stress is not a main cause of high blood pressure, it can make high blood pressure worse. Perhaps the most important aspect of stress is that it may lead to such behaviors as overeating, smoking, or alcoholism, which do contribute to high blood pressure.

Summary

Again, we wish to emphasize that the *goal* of our program is not just to get your blood pressure down but to correct the imbalance in your body that caused the problem in the first place. This will also make you feel more healthy and live longer.

If this program doesn't decrease your blood pressure right away, don't get discouraged. Stay with it. It will probably take weeks—and it may take months—for your blood pressure to respond to the program, especially if you've had hypertension for several years.

Remember, lowering blood pressure with drugs does not always lead to better health or a longer life. On the other hand, evidence from studies of experimental animals indicates that even if your blood vessels have become so damaged that your blood pressure can't come down, our program can still extend your life. So stick with the program even if your blood pressure doesn't come down. After all, what you really care about is your sense of well-being and your living a long, healthy life.

You *can* reload the dice; you can change the odds of your suffering or dying from high blood pressure.

You are the one who is ultimately responsible for your own health. To keep on top of this program, you must follow your own progress, using the progress chart in Part IV.

CHAPTER 9

Step One: See Your Doctor

The very first step you should take is to see your doctor.

Please do not go off half-cocked with the other steps of our program before you do this. The results could be disastrous if you do. Your doctor needs to examine you to verify that you do indeed have high blood pressure, and, if you do, to determine just what type of high blood pressure it is.

Then, if certain types of hypertension are ruled out, your doctor should

- Advise you about any changes in whatever drugs you may currently be taking.
- Evaluate your risk of coronary artery disease to determine the type and amount of exercise that is safe for you.
- Monitor your progress with our program as a whole.

Get a Complete Physical Exam

Your doctor should carefully evaluate your blood pressure and test for other specific disease conditions that may cause high blood pressure. In order to get a complete picture, your physician will have to perform specific tests and will have to see you regularly.

Do You Have High Blood Pressure?

On three separate visits, your doctor should measure your blood pressure while you are relaxed and not talking, at least twice during each visit and at least once on both arms. According to the Joint National Committee's 1984 Report, you have high blood pressure, or hypertension, if your systolic blood pressure is greater than 140 mm Hg and/or your diastolic blood pressure is greater than 90 mm Hg. But keep in mind that insurance statistics show that a diastolic blood pressure over 80 is actually bad for you (see p. 10).

What Type Do You Have?

Once your doctor has verified that you have hypertension, he or she will need to consider other specific disease conditions that may have caused it by taking a comprehensive health history and by performing certain tests, including testing your kidney and heart.

Although high blood pressure itself is bad, it is also a symptom, or a sign, of abnormal body function. Although the abnormality in body function is almost always caused by a nutritional imbalance such as a low *K Factor* or calcium deficiency in the food we eat, it is sometimes (in less than 5 percent of cases) a symptom of other disease conditions, such as kidney disease or adrenal gland tumor. When high blood pressure is due to another disease, it is called *secondary hypertension.* Before you embark on our program, your doctor will need to rule out the possibility that you have secondary hypertension.

SECONDARY HYPERTENSION. Secondary hypertension is caused by such conditions as:

○ Kidney disease.
○ Narrowing of the artery to a kidney.
○ Primary aldosteronism.

- Renin-secreting tumor.
- Cushing's syndrome.
- Congenital adrenal hyperplasia.
- Coarctation (narrowing) of the aorta.
- Pheochromocytoma.
- Contraceptive, or estrogen, therapy.
- Reaction to appetite suppressants.
- Reaction to decongestants.
- Rigidity of the arteries due to arteriosclerosis.
- Leakage of the aortic heart valve.
- Block of electrical signaling between the upper chambers (atria) and lower chambers (ventricles) of the heart.
- Conditions involving increased blood output from the heart, including thyrotoxicosis.
- Severe anemia.

The last five are characterized by an increase in systolic blood pressure and so are sometimes also called *systolic hypertension.*

We must emphasize that our program will not help those people whose high blood pressure is due to secondary hypertension. Each of the possible causes of those types of high blood pressure requires specific diagnosis and treatment, which may include surgery.

PRIMARY HYPERTENSION. The vast majority of people with high blood pressure, however—more than 95 percent of cases—have *primary hypertension* (or *essential hypertension,* which is what your doctor probably calls it).

If your doctor determines that you do not have secondary hypertension, you are one of the 95 percent who have primary hypertension. And it is you, your children, and your doctor for whom this book has been written. This book shows how simple—and safe—modifications in your life-style, especially in what you eat and in how you prepare it, can lower your blood pressure and restore your health or prevent high blood pressure from developing in the first place.

You should do something about your blood pressure, because your chances of dying are significantly increased—on the average, doubled—compared with people in your age group with normal blood pressure.

Fortunately, it is primary hypertension that can be helped by the *K Factor.*

Work with Your Doctor

Although it is essential that you consult with your physician, you must realize that in the final analysis, you are the one responsible for your health. When it comes to preventive medicine—and keeping you from having a stroke or heart attack is legitimately called preventive—we and others in the health professions can only provide you with the information. *You* must put it into practice.

Many doctors, and many laypersons as well, realize that achieving health and maintaining it require a transformation of the typical physician-patient relationship into a physician-partner collaboration. For this to work, the "patient" needs to take greater responsibility, and the physician needs to approach the "patient" as a co-worker.

We suggest that you take this book to your doctor and ask for his or her cooperation. If your doctor will not cooperate—that is, will not consider the *K Factor* approach—seek a second, or even a third, opinion.

You should work with your doctor as a team. In the interest of facilitating this physician-partner collaboration, the rest of this chapter will provide you with:

○ Some idea of what to expect when you visit your doctor.
○ Some timely warnings about discontinuing any drug therapy you may currently be following.
○ Some information about evaluation of exercise risk.
○ Some suggestions for evaluating your progress with our program.

What to Expect When You Visit Your Doctor

In the section "Do You Have High Blood Pressure?" we discussed the blood pressure measurements your doctor needs to take. But your doctor needs to perform several other tests as well, in particular, to rule out secondary hypertension. For example:

○ Routine urinalysis.
○ Test for blood hemoglobin and hematocrit.
○ Test for serum levels of potassium, glucose, cholesterol, urea nitrogen (BUN), and creatinine.
○ Electrocardiogram.

You may need to fast before the test for serum levels of glucose.

In addition, your doctor may want to do a chest X ray and possibly a test called an *intravenous pyelogram* to look for obstruction of the urinary tract, a cause of kidney disease. Depending upon the results of these tests and the history and physical exam, other diagnostic tests may be performed.

Changes in Drug Therapy

Stopping drugs should be done *only* under your doctor's supervision. The actual change can be dangerous.

NEVER WITHDRAW ANY DRUG SUDDENLY.

This should be emphasized. Any sudden change can be dangerous. For example, sudden withdrawal of Clonidine can precipitate a rebound hypertension. If you have angina, a sudden withdrawal of beta blockers can precipitate anginal attacks.

A note of caution about potassium-sparing diuretics: If you are taking a potassium-sparing diuretic, be sure to consult with your doctor about whether the *K Factor* program should be used with these drugs. In any case, until further research is done, you should not take any potassium-containing pills or potassium-containing salt substitutes while you are on potassium-sparing diuretics.

Getting a Checkup Before Starting Your Exercise Program

Before you begin a new exercise program (Step Three) or make any changes in one you're already in, have your doctor measure your blood cholesterol and, if possible, blood tri-glycerides.

You really should get a stress test if:

∘ You are over 40.
∘ You have at least one other major coronary risk factor:
  1. You have a blood cholesterol level greater than 200 mg/ml.
  2. You are (or have been) seriously overweight.
  3. You smoke cigarettes.
  4. You have diabetes mellitus.
  5. You have a family history of coronary disease by age 50.
∘ Your blood pressure is over 145/95.
∘ You have known cardiovascular, lung, or metabolic disease.

It's not a bad idea to get one even if you are under forty.

By "stress test," we are not referring to the Master Two-Step Test but to a multistage stress test that utilizes a treadmill or a stationary exercise bicycle. In the multistage test, your elec-trocardiogram (EKG) and blood pressure can be taken continu-ously while you exercise and as the level of exercise is increased.

An EKG is a tracing of the electrical activity of the heart. You may already have had one taken at rest. If a resting EKG shows abnormal electrical activity, you need careful consultation with your doctor about whether and how you should begin an exer-cise program. If coronary artery disease has caused your heart any problems, a resting EKG may show signs of this.

However, a resting EKG often fails to show signs of coronary disease and so provides no assurance that you are not about to have a heart attack. On the other hand, abnormalities in the EKG are much more likely to show up during exercise, so a properly conducted treadmill EKG (the stress test) offers much better evidence. We discuss the value and limitations of the treadmill stress test in more detail in Chapter 11 and in Part VII.

The treadmill stress test also gives some idea of how hard you can exercise safely. Let's say you get your heart rate up to 150 and the electrical tracing (EKG) is still normal. Although it is not a guarantee, that provides an indication that so long as your heart rate is not higher than 150 when you exercise, you are unlikely to have a heart attack.

But even the exercise EKG isn't infallible, unfortunately. Your coronary arteries could be almost two-thirds closed with cholesterol deposits and you might still pass the stress test—especially if it is not conducted according to the guidelines set by Dr. Kenneth Cooper. But among the simple and safe methods, it's the best we have for evaluating your cardiac health. Remember the running guru, Jim Fixx? If he had taken recent advice to have a stress test, there is a good chance he would be out there today slowly jogging, or at least walking. Fixx had once been overweight and had a family history of heart trouble—both factors that increase the chance of having a heart attack.

Especially for people new to regular aerobic exercise, we advise the stress test to help rule out coronary artery deficiency before you begin anything more than walking.

Even if you *have* been exercising regularly, you should get a physical reevaluation every year or two. And it doesn't hurt to get a stress test every few years, especially if you are going to change the amount of your exercise.

Following Your Progress

In order to maximize your chances of success, you will need not only to work with your physician but to follow your own progress. To do this, you need to learn to take your own blood pressure (as we explain in Chapter 16). Using the progress sheet we provide in Part IV and at the back of the book, keep a weekly record of your blood pressure, morning pulse, weight, amount of exercise, and dietary *K Factor*.

CHAPTER 10
Step Two: Eat Right

The diet of our remote ancestors may be a reference standard for modern human nutrition and a model for defense against certain "diseases of civilization."

—Eaton and Konner[1]

Cutting back on table salt, losing excess weight, and getting regular exercise—all steps recommended by the Joint National Committee in its 1984 Special Report—are essential steps for treating primary hypertension.

But are they enough?

The answer is no, because they do not address the need for a dietary balance we inherited from our remote ancestors: a balance between sodium and other minerals, such as chloride, magnesium, calcium, and especially *potassium*. Your high blood pressure is really an outer symptom of an abnormal balance in your body's cells. Establishing the proper balance of these elements—especially the ratio of potassium to sodium (the *K Factor*)—will usually lower your blood pressure, improve your health, and increase your life span *even if your blood pressure does not return to normal levels!*

To be successful, you must eat food that is richer in potassium and lower in sodium; the *K Factor* should be at least 3 (three times as much potassium as sodium). This oughtn't to be very difficult. When food comes directly "off the vine" or "off the hoof," it has a *K Factor* of at least 5. The diet of our remote ancestors had a *K Factor* of about 16! Unsalted fruits and vegetables generally have a *K Factor* of at least 20 and often well over 100. But because of common mistakes we make in preparing our food, the *K Factor* of the average American diet is less than 1— only 0.4.

In this chapter, essentially the heart of our recommended program, we are going to show you how you can actually eat your way out of high blood pressure—or at least into improved health and longer life. As we will show, you don't have to give up many of your favorite foods; by following our simple suggestions for preparing your meals, you will be able to reap the benefits of our program with very little effort.

We will start in the supermarket, focusing on foods to avoid and foods to select. Then, when you have the right foods at home, we will show you the best ways to prepare them so that your meals have a high *K Factor*, so that your body is in balance. At the end of this chapter, we will give you some tips on what to avoid and what to select when you are eating out.

Selecting Your Foods: In the Supermarket

For the one out of three people who have the genetic tendency, the following food shopping list is a sure way to high blood pressure and its consequences:

A BAD SHOPPING LIST

Smoked ham

Franks

Pork sausage

Bacon

Bologna

Olives

Frozen chicken (breaded and seasoned)
Canned peas, canned corn (unless unsalted)
Canned tomatoes (unless unsalted)
Tomato juice (unless unsalted)
Frozen french fries (salted)
Spam
Butter
Creamed cottage cheese
Cream
Sour cream
Ice cream
Most cheeses
Soy sauce
Table salt (NaCl)
Potato chips (unless unsalted)
English muffins
Dill pickles
Frozen dinners
Frozen pizza

What? Are some of these items among your favorite foods? Are we proposing another rigid diet, like all the other diets? Don't you have enough restrictions in your life already? Do we expect you to starve, or to eat only tasteless food?

Not at all. The suggestions we make are not only good for you; they are excellent tasting as well. Mother Nature gave us foods that are fine for us. Foods with a high *K Factor*—that are also generally high in magnesium and low in fat—are plentiful, tasty, and healthy.

Hard to believe? At the end of this section, there will be another shopping list, an alternative to the foregoing one. This one will contain foods that are tasty *and* healthy. But first, we want to present you with simple nutritional principles so that you can write your *own* healthy shopping list!

In most cases, it's not the food that's harmful—it's what we do to it that hurts us. That means you can eat almost whatever type of food you like, provided the *K Factor* hasn't been lowered in the manufacturing plant (or, later, in your own kitchen). So the success or failure of our program begins in the supermarket.

The following are key points in selecting food that can lower your blood pressure to normal levels and make you feel better and live longer:

- ○ Select foods with a high *K Factor*.
- ○ Select foods with enough calcium and magnesium.
- ○ Select nonfat foods.

Select Foods with a High K Factor

In food shopping, put your emphasis on whole grains, fresh vegetables and fruits, and nonfat dairy products. Deemphasize most processed foods, fast foods, and "junk" foods.

Although there are a few details to learn, the following three simple steps—the *magic three*—will take you most of the way to your goal of a high–*K Factor* diet:

1. Avoid commercially prepared foods containing added sodium, such as most canned foods and junk foods.
2. Don't buy table salt (sodium chloride). (We'll suggest alternatives later.)
3. Buy foods that naturally have a high *K Factor*, such as fresh fruits, vegetables, and grains.

1. Avoid commercially prepared foods with added sodium. Cut out most canned food and most "junk food" unless it is clearly labeled unsalted or no added salt (not just low salt). Stay away from commercial frozen dinners or combination foods. Although some are now low in fat, we have not been able to find any that are low enough in salt; many of them are also high in fat. Stay away from fast foods, most of which are loaded with sodium and fat.

COMMERCIAL FOOD PROCESSING. Over the past several decades, Americans have used more and more canned and otherwise processed foods. Before canning, the food companies may put some vegetables into a salt brine to separate the ripe ones, which float, from the overripe ones, which sink. Canned whole tomatoes and some canned or frozen fruits may be bathed in a solution of sodium hydroxide to remove their peel. The canning process usually involves boiling the food, which leaches out the potassium. The tasteless result is then flavored with sodium chloride. All this tends to replace the potassium with sodium. So with too little potassium and all the added sodium, most processed food has a very low *K Factor*.

PROCESSED VEGETABLES AND FRUITS. Whereas fresh peas contain almost no sodium and have a *K Factor* of 160, most canned peas contain very large amounts of sodium and have a *K Factor* of only 0.4. So canned peas have a *K Factor* that is three hundred times lower than fresh peas. The same large decrease in the *K Factor* is usually found in canned corn and beans as well. Pass up most canned food. To take just one example: Campbell's Cream of Mushroom Soup contains 825 milligrams of sodium per serving. But Campbell's *also* makes some low-sodium soups with only about 100 milligrams of sodium per can.

Much frozen food should also be avoided. Plain frozen peas may not have sodium added, but those frozen with prepared sauce usually do. Your job is to learn to pick and choose. For example, the amount of sodium in frozen apples ranges from 2 to 200 milligrams per 100 grams. Watch out for frozen green beans in butter sauce; not only do they have a lot of fat, they have 255 milligrams of sodium per ½ cup serving. Some frozen lasagna has 855 milligrams of sodium per package. One-half of a small frozen pizza may have 1000 milligrams of sodium.[2] That's eleven times your minimum daily requirement, and half of your *maximum* daily allowance!

PROCESSED MEATS. Sodium salts are added to processed meats. Although most fresh meats have a reasonably high *K Factor*, processed meats, including hot dogs, pork sausage, bacon, smoked ham, and cold cuts such as bologna and salami not only have unacceptably low *K Factors* but are also high in fat. Spam has 1025 milligrams of sodium per 3-ounce serving. Ordinary

fresh beef may be 30 percent fat, even with the visible fat
trimmed off. Compare this to the wild animals our ancestors ate,
which were less than 5 percent fat.[3] Fish, skinned chicken, and
turkey have less fat than beef and pork. Thus unsalted turkey or
chicken breast, or unsalted water-packed tuna, make good sandwich meats. We also provide a recipe for a healthy luncheon loaf
that you can make at home. A thin slice of roast beef is okay
occasionally.

BREADS. Unless they are marked low salt, beware of most commercially baked breads. As you can see from the table in Chapter 13, most commercially prepared English muffins have an
unacceptably low *K Factor* of about 0.1. Some bakeries are making unsalted bread, or you can bake your own without salt. Yeast
does not need added salt. We will show in the menu plans that
you can get away with a couple of slices of commercial (whole
grain) bread if you're sensible about the other foods you eat.

DESSERTS. Unfortunately for those of you with a sweet tooth,
most commercially prepared desserts have a low *K Factor*. Besides, sugar is bad for your teeth and it may overstimulate the
secretion of insulin, a hormone that stimulates both appetite
and the conversion of calories to fat. So most commercially prepared desserts should be avoided.

Fortunately, there are some exceptions. Featherweight, for instance, makes a no-sugar, no-salt chocolate pudding. Also, packaged gelatin dessert mixes have only moderate amounts of sodium. At home, with some flavorful fruit juice and plain gelatin,
you can make no-sodium ones. For added interest, whip the
gelatin when it has just begun to harden and add some fruit. You
can even add a dollop of "whipped cream" made by beating
together equal parts of powdered milk and water, with a few
drops of lemon juice and vanilla and artificial sweetener.

Rice or tapioca puddings and cornstarch-based puddings can
be made without salt. Since angel-food cake and meringues are
made with egg whites and not yolks or shortening and can be
made without salt, they are also good. If you hanker for cheese-
cake, try avoiding the fat this way: Dissolve a package of lemon

Jell-O in 1½ cups of hot water, then cool until slightly firm, then whip. Put a pint of cottage cheese through a sieve or puree it in the blender, then add to the whipped Jell-O, sweeten to taste, add a few drops of vanilla, and pour into a cake pan and leave in the refrigerator until firm.

Except for the sugar, sherbets or fruit ices are healthy low-salt, low-fat desserts. If you like fresh fruits, which have a high *K Factor*, these are excellent for dessert.

Surprise—we saved the best for last: you can make a hot fudge banana split (with nuts, no less) that has only 29 percent of the calories from fat and a *K Factor* of about 8! Split one banana, use one cup of ice milk (*not* ice cream), top with 1 tablespoon cocoa powder dissolved in about 2 ounces boiling water (no sugar and you don't need sweetener), and sprinkle with ¼ ounce walnuts. Don't eat this *too* often, though, because it does have 365 calories and there's a good deal of sugar in the ice milk.

JUNK FOODS. The term *junk food* is no misnomer. Junk food not only contains too much sodium but also too much fat. Avoid all salted nuts, potato chips, and most crackers (Ritz crackers, for example, have 200 milligrams of sodium per 1-ounce serving). Some low-salt whole grain crackers are available, such as: Health Valley's Stoned Wheat, and Herb Stoned Wheat crackers.

CAUTION: "LOW-SODIUM" IS NOT SODIUM-FREE. Campbell's "low sodium" Chicken Noodle Soup has 90 milligrams of sodium per 10¾-ounce portion. This is much better than the regular Chicken Noodle Soup, which has 825 milligrams per portion, but it is still enough sodium to make a significant impact on your daily total. If you like, eat the low-sodium soup—but keep the sodium low in the other things you eat that day.

On the other hand, some newer canned foods are really low in sodium.

OTHER FOODS TO AVOID. Most people would recognize the following foods as salty: olives, anchovies, canned sardines, commercially prepared dill pickles (but see our recipe), soy sauce, and bacon. Other high-salt foods include most breads, cheeses, most peanut butters, canned tomato juice (unless it's unsalted), V-8 juice (unless it's the low-salt variety), creamed cottage cheese, instant pudding, and most instant hot cereals (most of the regular hot cereals are excellent if you don't add salt). Most cold cereals should be avoided as well; for example, Wheaties has 365 milligrams of sodium per 1-ounce serving. But several low-salt brands, such as Nabisco Shredded Wheat, are very good. Club soda has 93 milligrams of sodium per 12 ounces, low-sodium sparkling water has almost none.

SOFTENED WATER. Most water softeners work by replacing calcium, magnesium, and other minerals that make water "hard" with sodium; thus, "softened" water is loaded with sodium. Not only that, the magnesium and calcium that are removed would have been good for you. If you have a water softener, make sure it is hooked up only to the hot-water side of your plumbing and that you avoid using hot water for cooking or drinking. You might also want to check to see if your local water supply has a significant amount of natural sodium.

OVER-THE-COUNTER DRUGS. Finally, watch out for nonprescription drugs. According to *Consumer Reports*, Vicks' Formula 44 has 105 milligrams of sodium per 2-teaspoon dose. Rolaids Antacid has 70 milligrams per two-tablet dose. Alka-Seltzer has 592 milligrams per two-tablet dose; this is one-half the maximum daily allowance of sodium in our recommendations! So if you're getting an over-the-counter medicine, first read the label or ask your pharmacist.

THE GOOD NEWS. Fortunately, not all food processing lowers the *K Factor*. Bulk-packaged oatmeal, cream of wheat, and other hot cereals cooked without salt have a high *K Factor*. Beware, though: while individual serving packets of instant hot cereal are convenient, they are likely to be presalted. Several types of dry breakfast cereals, including puffed wheat, puffed rice, shredded wheat, and some of the granolas, are unsalted and have a high *K Factor*. Unfortunately, many of the granolas contain saturated fats such as palm or coconut oils.

Gradually, food companies are responding to the demand for

low-salt, healthy foods. Campbell's, Hunt's, Del Monte, several of the supermarket chain brands, and others have come out with a variety of unsalted canned foods. Herb-Ox makes very good salt-free chicken and beef instant broths, which can be used in soups and also as a seasoning in a wide variety of dishes. More unsalted food products are appearing on the market every day.

Remember your goal: good health. It's worth the effort to look for unsalted prepared foods. Ask the store manager to order them if you can't find them.

Study the table in Part IV and avoid the items in italics except on rare occasions, go for the boldfaced items, and use your judgment on the others (they are okay in moderation). If you shop around, it is possible to buy unsalted mustard, catsup, low-fat cheeses, potato chips, crackers, and so on.

Most cheeses have added sodium salt, but unsalted cheese can be obtained at health food stores and some supermarkets. Unsalted Swiss cheese tastes just as good as the regular Swiss: A single thin slice is flavorful and won't add too much fat to your diet. Ricotta and dry curd cottage cheese (not creamed) have less sodium than creamed cottage cheese and are low in fat as well.

Del Monte Low-Salt Whole Kernel Corn has only 5 milligrams of sodium per one-half cup—much better than the regular Del Monte Kernel Corn, which has 115 milligrams of sodium per serving.

Nonfat dry milk, cornstarch, low-sodium baking powder, gelatin, and quick-cooking tapioca are good items to have on hand. Several old standby products never did have salt. Tomato paste is still your old friend and, when diluted, will do many of the things tomato sauce will do. In recipes calling for tomato sauce, you can still add the herbs, wine, mushrooms, green pepper, onion, garlic—everything tasty but salt.

How Can You Tell? How can you determine the *K Factor* in processed foods? Only if the label lists both the potassium and the sodium content. If it does, divide the milligrams of potassium by the milligrams of sodium to get the *K Factor*. It's as simple as that. A glance will tell you if the *K Factor* is over 1 (if there is more potassium than sodium). Until the amount of potassium is listed on all labels, your best bet is to *avoid foods with more than about 100 milligrams of sodium per serving.*

Although there are signs that this will change, much of the time, only the sodium content is listed. In fact, about two-thirds of the time, neither is listed. Unless the manufacturer makes a low-sodium claim on the label, the U.S. Food and Drug Administration (FDA) doesn't require the sodium content to be stated. It's purely up to the manufacturer. Potassium content is entirely up to the manufacturer in all cases.

The FDA has proposed labeling food products not with sodium content but, instead, with the less informing terms *sodium free* (meaning less than 5 milligrams of sodium per serving), *low sodium* (35 milligrams or less per serving), *moderately low sodium* (140 milligrams or less), and *reduced sodium* (the original sodium in the product has been reduced by 75 percent or more). We think this is a backward step. It would keep important information from you, the consumer. Write to your congressional representative and ask for legislation that requires food manufacturers to list the actual sodium and potassium contents of processed foods.

2. **Use substitutes for salt.** As you should recognize by now (and see Chapter 21), you just do not need table salt (sodium chloride). It doesn't belong on your table or in your cooking. Food in its natural state has plenty of sodium—all you need. So don't buy table salt, and get rid of the supply you already have at home.

POTASSIUM-CONTAINING SALT SUBSTITUTES. At the table and in your cooking, potassium-containing salt substitutes can be used instead of table salt.

We recommend that the increase in potassium intake be achieved primarily through a return to a more natural diet. The natural potassium in food is generally safe because it is absorbed slowly and because it occurs mostly as organic salts rather than as potassium chloride. But moderate use of commercially available potassium-containing salt substitutes helps increase the *K Factor* in your diet, both by replacing salt (sodium chloride) and by increasing potassium.

These salt substitutes are commonly available on grocery shelves. Be aware that some contain sodium: read the label.

Do read the precautions on the label, and also consult with your doctor before using a salt substitute, as too much potassium could cause problems if you are taking a potassium-sparing diuretic or if you have kidney or heart disease.

OTHER WAYS TO SEASON WITHOUT SALT. But there are other ways around salt besides just salt substitutes. Vegit is a versatile seasoning, Lawry's Seasoned Salt-Free adds more familiar flavor to many saltless dishes, and Mrs. Dash adds a peppery note where appropriate. Mrs. Dash steak sauce is a tangy blend of herbs and spices that is good on many things other than steak, for example, Chinese cabbage, rice, spaghetti, and vegetables. Bitters is a neglected but very useful addition to many salt-free dishes. Bell's poultry seasoning can be used for more than stuffing a turkey; many meats profit from the touch of sage it provides. Worcestershire sauce is relatively low in sodium. Lemon and its juice are very useful for many things besides fish. Lemon juice dresses salads, with or without a little oil.

Curry is certainly an authoritative flavor, as are chili and Tabasco. Dry mustard enlivens many things, especially salad dressings and sauces for vegetables. Horseradish can be found fresh in some markets (caution: the jars of prepared horseradish usually contain salt).

It's amazing how much savory flavoring onion or garlic, sautéed in a little unsaturated oil, can provide a dish. Without salt, in any recipe, the flavors of onion and garlic—and most other spices as well—will be more pronounced.

AVOID BAKING SODA AND BAKING POWDER. Actually, salt (sodium chloride) is not the only sodium compound you should avoid. Common baking soda is sodium bicarbonate, which is also one of the ingredients of baking powder. Remember, you're cutting sodium, so don't use ordinary baking powder in things you bake. Low-sodium baking powder, such as Golden Harvest, is available at health food stores. (This brand contains potassium bicarbonate and thus actually helps to boost your *K Factor*.)

3. **Buy foods with a naturally high *K Factor*.** The third point of the magic three is to buy foods that naturally have a high *K Factor*. These include fresh vegetables (including potatoes), fresh fruits (not just bananas), skim or low-fat milk and yogurt, grains (including rice), chicken, fish, lean meat—in fact, almost any food that has not had its naturally high *K Factor* diminished in commercial processing.

POTATOES—THE PERFECT FOOD. The lowly potato, as it comes out of the ground, is excellent. Why? Not only do potatoes have a potassium-to-sodium ratio of about 130 to 1, or a *K Factor* of 130, but in addition, only 1 percent of their calories come from fat. The potato has gotten an undeservedly bad reputation. Too many people think potatoes cause weight gain, but it's not the potatoes—it's the grease they're fried in or the gravy, sour cream, or butter they're topped with.

It's been said that milk is a perfect food, but in fact, potatoes are even better in several respects. For example, milk's *K Factor* is only 2.8, and 50 percent of the calories of whole milk comes from fat, compared to potatoes with a *K Factor* of 130 and 1 percent fat.

Table 3 shows the percent of an adult woman's National Academy of Sciences Recommended Dietary Allowances (RDA) of vitamins and minerals she would get if she ate all her daily 2000 calories as milk (3 quarts of whole milk or 6 quarts of skim milk) or as 4.6 pounds of potatoes (11 medium-size potatoes).

A pure whole milk diet would be deficient in vitamin B_1, but a skim-milk diet of the same number of calories would not, because skim milk is fortified with extra vitamin B_1. A milk diet (either kind) would be deficient in niacin, vitamin C, and iron. A pure potato diet would be deficient in vitamin A, vitamin B_2, some essential amino acids, calcium, and iron (the latter is true only for women).

Each has ample supplies of what the other lacks; in essence,

TABLE 3.

Vitamin or Mineral	Percent RDA from 3 quarts whole milk	Percent RDA from 6 quarts skim milk	Percent RDA from 4.6 pounds potatoes
Vitamin A	114	294	trace
Vitamin B$_1$	91	212	220
Vitamin B$_2$	443	667	75
Niacin	23	36	282
Vitamin C	51	78	717
Calcium	443	876	24
Phosphorus	384	725	175
Iron	trace	13	84*

*For males, it would be 151 percent.

they are complementary. A supergood combination is a baked potato with low-fat yogurt on it.

OTHER HIGH–K FOODS. Pasta (spaghetti, linguine, elbow macaroni, spiral and flat noodles) is excellent, since it is low in sodium and fat and high in potassium, complex carbohydrates, and fiber. Since you should get most of your calories from complex carbohydrates, you can eat pasta as often as you like—just watch what's in the sauce and remember not to salt the cooking water.

All legumes have a very high *K Factor.* These include dried pinto, red, black, navy, garbanzo (chick pea), and kidney beans as well as dried lentils and split peas. An added bonus is that legumes are cheap and easy to store.

Virtually all fresh fruits are excellent sources of potassium— not only the famous banana, but oranges, grapefruits, grapes, pears, peaches, apricots, pineapples, mangoes, and plums. And remember the Japanese study we described in Chapter 4 that showed that six apples a day keeps both the doctor and high blood pressure away! If you like them, dried fruits, including raisins, dates, pears, apples, bananas, peaches, and apricots, are handy to have for snacks and for cooking.

Fortunately some freezer foods do not have added sodium and offer the convenience of immediate availability. We suggest frozen vegetables, fruits, and fruit-juice concentrates (orange juice has a very high *K Factor*).

If you read about nutrition, you may worry that a plan that excludes most red meat might be deficient in iron, but many other foods are rich in iron. You can meet your iron needs by eating the dried fruits we just listed or sunflower seeds, oysters, clams, peas, or beans. Most of these also have a very high *K Factor*. Multivitamin supplements containing iron offer another option. Since women require more iron than men, we recommend that all premenopausal women take daily iron supplements.

Rice, especially brown rice and wild rice, is very good, as are barley, bulgur wheat, buckwheat, and bran. Flour, especially whole wheat and potato, is good and can be used in many ways.

For snacks, popcorn can't be beat if it's prepared as we describe under Snacks. Provided they aren't covered with fat or salt-containing batter or sauces, chicken breast, turkey breast, and fish (lean white fish such as bass, cod, halibut, salmon steaks, red snapper, and sole) are good for you and good to have on hand. Eating seafood is especially important. Since you will be eliminating all table salt, including iodized salt, you could develop an iodine deficiency. Seafood—from the ocean—is a good source of iodine. On top of that, seafood is rich in "omega-3" polyunsaturated fatty acids that lower your risk of heart attack.[4]

Select Foods with Enough Calcium and Magnesium

Adults need about 400 milligrams (mg) of magnesium and at least 1000 mg of calcium each day, according to the current U.S. RDA (Recommended Dietary Allowances set by the U.S. Food and Drug Administration, based on the 1980 National Academy of Sciences Report). The U.S. RDA for pregnant women is 1300 mg for calcium and 450 mg for magnesium. Some nutritionists recommend up to 1500 mg of calcium a day (especially for postmenopausal women) and 500 mg of magnesium for all adults and even more for pregnant or older women. There is evidence that a deficiency in either calcium[5] or magnesium[6] can contribute to the development of hypertension, especially hypertension associated with pregnancy.

Calcium is found primarily in dairy products. Skim milk or low-fat or no-fat yogurt are excellent low-calorie sources of calcium. They also have a relatively high *K Factor* (about 3). However, beware of cheese, which usually contains a lot of added sodium as well as a lot of fat; the payoff in calcium isn't worth it in this case. As we said before, unsalted Swiss cheese (which can be obtained at health food stores and some supermarkets), ricotta, and dry cottage cheese are acceptable. Many people who can't digest the lactose in milk do fine with yogurt. You can now buy lactose-free milk in many groceries.

We believe that getting enough magnesium is especially important for preventing and alleviating high blood pressure. Fortunately, foods that have a high *K Factor* tend to have adequate amounts of magnesium as well. Nuts, whole grains, beans, shrimp, bananas, and green leafy vegetables are among the good sources of magnesium. Go easy on the nuts, however, for they are high in fat. Eating a *few* nuts is okay, since some of the fats are unsaturated, especially in walnuts. Chestnuts are low in total fat.

Select Nonfat Foods

In this chapter, we are discussing foods you should buy and eat as well as those you should avoid, and our focus now is on the fat content of foods and its relationship to hypertension. Chapter 7 explores the relationship of obesity itself, often the result of overindulgence in fatty foods, to hypertension.

We believe it is important to decrease your dietary fat intake to no more than 20 percent of the calories you take in each day. There is evidence (discussed in Chapter 8) that a diet low in fat, and the majority of that fat polyunsaturated (that is, liquid vegetable oils), can lower high blood pressure. But the main reason for keeping fat low is to prevent heart attacks, atherosclerosis, and cancer.

A ten-year study, recently completed under the direction of the National Heart, Lung and Blood Institute, clearly shows that reducing blood cholesterol (by avoiding the cholesterol and saturated fats from animal fat) greatly decreases the chance of having a heart attack or other complications caused by atherosclerosis (deposits of fat in the arteries).[7] The American Heart Association (AHA) now recommends that in addition to decreasing dietary cholesterol, we should keep our consumption of fat to no more than 30 percent of our total calories. If you are an American male, the chances are 1 in 2 that your blood cholesterol is elevated (above 200 milligrams of cholesterol per 100 milliliters of blood). If you are one of those with elevated blood cholesterol, the AHA recommends you cut the fat intake down to 25 percent, or even 20 percent. The AHA also recommends that more than half of all the fat you do eat should be polyunsaturated, such as that found in liquid vegetable oils. Because of all the bad things about fat and the fact that you don't need very much, we believe everybody should shoot for that 20-percent limit on fat.

Butter, sour cream, and cream are almost pure fat. On top of that, the usual salted butter also has a high sodium content. So these three items are to be avoided if at all possible. At first thought, that might seem difficult—but don't worry, we'll show you healthy and tasty substitutes.

You do not need oil for salad dressings, as we explain later in this chapter. But for those of you who insist on dressings with some fat, use polyunsaturated oils. For table use, safflower oil is highest in polyunsaturates and is a nice light oil for salad dressings. Buy it in small quantities and refrigerate it to keep it fresh. For a butter flavor, soy oil is available with butter flavoring to use in cooking. Look for it in the popcorn section of your grocery store.

Butter Buds are virtually fat free and taste remarkably like real butter, but unfortunately they do contain added sodium (perhaps the manufacturer will get wise and leave out the salt in the future).

Nonstick Teflon cooking ware or sparing use of Pam can reduce or eliminate the need for fat in your cooking. However, a small amount of oil can greatly improve some recipes without adding undue fat. For high-temperature cooking, such as deep-frying and wok cooking, try corn oil: while not quite as high in polyunsaturates as safflower oil, it does have a higher smoking point. But limit the amount of deep-fried foods you eat, and drain them well before eating.

In general, the longer the shelf life of a fat at room temperature, the higher it is in saturated fat and therefore the worse it is for your heart and circulatory system. Lard and hydrogenated vegetable oils (the ones that are solid at room temperature), palm oil and coconut oil, keep without refrigeration for many months, but unfortunately they're the ones that are bad for you. The liquid oils we recommend instead should be fresh; don't buy the giant economy size, and throw away any rancid oils.

Keep in mind that cake and muffin mixes also contain fats. They keep a long time on the grocer's shelf, a clue that the fats are saturated. These mixes are also high in sodium.

Several studies have shown that the "omega-3" polyunsaturated fatty acids that are found in fish oils are especially beneficial in helping to reduce blood pressure,[8] blood cholesterol level,[9] and the risk of heart attack.[10]

Shopping Lists

The following food shopping lists are alternatives to the one at the beginning of this chapter. With lists like these, you will be selecting foods that prolong your life and keep your palate happy.

VERY GOOD SHOPPING LIST

Chicken or turkey breast

Fresh fish (or frozen without salt)

Clams or oysters

Apple juice

Canned fruit without added sugar

Tomato paste

Dry pasta (spaghetti, noodles, etc.)
Fresh potatoes
Fresh peas, beans, corn
Fresh romaine, escarole
Fresh spinach
Fresh green or red peppers
Fresh mushrooms
Fresh lemons, oranges, and apples
Fresh bananas
Frozen orange juice concentrate
Dried dates and apricots
Raisins
Brown rice
Dried beans, lentils, peas
Flour
Bulgur wheat
Fresh-ground peanut butter (unsalted)
Safflower oil (small bottle)
Skim milk
Low-fat yogurt
Ricotta cheese
Matzo crackers (no salt, egg, or fat)
Unsalted Swiss cheese
Orange sherbet
Low-sodium baking powder
Unsalted mustard
Sunflower seeds
Curry powder, chili powder
Fresh horseradish
Onions, garlic

VERY GOOD SHOPPING LIST WITH BRAND NAMES

Breakfast Foods

Soy-o Low Sodium Pancake Mix

Sunshine Bite Size Shredded Wheat (unsalted)

Nabisco Shredded Wheat (unsalted)

Quaker Shredded Wheat (unsalted)

Kellogg's Puffed Rice or Puffed Wheat (unsalted)

Malt-O-Meal Puffed Rice or Puffed Wheat (unsalted)

Quaker Puffed Rice or Puffed Wheat (unsalted)

Quaker Oats (when cooking hot cereals, do not add salt as per instructions on the package)

Wheatena

Nabisco Cream of Wheat

Any other unsalted brands

Breads and Crackers

Mrs. Wright's Low-Sodium Breads

Stop & Shop No Salt Added Breads

Manischewitz Matzo Crackers

Devonsheer Unsalted Melba Rounds

Health Valley "No Salt Added" crackers

Featherweight Unsalted Crackers

Any brand labeled "no salt added"

Seasonings and Sauces

Hunt's No Salt Added Ketchup, Tomato Paste, and Tomato Sauce

Del Monte No Salt Added Catsup

Vegit, Mrs. Dash, or Bell's seasonings

Regina Wine Vinegar (or other brands)

Dia-Mel low sodium creamy garlic salad dressing

Contadina No Salt Added Tomato Paste

Sano's No Salt Added Spaghetti Sauce

Ocean Spray Cranberry Sauce or Cran-Orange Relish

Angostura Bitters

Any brand labeled "no salt added"

Canned Fish

Star Kist Diet Pack Chunk Light Tuna in Water

Chicken of the Sea Dietetic Albacore Chunk White Tuna in Water

Health Valley No Salt Added Pink Salmon

Any brand labeled "no salt added"

Soups

Health Valley No Salt Added Soups

Campbell's Low Sodium Split Pea, Cream of Mushroom, Chunky Vegetable Beef, Corn, or Tomato Soups

Any brand labeled "no salt added"

Other

V-8 Low Sodium Vegetable Juice

La Choy Water Chestnuts (canned)

Libby's Solid Pack Pumpkin (canned)

Health Valley Spicy Vegetarian Chili and other food products

Golden Harvest unsalted food products

Any brand of dry ("instant") potatoes *(but do not add salt as per instructions)*

Any brand of canned or bottled fruit or fruit juices (apple sauce or juice, pineapple, etc.)

Any brand of canned vegetables *if labeled "no salt added"*

MODERATELY GOOD SHOPPING LIST WITH BRAND NAMES

Dia-Mel Pancake Mix

Featherweight Pancake Mix

Health Valley Pancake Mix

Nabisco Low Salt Triscuit

Nabisco Holland Rusk or Zweiback

Ralston Purina Graham Crackers

Kraft Pure Prepared Mustard, Horseradish Mustard, or Prepared Horseradish

Tabasco Sauce

Dia-Mel Mayonnaise

Campbell's Low Sodium Chicken Soup with Noodles or Chunky Chicken Vegetable Soup

Star Kist Select Chunk Light Tuna in Water with 60 percent Less Salt

SHOPPING LISTS FOR DECREASING BLOOD PRESSURE. Feel free to eat anything on the very good shopping lists. The items on the moderately good list contain a moderate amount of sodium. They should be eaten in moderation. On the day that you get stuck with a meal with a low *K Factor*, however, eat only items on the very good lists or boldfaced items from the table in Chapter 13 for the rest of the day.

Again, the key to our approach is what you eat and how it's prepared. We want to emphasize that this program is not only good for your blood pressure but it should decrease your chances of having a heart attack as well, since it automatically cuts the fat you eat to levels at or below those recently recommended by the American Heart Association in order to prevent heart attacks. Not only that, but it turns out that low-fat, high-fiber eating programs such as ours probably decrease your chances of getting some kinds of cancer.

Our program is good for your blood pressure, good for your heart, and helps prevent some types of cancer. So it's your choice. You will live with the consequences. You can either adopt this eating program or go ahead eating your way into not only hypertension but into heart attacks and perhaps into cancer. You can eat to live and be healthy, or you can eat so you will ruin your health, live poorly, and maybe die before your time. If you want to live longer and not only enjoy good health but enjoy your food, read on.

Preparing Your Meals: In the Kitchen

Now that you've selected your foods in the grocery store, it's time to use them in preparing healthy—and appetizing—meals. Once you understand the simple principles we'll describe, it's easy. Because this eating program is based upon natural principles, it will allow you to eat almost any food you want, provided it is prepared correctly. So once you've made the change, you'll forget you ever ate food prepared the wrong way—the way that leads to high blood pressure.

In this section, we'll discuss how you can plan your meals to obtain the highest possible *K Factor*, thereby reducing (or avoiding) high blood pressure. We also offer you some tips in food preparation to ensure that foods with a naturally high *K Factor* do not lose potassium in cooking.

At the end of this chapter, we provide four weeks' worth of specific menus to get you started, followed by some recipes used in the menu plan. We'll also provide you with general suggestions for planning your menus.

Before looking at the specific suggestions for a month's worth of meals, consider the following general guidelines for breakfasts, lunches, dinners, and snacks.

Breakfast

Nutritionists say that breakfast is the most important meal of the day, since you have been the longest without food. A recent study done in Minnesota indicates that this is especially true if you are overweight. A large number of overweight women who volunteered for this study were randomly divided into two groups. Both groups ate exactly the same foods, totaling 2,000 calories, every day. One group ate all their food in the morning, the other group ate all their food in the evening. Almost all the women in the first group lost weight, whereas the women in the second group either gained weight or maintained the same weight they started with. This is because activity gears your metabolism to burn calories, whereas rest gears your body to store calories as fat. So don't skip breakfast!

For breakfast, always have fruit and/or fruit juice. Fresh whole fruits are best. If you use canned tomato or V-8 juice, use a brand that doesn't have added salt. In the menus that follow, we often list orange juice because it's easily available year-round, but substitute fresh fruit when possible. Low-fat yogurt with fruit or preserves stirred into it makes an excellent breakfast.

If you have toast, use unsalted bread. (If you can't find it in a health food store or in the supermarket, you can make it at home.)

If you make hot cereal, don't add salt. Use cinnamon or a salt substitute if it tastes too flat to you. Because of the saturated fat problem, we recommend 1-percent fat, ½-percent fat, or—best of all—skim milk on your cereal. Almost any fruits are good on cereal—bananas, strawberries, blueberries, peaches, apricots, dates, raisins. For more sweetening, add Equal or a small amount of brown sugar, molasses, or maple syrup. The last three have more flavor than white sugar and provide some minerals as well, but nevertheless are primarily sugar (sucrose) and should be used sparingly.

One suggested feature of our menu plan is the breakfast potato, which is rich in potassium and low in fat. Having a potato for breakfast is actually an old American practice first used by farmers and cowboys, and it is still popular in the South and parts of the West. An interesting breakfast variation is our modern version of the potato pancake. Simply shred one or two potatoes without peeling, add some minced onion, and fry in a pan coated with Pam or a thin layer of unsaturated cooking oil. Serve with applesauce or yogurt.

George even enjoys a baked potato with yogurt for breakfast. Remember, potatoes and milk complement each other's nutritional deficiencies.

Lunch

For lunch, frequently include fresh fruit. Raisins, dates, dried apricots, or other dried fruits make a nice addition. Since unsalted nuts are loaded with potassium (Planters markets several varieties), they make a good choice, but take it easy, because they do contain a lot of fat.

Whenever possible, use unsalted bread for sandwiches. Between the slices, use lettuce or sprouts, unsalted mustard, and unsalted tuna (from the health food store), or chicken, or turkey.

A healthy alternative to cold cuts is our luncheon loaf (see recipes). As we mentioned earlier, a thin slice of unsalted Swiss cheese or a moderate layer of unsalted peanut butter is okay.

Salads are excellent for lunch. If you brown-bag it, try carrot sticks, florets of broccoli or cauliflower, radishes, or slices of zucchini; they're all refreshing and rich in potassium. If you don't carry your lunch, head for the salad bar for lots of almost any raw vegetables and fruits. But do watch out for pickled vegetables, which have an alarming amount of salt, and for dressings, which are usually salty and loaded with fat. Be a purist and use vinegar or lemon juice with a small amount of unsaturated oil such as safflower oil, sunflower seed oil, or olive oil (or even better, skip the oil).

Soups that do not contain cream or whole milk or added table salt are excellent. They tend to be low in calories yet filling as well as tasty and nutritious.

Dinner

What if your hectic schedule leads you to arrive home late, too bushed to cook? Are high–*K Factor* meals out of the question? By no means! It takes just a bit more time than using a frozen dinner. Broil lean meat, or broil or steam fish. Microwave potatoes in five to ten minutes. Pasta cooks quickly; add herbs instead of salt to the cooking water. Combination meals can be thrown together in minutes with leftovers and previously cooked rice. You'll have a meal in short order.

Keep fresh fruits and vegetables in your refrigerator for quick salads. Some unsalted canned vegetables, including beets, corn, and sweet potato, are still tasty. However, beans are not very tasty when unsalted, so add spices and a little salt substitute. Frozen vegetables (without prepared sauces, which are invariably salty) can be heated in very little time, especially in a microwave oven.

Many traditional recipes work very well with the simple omission of salt. With any recipe, this is worth a try.

Onion can be the cook's best friend. When in doubt about how to prepare a good salt-free meal, fry a few slices of onion in a little unsaturated oil or Pam in a pan, and the aroma will give you confidence that the rest of the meal will materialize. This is also a boon for the spouse who arrives home first, so the one who arrives home second, starving, will find olfactory comfort wafting from the kitchen to the hall, driveway, or sidewalk. Garlic is as useful as ever, and the whole array of fresh and dried herbs and spices can provide new sodium-free excitement.

Remember, potatoes aren't fattening as long as you don't use fatty toppings like butter or sour cream. You can make a topping that tastes almost the same as sour cream by using low-fat yogurt with a touch of lemon blended in.

Use more fish and poultry, which are also excellent sources of complete protein, as you cut down on the sodium and fat in meats, eggs, and cheese. Vegetables and whole grains also provide protein. For example, legumes (beans, peas, and lentils) have almost as much protein as an egg.

In order for your body's cells to make proteins, all the essential amino acids must be present at the same time. Because plant proteins are sometimes low on one or more of the essential amino acids, the building blocks of proteins, it is good practice to combine two or more types of vegetables or grains in a meal to make a more complete mixture of amino acids. Rice and beans are the classic example. The essential amino acids that are low in the rice are plentiful in the beans, and vice versa. Other good protein pairs include corn tacos with beans, chili with corn bread, or skim milk on rice pudding.

It's not necessary to worry about this with each meal, because no plant protein is totally deficient and some amino acids are present in your intestine and blood to help tide you over until the next meal. However, if you were to regularly eat only one thing, such as rice, you would have to eat an awful lot to get enough of each essential amino acid.

For a complete explanation, see *Diet for a Small Planet* by Frances Moore Lappé (Ballantine Books). In this book, Frances Lappé points out that, provided you don't eat only one single food or a diet that is almost completely fruits, sweet potatoes, or junk food, it is almost impossible not to get enough protein if you eat enough calories to maintain your ideal weight. For example, per calorie, spinach is 49 percent protein—more than a cooked hamburger patty, which on a calorie basis is only 39 percent protein (and 58 percent fat). Spinach is also rich in mag-

nesium. Perhaps Popeye knew what he was doing after all!
(One word of caution: spinach contains oxalic acid, which ties up calcium so that you can't absorb it. You can neutralize the oxalic acid by adding calcium when you cook spinach (milk, for example). Also, since spinach is low in calories, you won't get much protein from a normal portion.)

Snacks

The bad snacks are the ones that are high in fat, salt, and/or sugar, such as commercial doughnuts, ice cream, fatty cheeses, candy bars, salted potato chips. Good snacks should not have added salt or sugar and should be low in fat.

Don't despair—popcorn can be great for you! If possible, use a hot-air popper or use a very small quantity of butter-flavored oil. Flavor with brewer's yeast, no-salt seasoning, or a potassium-containing salt substitute instead of table salt. Butter Buds can provide a butter flavor with almost no fat but unfortunately does contain some salt, so use sparingly if at all. Prepared this way, popcorn is not only tasty but low in fat while high in fiber and complex carbohydrates.

Because of their high *K Factor*, fruits or raw vegetables make excellent snacks. Unsalted nuts have a very high *K Factor*, but go lightly because of their high fat content. Unsalted pretzels, low-fat crackers, corn or flour tortillas (buy them fresh and toast them) all make healthy snacks (unsalted or salted with salt substitutes, of course). To make a dip for your crackers, chips, or tortillas, mix some unsalted hot pepper sauce and/or some unsalted fresh horseradish into some low-fat yogurt.

Eat snacks early in the day, so you will burn off the calories. Eating just before bed is probably the worst time, because most of the calories may end up as fat.

Selecting Your Meals: In the Restaurant

Obviously you will need to select foods high in the *K Factor* when you are dining out just as much as when you are shopping in the supermarket. Since you cannot control how the food has been selected or prepared in a restaurant, you need to be especially wary. While you are somewhat at the mercy of our habits of food preparation, there *are* some things you can do.

First we'll give you a few specific examples of good things to order:

- For breakfast: fresh fruit (orange, grapefruit, melon, banana, etc.) and pancakes (no butter, light on syrup), oatmeal, poached egg white on whole wheat toast, or shredded wheat.
- For lunch: turkey breast sandwich on whole wheat bread with no salt, no pickle, but lots of tomato and lettuce, or salad in a pita bread pocket (preferably whole wheat).
- For dinner: fish, other seafood, white meat of chicken or turkey, or go vegetarian.
- For a beverage: skim milk, low-salt sparkling water (e.g., Perrier) with lemon or lime, or fruit juice.
- For dessert: fresh fruit (apple, berries, peach, pineapple, mixed fruit cup, melon, etc.).

If your physician has okayed your use of a salt substitute, take it with you when you eat out, and use it instead of table salt.

A number of restaurants are now specializing in the preparation of "heart-healthy" meals, which are low in salt and fat. The American Heart Association is encouraging restaurants to do this through their "Creative Cuisine" program; call your local affiliate to see what's available in your area.

Other than fast foods, all cuisines offer some choices with a high *K Factor*. Be selective and give some thought to the foods as well as the method of preparation. Don't despair if nothing you can order is low in sodium. You can ask the chef not to add salt and to go light on fat. Be creative about balancing the meal: If the filet of sole has a delicious sauce that contains sodium, balance it with a high-potassium salad and a baked potato topped with a grind of pepper and yogurt or cottage cheese (if the restaurant has it; you'll have to ask). When you order, consider how the food is prepared. Boiling causes the potassium to leach out of foods, whereas steaming, baking, and stir-frying produce no significant drop in the *K Factor*.

Beware of fast foods: Almost all are high in sodium chloride and in fat. But don't just give up if you're trapped at a fast-food restaurant—you can ask the chef not to add salt! Even McDonald's will make unsalted fries on request. Salad bars are now available at many Burger King and Kentucky Fried Chicken franchises (if you order chicken, though, don't eat the skin: you'll be able to eliminate most of the salt and fat). A few pizza parlors now offer low-salt pizza with whole wheat crust and healthy toppings such as tuna, mussels, chicken, or vegetables.

On the other hand, don't overcerebrate. Enjoy!

Getting the Family to Go Along

If you are starting the high–*K Factor* diet because you have high blood pressure, it is a good idea for you to encourage your children to adopt the same diet. Since the tendency for high blood pressure is inherited, your children are likely to develop high blood pressure when they reach your age if they continue eating the usual American diet. Not only that, there is some evidence that even in people who have inherited the tendency, eating excess salt in childhood may reset their system to make them even *more* sensitive to salt in adulthood. You can prevent this by starting them on the proper diet now.

If your children live at home, they probably eat the same food you do. George has found that his teenagers have gotten accustomed to high–*K Factor* low-fat foods, and they like most of them. Healthy snacks are on hand, so they can get their caloric needs with things like unsalted whole wheat bread, sliced turkey, locally ground unsalted peanut butter, low-fat yogurt, a variety of fruits, oatmeal-raisin cookies, ½-percent fat milk, cider, orange juice, cranapple juice, and the like.

If your spouse doesn't have high blood pressure, he or she will probably want to eat the same food you do just to share the experience. The diet we are recommending has added appeal since it is not only good for keeping your blood pressure down but also helps prevent coronary artery disease as well as some types of cancer. Although he is genetically resistant to hypertension, Dick eats a diet with a high *K Factor* that is low in fat because of basic research that hints that a low *K Factor may* affect cell division and might possibly be a factor in some cancers. Even if you are resistant to hypertension, why stress your system with a *K Factor* only a tenth of what it should be?

Cooking Tips

The recommended recipes specify that:

- All cooking be done without salt.
- All vegetables be steamed, baked, or microwaved rather than boiled.
- All meats have as much fat removed as possible.

Detailed methods are discussed with each recipe.

As we have said, many familiar recipes taste just as good without added salt. Salt-free bread is just one example. Simply omit the salt from a standard recipe. It is a mistaken notion that yeast needs added salt to work: We have made some delicious bread without salt. Many of the quick breads (coffee cakes, muffins, cornbread) can be made with a low-sodium baking powder, such as the one made by Golden Harvest. Follow directions on the label: one and a half times the usual quantity of baking powder may be required.

If you must add salt during food preparation, use a *salt substitute*.

In the few cases in which leaving out salt makes the recipe unpalatable, some modifications are in order. The list of salt-free cookbooks increases almost daily. *Craig Claiborne's Gourmet Diet*, by Craig Claiborne with Pierre Franey (Ballantine Books, 1980), is good. An excellent guide for changing sodium-potassium balance is *How to Up Your Potassium*, by Corinne Azen Krause (William G. Johnston Company, 1979). If you can't find the latter in your bookstore, write to Potassium Cook Book, 7 Darlington Ct., Pittsburgh, PA 15217. The American Heart Association has published a good cookbook titled *Cooking Without Your Salt Shaker*.

Boiling is out, but broiling, steaming, stir-frying, baking, or using a microwave oven are in. Boiling not only causes food to lose vitamins but really lowers the *K Factor*. For example, raw potatoes have a *K Factor* of about 130. If the potatoes are boiled in even slightly salted water, the *K Factor* drops from about 130 down to between 1 and 3.[11] The same holds true for carrots, beans, and peas. Vegetables cooked in the microwave oven are crisply appealing as well as rich in vitamins and minerals. Since some nutrients and flavors do escape when you steam vegetables, save the small quantity of water remaining for a soup stock.

Since many traditional protein sources are high in saturated fats, we emphasize proteins from plant sources. When you do use meats, trim or skin off as much fat as possible.

Starting the Menu Plan

In this section we provide you with twenty-eight days of menus. There are two reasons for this:

○ It is very important that you do not change your eating style suddenly—*this could be dangerous*. The menus for the first week are scientifically designed to provide a progressive increase from the *K Factor* of the average American to a more reasonable level.

○ The menu plan provides security and peace of mind by showing you exactly what to do until it becomes second nature.

No matter how desirable, any change can be dangerous if it is made too quickly. If you turn the wheel of your car too fast, if you lose weight too fast, if you increase the amount of exercise you do too fast—all these sudden changes can get you in trouble. This is also true when increasing your *K Factor*. Remember, if you're like the typical American, your dietary *K Factor* is only about 10 percent of the minimum it should be. Paradoxically, when your body is deficient in potassium, it cannot tolerate as much as it would normally.[12] So it's necessary to build up slowly for about a week.

Therefore, we recommended in the beginning of the book that you take a week to eliminate the salt you add at the table. *Now* you should stop adding salt in the kitchen as well as at the table. Over the first week of menus, we gradually increase your *K Factor* from just under 1 to almost 4. *It is essential that this first week of menus should be taken in order and not repeated.* If you have already been on a *low* salt diet, you should start at day 3 or later. Otherwise you'll be taking a step backwards.

This menu plan provides about 2,000 calories per day, approximately the amount required for maintaining constant weight for an average middle-aged woman. Larger women and men and more active people will generally need to eat more. Smaller women, less active or older people, those who are reducing, or those whose metabolism is geared for storing fat will need to eat less. You can adjust for your particular caloric requirements by increasing or decreasing the portion sizes. Obviously the sensible serving size for a petite great-grandmother and for a high school athlete are two very different things.

The last three weeks of menus we present contain adequate vitamins, minerals, and amino acids.* So if you follow a similar plan, vitamin or mineral pills will not be necessary, with the exception of iron. Our menus contain sufficient iron for men, but several days are short of meeting the U.S. RDA for women (18 mg, as opposed to 10 mg for men). Therefore, women should take daily iron supplements.

We've summarized each day's plan in terms of total calories, percent of calories from fat sources, total potassium, total sodium, and, finally, the potassium-to-sodium ratio (the *K Factor*).

The nutritional summaries given at the end of each day's plan allow for typical commercial bakery bread (except where specified otherwise), but you can probably find low-sodium bread instead or bake your own, and thus lower your total sodium intake for the day. (We offer some bread recipes at the end of the meal plan.)

---

*These were checked using food tables and the Nutritionist III computer program by N-Squared Computing Co., Silverton, Oregon 97381. The U.S. RDAs for all major vitamins, essential amino acids, iron, magnesium, and calcium were exceeded on the weekly averages (see text regarding iron for women). Only a few individual days were short on one vitamin, which was more than compensated for on the next day.

Most of the fat you see listed is from plant sources and is high in polyunsaturates.

An asterisk indicates that the recipe is provided in the alphabetical list at the end of this chapter. If you want additional recipes that emphasize reducing the fat in your diet and increasing unsaturated fats, a good one is *The American Heart Association Cookbook*, published by Ballantine Books. We also recommend the new booklet *Eating for a Healthy Heart*, which is available from your local affiliate of the AHA.

These meal plans are suggestions. Feel free to make substitutions following our guidelines. The snacks as listed can be shifted to the time of day you need them most; just remember, you're likely to store calories as fat at the end of the day. They can also be eliminated if you need a much lower caloric intake. Conversely, if you need more calories, enlarge the portions.

Points to Keep in Mind

In the plan, you'll find ideas for saving a day's plan from sabotage by occasional low–*K Factor* binges. Specific suggestions are given for such days. Remember: *the first seven days' menus should be taken in order*, since they are planned to increase your *K Factor* at a rate designed to allow your body's cells sufficient time to adapt.[13] Do not return to menus of the first week after you have completed it. In the last three weeks, you may shift days around, since all the days have healthy *K Factor*(s). Several items in the last three weeks (beginning with day 18) have asterisks (*) in front of them. For these foods, recipes can be found in alphabetical order at the end of this chapter. When an alternative is listed, nutritional data apply to the first choice. Eating the alternative food will mean little, if any, significant change in the day's nutritional totals.

Remember: No salt should be added in the kitchen or at the table for any of these menus (and for the rest of your life).

The Plan

THE TRANSITION PERIOD

First Week: Eliminate salt at the table *and* in cooking.

Second Week: Now, start the transition week of menus on day

one—*do not repeat these menus*. If you've been on a low sodium diet, start with day 3. Keep days 1 through 7 *in order*.

THE PERMANENT PLAN

Third, Fourth, and Fifth Weeks: Now, starting with day 8, your food has a *K Factor* of at least 4. From now on, you can repeat, or exchange, days in the menu plan. By the end of the fifth week, you should be able to plan your own menus so that your *K Factor* is above 4.

Day 1

BREAKFAST

8 ounces orange juice (from frozen concentrate)
1½ ounces cold cereal (Grape Nuts Flakes or your choice)
8 ounces whole milk
1 corn muffin

LUNCH

Lean hamburger on roll (catsup, 2 slices pickle—make the pickle your last)
Pretzels, 1¼ ounces (adieu to these)

SNACK

1 slice coconut custard pie

DINNER

Fish and chips dinner, 10 ounces
Broccoli with cheese sauce, ½ cup
Instant butterscotch pudding, ½ cup

Calories (total for the day): 2,000

Fat (total for the day): 74 g

Calories from fat: 37%

Potassium (total for the day): 2,800 mg

Sodium (total for the day): 4,200 mg†

---

†If you are a heavy salt user, we are tapering your sodium down gradually. If you are already on a low salt diet, you should enter the menu program at day 3. This day's total was calculated using values for a frozen fish and chips dinner, which definitely has too much sodium in it for later in the program.

K Factor for the day: 0.7 (potassium to sodium ratio = 0.7 to 1)

Note: Calories are rounded to the nearest 50; sodium and potassium are rounded to the nearest 100 mg, except to the nearest 50 if under 1,000.

Do not repeat this day.

Day 2

BREAKFAST

8 ounces orange juice

1½ ounces shredded wheat

1 teaspoon sugar

½ cup whole milk

English muffin (or buttermilk biscuits from packaged refrigerated dough would have about the same *K Factor*, but the fat content would be higher)

1 tablespoon jam

LUNCH

1 bagel (or hard roll)

1 ounce lox (smoked salmon, or use other lean meat)

1 tablespoon cream cheese

4 ounces apple juice

SNACK

1 oatmeal cookie and an apple

DINNER

Zucchini lasagna, 11 ounces

"Boil in bag" green beans, onions and bacon bits, frozen vegetables (½ cup)

2 hard rolls (bakery type)

4 ounces whole milk

1 cup cherries (frozen, sweetened)

Calories: 2,000

Fat: 34 g

Calories from fat: 15%

Potassium: 3,100 mg

Sodium: 3,500 mg

K Factor: 0.9

On this day, you have eaten slightly less potassium than sodium; if the amounts were equal, their *K Factor* would be 1. The ratio, or *K Factor*, of 0.9 is slightly higher than yesterday's ratio. Each day during this first week, you will see a gradual increase. This small daily increase gives your system a chance to readjust. Remember, this slow increase is very important.

Do not repeat this day.

Day 3

BREAKFAST

8 ounces orange juice

1 egg, scrambled (no salt, no butter; oil the pan sparingly)

1 breakfast patty (sausage substitute)

2 slices whole wheat toast, no butter

1 tablespoon jelly

LUNCH

Turkey pastrami sandwich (1 ounce of turkey or other lunch meat, lean as possible), unsalted mustard, extra lettuce

1 medium-size kosher dill pickle

8 ounces skim milk

SNACK

Strawberry shake

DINNER

3½ ounces chicken, fried, without skin

Frozen spinach, rice and mushrooms, no sauce, ⅔ cup

Medium baked potato

1 roll

Lime ice served on a split banana

Calories: 1,950

Fat: 39 g

Calories from fat: 16%

Potassium: 3,300 mg
Sodium: 2,700 mg
K Factor: 1.2

Today your foods have slightly more potassium than sodium, giving you a *K Factor* greater than 1. By the end of this week, your system will have had a chance to adjust to the higher *K Factor* and you will be eating menus with a healthy *K Factor* of 4 or above.
Do not repeat this day.

Day 4

This is an example of a day on which you might be eating a Mexican (or other) dinner that is high in sodium. By keeping the sodium low at breakfast and lunch, you can eat the Mexican dinner without ruining your progress.

BREAKFAST
8 ounces orange juice
¾ cup oatmeal, cooked without salt
10 chopped dates cooked with the oatmeal
8 ounces skim milk

LUNCH
Very large fruit salad with lots of greens, dressed with lemon juice or orange juice
Iced tea

DINNER
Mexican combination platter (16-ounce frozen dinner or at restaurant)
2 glasses of beer (or soft drinks)
1 cup lime ice

Calories: 1,950
Fat: 39 g
Calories from fat: 18%
Potassium: 3,200 mg

Sodium: 2,100 mg

K Factor: 1.5

Do not repeat this day.

Day 5

BREAKFAST

8 ounces orange juice

½ cup stewed prunes (cook without sugar and mix with cereal)

¾ cup Cream of Wheat, cooked without salt

8 ounces skim milk

LUNCH

Tuna salad, made from 3¼ ounces water-packed unsalted canned tuna, plenty of lettuce, small amount of mayonnaise, preferably unsalted

1 apple

2 slices canned Boston Brown Bread (or low-sodium whole wheat bread)

8 ounces skim milk

SNACK

Freeze-type citrus drink, made with fruit ice, not ice cream

DINNER

Frozen 11¼-ounce pork loin dinner or Swiss steak

Large salad of greens and tomato, dressed with wine vinegar and a sprinkle of sugar if you like

8 ounces skim milk

1 cup sliced peaches

Calories: 2,100

Fat: 38 g

Calories from fat: 16%

Potassium: 4,100 mg

Sodium: 1,900 mg

K Factor: 2.2

Do not repeat this day.

Day 6

Here is an example of a day with steady progress in spite of a piece of sweet potato (or similar) pie.

BREAKFAST
8 ounces tangerine juice
¾ cup Maypo (or oatmeal) cooked without salt, 10 chopped dates added for flavor
8 ounces skim milk

LUNCH
Large fruit salad with 1 cup cottage cheese and lemon/honey dressing

SNACK
1 slice sweet potato pie

DINNER
Curried fish (3½ ounces) and ⅘ cup of rice, cooked without salt, ⅔ cup of raisins added
⅔ cup green beans, steamed, no butter
8 ounces skim milk

Calories: 2,000
Fat: 27 g
Calories from fat: 12%
Potassium: 4,300 mg
Sodium: 1,600 mg
K Factor: 2.7

Do not repeat this day.

Day 7

BREAKFAST
8 ounces orange juice
¾ cup oatmeal, cooked without salt
Banana or melon in season
8 ounces skim milk

LUNCH
Chef's salad: all types of raw vegetables, greens, sprouts,

strips of Swiss cheese (1 ounce), and slices of hard-boiled egg; oil and vinegar dressing
8 ounces skim milk
1 cup of grapes (or similar fruit)

SNACK
Mixed dried fruit

DINNER
Noodles Romanoff from mix (¼ package) or spaghetti with meatless tomato sauce
Baked acorn squash, brown sugar, no butter
⅔ cup asparagus with lemon
8 ounces skim milk

Calories: 1,900
Fat: 45 g
Calories from fat: 21%
Potassium: 5,000 mg
Sodium: 1,300 mg
K Factor: 3.8

You have now completed the week of "break-in" menus to gear your body up for food with a naturally high *K Factor* of 4 or more.
Do not repeat these days.

From now on (days 8 through 28) you can change the order or repeat days as you choose.

Day 8

BREAKFAST
8 ounces orange juice
3 pancakes, made with no salt and using low-sodium baking powder (just whisk together 1 egg, 1 cup of water, and 2 tablespoons oil; then add ¼ cup nonfat dry milk, a rounded tablespoon of low-sodium baking powder, and about 1½ cups flour. Makes about 8)

2 tablespoons maple or other syrup
8 ounces skim milk

LUNCH
2 cups bean soup made from dry or unsalted canned beans, using low-sodium beef bouillon
2 pieces cornbread
8 ounces skim milk

SNACK
Dried apricots, 10 halves

DINNER
3½ ounces veal, cooked without butter
⅔ cup peas and carrots, steamed, unsalted, no butter
Green salad, Italian dressing used sparingly
8 ounces skim milk
⅔ cup strawberry ice milk

Calories: 2,000
Fat: 52 mg
Calories from fat: 23%
Potassium: 4,800 mg
Sodium: 1,200 mg
K Factor: 4.0

Day 9

Today you'll be able to accommodate a commercial super hamburger with all the fixings and still achieve a *K Factor* of over 4. For instance, you might be going on an outing with the children.

BREAKFAST
½ grapefruit
2 ounces shredded wheat
1 banana
8 ounces skim milk

LUNCH
Super hamburger (e.g., McDonald's Big Mac)

French fries without salt (ask for them that way—you may
have to wait a few extra minutes for a special order, but it's
worth it)
8 ounces orange juice

DINNER

1½ cups beans (cooked from dry beans, no salt, add molasses
and dry mustard for flavor, tomato paste, unsalted flavor-
ings)
2 corn muffins, made with low-sodium baking powder (whisk
together 1 egg, 1 cup water, 3 tablespoons oil, then add ¼
cup each of sugar and nonfat dry milk, then 1 cup each of
flour and cornmeal, and 2 tablespoons low-sodium baking
powder; stir and bake in preheated oven at 425 degrees for
about 15 minutes)
⅔ cup frozen broccoli, cauliflower, and red pepper, steamed,
no sauce

Calories: 2,050

Fat: 60 mg

Calories from fat: 26%

Potassium: 6,600 mg

Sodium: 1,400 mg

K Factor: 4.7

Day 10

BREAKFAST

8 ounces orange juice
1 cup whole wheat cereal (Ralston, Wheatena, Maltex), cooked
without salt
1 banana (on cereal)
8 ounces skim milk

LUNCH

Sandwich of sliced turkey (2 ounces) on low-sodium bread,
lettuce and cranberry sauce, with a little mayonnaise
8 ounces skim milk

DINNER
    4 ounces steamed fish
    1 cup brown rice
    ½ cup chopped spinach
    Salad of ½ avocado with grapefruit sections
    2 whole wheat muffins
    1 cup mixed frozen fruit, sweetened

Calories: 1,900

Fat: 36 g

Calories from fat: 17%

Potassium: 4,900 mg

Sodium: 1,200 mg

K Factor: 4.1

Day 11

BREAKFAST
    ½ grapefruit
    ¾ cup Cream of Wheat, no salt, with ⅔ cup raisins
    8 ounces skim milk

LUNCH
    Sandwich of tuna salad using low-sodium, water-packed tuna
    8 ounces skim milk
    1 apple

SNACK
    3½ ounces mixed dried fruit

DINNER
    6 ounces lean club steak
    Medium-size sweet potato, baked
    ½ cup succotash, no salt or butter
    8 ounces skim milk
    1 cup strawberries, sweetened

Calories: 1,950

Fat: 21 g

Calories from fat: 9%

Potassium: 5,100 mg

Sodium: 800 mg

K Factor: 6.4

Day 12

BREAKFAST

8 ounces orange juice
½ ounce Kellogg's Puffed Rice
1 banana
8 ounces skim milk

LUNCH ·

1⅓ ounces lentil soup, made with dry lentils, chopped carrot, low-sodium broth†
1 slice Boston Brown Bread, canned (or French-, Vienna-, or Italian-style bread)
1 ounce Swiss cheese
1 cup red-cabbage-and-apple salad
8 ounces skim milk

SNACK

1 soft ice cream cone

DINNER

16 ounces eggplant-and-rice casserole, using unsalted canned tomatoes
2 whole wheat rolls, no salt
¾ cup brussels sprouts
8 ounces skim milk
1 cup frozen cherries, sweetened

Calories: 2,050

Fat: 26 g

Calories from fat: 11%

---

†Unlike other legumes, lentils don't require long soaking; simmer the soup that day to use, or simmer it one day and reheat when you need it.

Potassium: 4,600 mg

Sodium: 1,000 mg

K Factor: 4.6

Day 13

BREAKFAST

    8 ounces grapefruit juice

    1 cup shredded wheat

    1 cup strawberries

    8 ounces skim milk

    1 slice whole wheat toast, low sodium

    1 teaspoon jelly

LUNCH

    Low-sodium canned soup (see list p. 133)

    1 ounce Swiss cheese

    2 zwieback

    8 ounces skim milk

SNACK

    1 cup fruit-flavored low-fat yogurt

    5 dried peach halves

DINNER

    ½ chicken breast, without skin, rolled in chopped walnuts (2
        tablespoons) and baked

    1 medium-size baked potato, no salt or butter

    ⅔ cup turnips

    Salad of fresh spinach and mushrooms, oil/vinegar dressing

    8 ounces skim milk

Calories: 2,050

Fat: 37 g

Calories from fat: 16%

Potassium: 4,900 mg

Sodium: 950 mg

K Factor: 5.2

Day 14

Some days it seems a social necessity to eat a friend's master-piece dessert, such as a rhubarb pie, but with judicious choices made earlier in the day, you can avoid disaster and maintain a *K Factor* of 5.

BREAKFAST

½ grapefruit

1 cup Cream of Wheat, cooked without salt, ⅔ cup raisins added

8 ounces skim milk

LUNCH

2 blueberry muffins, made with low-sodium baking powder (or 4 graham crackers)

1 cup low-fat yogurt

3 medium-size fresh apricots or 1 large peach

DINNER

Noodles (2 ounces dry) and goulash, made with 3½ ounces chicken previously simmered and chilled, with fat and skin removed, then simmered again with paprika, carrots, cabbage, a little yogurt at serving time

Beet salad, using ¾ cup canned unsalted beets, lettuce, and onions

8 ounces skim milk

SNACK

1 slice rhubarb pie

Calories: 2,000

Fat: 38 g

Calories from fat: 17%

Potassium: 4,300 mg

Sodium: 850 mg

K Factor: 5.0

Day 15

BREAKFAST

3 potato pancakes (see p. 136)

½ cup applesauce
1 cup low-fat yogurt

LUNCH
Salad of ½ cup pasta and ⅔ cup mixed vegetables (no pickled ones) and plenty of lettuce; 1 tablespoon blue cheese dressing
2 slices whole wheat bread
8 ounces skim milk

SNACK
*Prune-Pineapple Compote (1 cup)

DINNER
3½ ounces roast turkey without skin
½ cup mashed potato (no salt or butter)
Gravy made from chilled defatted meat drippings, thickened with a cornstarch paste and cooked without salt
½ cup rutabaga
⅗ cup peas
¼ cup cranberry sauce
8 ounces skim milk
1 cup stewed rhubarb or other fruit

Calories: 2,000
Fat: 21 g
Calories from fat: 9%
Potassium: 5,400 mg
Sodium: 1,000 mg
K Factor: 5.4

Day 16

BREAKFAST
8 ounces apricot juice
1 cup oatmeal with 10 chopped dates, cooked without salt
8 ounces skim milk

LUNCH
Banana (1 medium) salad, dressed with 1 tablespoon unsalted

peanut butter mixed with 1 tablespoon unsalted mayonnaise; lettuce
2 whole wheat rolls, made without salt
8 ounces skim milk

DINNER
3½ ounces codfish, or use other fish, or beef tongue with fat
removed by boiling and chilling
1 large baked potato
⅔ cup raw shredded parsnip salad, dressed with lemon juice,
sugar
⅔ cup frozen green beans with almonds
1 cup fruit-flavored low-fat yogurt

Calories: 2,000
Fat: 30 g
Calories from fat: 13%
Potassium: 5,600 mg
Sodium: 650 mg
K Factor: 8.6

Day 17

This day allows you to work around eating Wheaties or a
similar breakfast cereal containing salt. Although the cereal
contains over 500 milligrams of sodium, you save the day by
keeping the sodium low in everything else you eat.

BREAKFAST
8 ounces orange juice
1½ ounces Wheaties or corn flakes
8 ounces skim milk
1 peach

LUNCH
1 cup vichyssoise (for summer; if it's winter, make the same
thing and call it hot potato soup: Into 1 cup of boiling water,
stir one teaspoon each of low-sodium chicken bouillon

powder and dehydrated onion; 4 tablespoons each of nonfat
dry milk and potato flakes; season with a dash of bitters
and a sprinkle of white or black pepper; chill or use hot)
Raw spinach salad with added raw vegetables, 1 teaspoon oil,
and vinegar

SNACK
3½ ounces mixed dried fruit

DINNER
3½ ounces breaded veal cutlet
⅔ cup shredded steamed red cabbage
1 baked sweet potato
2 whole wheat rolls, unsalted
8 ounces skim milk
½ ounce rice pudding with raisins

Calories: 1,900

Fat: 23 g

Calories from fat: 11%

Potassium: 6,800 mg

Sodium: 1,700 mg

K Factor: 4.0

Day 18

BREAKFAST
½ grapefruit
⅔ cup shredded wheat
½ cup skim milk
1 medium-size banana

LUNCH
Sandwich of 2 slices whole wheat bread, ½ tablespoon unsalted mayonnaise, lettuce, and *Luncheon Loaf
1 apple
8 ounces skim milk
*Dill Pickles

SNACK
Mixture of chopped dried apricots, apples, peaches, and raisins, 5 ounces

DINNER
*Turkey and Water Chestnut Casserole, ⅛ recipe
1 cup cooked brown rice, without salt
*Carrots with Zing
Salad of lightly steamed peas, with lettuce and spring onions, with wine vinegar dressing (no oil)
8 ounces skim milk
1 cup cherries, in light syrup

Calories: 1,900

Fat: 17 g

Calories from fat: 8%

Potassium: 5,800 mg

Sodium: 1,000 mg

K Factor: 5.8

Day 19

BREAKFAST
6 ounces orange juice
2 cups puffed wheat (unsalted)
4 ounces skim milk
½ cup strawberries

LUNCH
Sandwich of 2 slices whole wheat bread, 1 tablespoon unsalted mayonnaise, tomato, and 1 ounce unsalted cheese
1 apple
8 ounces skim milk

SNACK
4 large fresh plums

COCKTAIL
*Zero Cocktail

DINNER
*Oriental Meatballs
1 cup brown rice, cooked without salt
Chinese cabbage, shredded, with *Sham Tonkatsu Sauce or
Mrs. Dash steak sauce
1 baked sweet potato
8 ounces skim milk
½ cup each applesauce and chopped dates

Calories: 2,000

Fat: 31 g

Calories from fat: 13%

Potassium: 5,100 mg

Sodium: 1,000 mg

K Factor: 5.1

Day 20

BREAKFAST
8 ounces orange juice
1 poached egg on 1 slice whole wheat toast, no butter
8 ounces skim milk (can be heated and poured on egg and
toast)
Second piece of toast
1 teaspoon jam

LUNCH
Chicken salad of 3½ ounces home-cooked chicken, defatted, ½
cup rice, and pineapple chunks (the fruit juice provides the
dressing)
2 whole wheat low-sodium muffins (or whole wheat bread)
8 ounces skim milk

SNACK
*Banana-Pineapple Yogurt Shake

DINNER
Fish creole (sizzle some chopped onion and green pepper in a

minimum of oil in a frying pan, then add unsalted tomatoes
and 3½ ounces fish; simmer gently until fish is opaque, add
hot pepper sauce or other seasonings to taste)
1 baked potato
1 cup cole slaw made with yogurt
2 slices fruit-nut bread (pumpkin, squash, etc., no salt)
8 ounces skim milk
1 cup fruit ice

Calories: 2,100

Fat: 41 g

Calories from fat: 18%

Potassium: 4,400 mg

Sodium: 1,000 mg

K Factor: 4.4

Day 21

BREAKFAST

8 ounces tangerine juice
1 cup oatmeal (or Maypo) cooked without salt, with 1 ounce
dates added for flavor
8 ounces skim milk

LUNCH

Mushroom omelet, made with 2 egg whites (discard yolks), 10
small mushrooms, 1 teaspoon unsalted butter, 3½ ounces
mung bean sprouts
8 ounces skim milk
1 apple

SNACK

Fruit-flavored "freeze" type drink

DINNER

Baked stuffed green pepper, using 3 ounces lean, well-drained
ground beef and 1 cup previously cooked rice
⅔ cup carrots, steamed
8 ounces skim milk

1 cup pineapple in juice

1 banana split, homemade, using 1 banana, 6 ounces ice *milk*, and 1 tablespoon cocoa powder mixed with hot water (for hot chocolate sauce), sprinkled with ¼ ounce walnut crumbs

Calories: 2,100

Fat: 34 g

Calories from fat: 15%

Potassium: 5,400 mg

Sodium: 900 mg

K Factor: 6.0

Day 22

Today you have lunch scheduled at a swanky restaurant. With care, you still end the day with a *K Factor* of over 5.

BREAKFAST

1 fresh orange

2 ounces shredded wheat

1 banana

8 ounces skim milk

SNACK

Mixed dried fruit and nuts

LUNCH

Broiled salmon steak

1 baked potato

4 ounces yogurt or cottage cheese on potato, rest for dessert

⅔ cup green beans

1 roll, no butter

Tea

DINNER

Meat substitute, canned or boxed (such as Reddi-burger, or "textured soy protein") cooked with 4 ounces diluted tomato paste and your choice of herbs

½ cup lima beans

Large salad of alfalfa sprouts, cauliflower, other raw vegetables, and crisp greens
8 ounces skim milk
8 ounces fresh pineapple

Calories: 1,900

Fat: 24 g

Calories from fat: 12%

Potassium: 6,200 mg

Sodium: 900 mg

K Factor: 6.9

Day 23

BREAKFAST
½ grapefruit
3 *Maple Bran Muffins
1 tablespoon preserves
8 ounces skim milk

LUNCH
1 cup gazpacho, made from fresh or unsalted canned tomatoes, cucumber, spring onions, green pepper
½ avocado, with lettuce and lime juice dressing
2 whole wheat rolls, low sodium
8 ounces skim milk
2 fresh plums

SNACK
8 ounces yogurt with fruit preserves

DINNER
5 ounces pompano en papillotte (or any fish): Take a square of
foil or parchment—even brown paper bag will do, with a
little oil on it—place a few slices of lemon and scallion in
the center, place fish on these, fold edges of package over
twice to seal, then bake. The juices stay in.
12 ounces potato casserole (thinly sliced potato, baked with
parsley and milk, onion, no salt or butter)
1 cup baked Hubbard squash

Salad of greens and alfalfa sprouts, wine vinegar dressing
1 cup mixed fruit

Calories: 2,100

Fat: 47 g

Calories from fat: 20%

Potassium: 7,000 mg

Sodium: 1,100 mg

K Factor: 6.4

Day 24

BREAKFAST
4 ounces stewed prunes
2 ounces shredded wheat
4 ounces skim milk

LUNCH
Sandwich of 2 slices whole wheat bread, tuna salad made
from water-packed unsalted tuna, chopped celery, ½ tablespoon unsalted mayonnaise
8 ounces skim milk
1 medium-size orange

SNACK
½ cup dried apricots

DINNER
*Pita (pocket bread) with garbanzos and *Tahini Sauce
*Tabouleh Salad
8 ounces skim milk
½ cup chopped dates

Calories: 1,950

Fat: 33 g

Calories from fat: 15%

Potassium: 4,700 mg

Sodium: 700 mg

K Factor: 6.7

Day 25

BREAKFAST
    ¼ cantaloupe
    3 potato pancakes (made without salt, see p. 136) and ½ cup
      applesauce
    8 ounces skim milk

LUNCH
    1 cup chunky chicken soup (canned, low sodium)
    2 slices *Rye Bread with 2 tablespoons jam
    1 banana
    8 ounces skim milk

SNACK
    1 large apple
    1 cup low-fat fruit-flavored yogurt

DINNER
    *Lentil Casserole (20 ounces)
    ½ acorn squash, baked, with 2 tablespoons maple syrup
    Tossed green salad with *Webb Dressing (1 tablespoon)
    8 ounces skim milk
    1 cup canned cherries, in light syrup

    Calories: 1,900

    Fat: 34 g

    Calories from fat: 16%

    Potassium: 5,600 mg

    Sodium: 750 mg

    K Factor: 7.5

Day 26

BREAKFAST
    6 ounces orange juice
    1 ounce (2 cups) unsalted puffed rice or puffed wheat
    1 banana (on cereal)
    8 ounces skim milk (on cereal)

SNACK
Popcorn, not more than 2 quarts, popped without oil
2 ounces mixed dried fruit

LUNCH
Sandwich of 2 slices *Rye Bread, 1 tablespoon unsalted mayonnaise, 1 slice ham (5% fat) or 1 slice other lean meat or poultry, lettuce
2 fresh apricots
8 ounces skim milk

DINNER
*Sole with Mushrooms (⅙ recipe)
1 cup rice
*Carrot Salad
⅔ cup green beans
2 whole wheat muffins
8 ounces skim milk
1 cup canned plums

Calories: 1,900

Fat: 23 g

Calories from fat: 11%

Potassium: 5,900 mg

Sodium: 900 mg

K Factor: 6.6

Day 27

BREAKFAST
½ grapefruit
*Coffee Cake (⅙ recipe)
Coffee

LUNCH
Sandwich of 2 slices whole wheat bread, *Luncheon Loaf, lettuce, ½ tablespoon unsalted mayonnaise
1 medium-size banana
8 ounces skim milk

SNACK
8 ounces pineapple (or other fruit) juice

DINNER
*Zero Cocktail
2 pieces chicken without skin, and *Barbecue Sauce
1 large potato, baked, with 2 tablespoons low-fat yogurt, chives
Salad of greens and shredded parsnips, dressed with lemon juice
8 ounces skim milk
½ cup apple crisp

Calories: 1,900

Fat: 29 g

Calories from fat: 14%

Potassium: 6,300 mg

Sodium: 900 mg

K Factor: 7.0

Day 28

BREAKFAST
1 cup blueberries
8 ounces skim milk
2 *Maple Bran Muffins

LUNCH
1 cup *Potato Salad
2 slices *Rye Bread, unbuttered
1 cup apricots in light syrup
8 ounces skim milk

SNACK
½ cup fruit ice

DINNER
*Moore's Lumberjack Chili (¼ recipe)
1 cup enriched white rice, cooked without salt
Veggies and dip (8 ounces low-fat yogurt with chopped cucumber and spring onions, used as a dip for raw carrots,

celery, cauliflower, broccoli, whatever; about 2 cups)
2 whole wheat rolls, low sodium if possible
Iced tea

Calories: 2,100
Fat: 31 g
Calories from fat: 13%
Potassium: 6,900 mg
Sodium: 1,300 mg
K Factor: 5.3

Note: All the data for calculating the nutritional summaries for each day were obtained from J.A.T. Pennington and H. Nichols Church, *Food Values*, Harper & Row, Publishers, New York, 1985; or the *Agriculture Handbook No. 8 Series*, U.S. Department of Agriculture, U.S Government Printing Office, Washington D.C.; or by using a personally edited version of the Nutritionist III computer software program by N-Squared Computing Co., Silverton, Oregon.

Recipes

Following are examples of some high–*K Factor* recipes that illustrate the principles we've just outlined. As you can see, almost any type of cuisine can be prepared so that it has a high *K Factor*. After a while, you should be able to modify your own recipes.

Since these recipes go with the menu plan, the portion sizes are adjusted to provide about 2,000 calories per day. If you need more than that, increase the portions accordingly.

Banana-Pineapple Yogurt Shake (SERVES TWO)
1 banana
½ cup pineapple (preferably fresh)
2–4 ounces low-fat or no-fat yogurt

4–6 ice cubes
1 teaspoon honey
½ cup orange juice or apple cider

Blend all ingredients in blender or food processor.

Calories per serving: 162

Fat per serving: 1.3 g

Calories from fat: 7%

Potassium per serving: 471 mg

Sodium per serving: 27.5 mg

K Factor: 17 (potassium to sodium ratio: 17 to 1)

Barbecue Sauce (SERVES SIX)

1 cup prune juice
⅓ cup unsalted catsup
2 tablespoons cider vinegar
1 tablespoon unsalted prepared mustard

Stir ingredients together and use for basting baked chicken or meats, or as an accompaniment.

Calories per serving: 37

Fat per serving: 0.07 g

Calories from fat: 0

Potassium per serving: 167 mg

Sodium per serving: 4 mg

K Factor: 42

Broths and Gravies

Any fat found in the pan after browning and draining the meat you cook can be mixed with a little very hot water, then poured off and refrigerated. The grease that congeals on top can be discarded (better thrown in the garbage than in your arteries), and the remaining liquid can be used as a seasoning broth for cooking rice, soups, vegetables—almost anything.

For a fat-free gravy, use 1 tablespoon of cornstarch per cup of liquid. Mix the cornstarch with a bit of broth to make a smooth paste, then stir it into the broth and heat. Stirring constantly, bring the broth to a boil and boil until thick—about 1 minute. Experiment with seasonings, and you will find that you have a nice gravy or a sauce to bind ingredients in a casserole.

Vegetable broths may be done the same way. While before you might have poured on the butter or sour cream to dress vegetables, you now can thicken some vegetable broths with cornstarch as directed and add lemon, herbs, and mushrooms, and have a sauce that will bind the vegetables rather than have them rolling around and looking lonely on the plate.

Carrot Salad (SERVES EIGHT)

6 to 8 medium raw carrots
2 tablespoons sugar
2 tablespoons lemon juice

Scrub carrots, scrape if necessary, then shred in processor or with a grater. Add sugar and lemon juice and mix.

Calories per serving: 41.4

Fat per serving: 0.1 g

Calories from fat: 2.1%

Potassium per serving: 223 mg

Sodium per serving: 29.5 mg

K Factor: 7.6

Carrots with Zing (SERVES EIGHT)

1 pound carrots, sliced
1 tablespoon butter-flavored oil
2 tablespoons brown sugar
1 teaspoon lemon juice
¼ teaspoon Tabasco sauce

Steam carrots until just tender. Make the sauce while they are steaming. Heat oil, brown sugar, lemon juice, and Tabasco together until bubbly. Pour over carrots and serve.

Calories per serving: 67

Fat per serving: 2 g

Calories from fat: 27%

Potassium per serving: 220 mg

Sodium per serving: 29 mg

K Factor: 8

Coffee Cake (SERVES SIX)
   4 large apples, quartered and sliced
   2½ tablespoons butter-flavored oil
   2 tablespoons chopped pecans
   1 teaspoon cinnamon
   ⅓ cup sugar
   1½ teaspoons baking powder (sodium-free)
   1 cup flour
   1 cup water
   3 egg whites

Preheat oven to 425°F. In an oven-proof pan, sauté the apples in oil until they begin to soften; set aside. Sprinkle pecans on apples. Mix cinnamon with sugar, sprinkle less than half on the apple-pecan mixture, and reserve remainder. Mix baking powder with flour; add water. Beat egg whites until stiff, fold gently into batter, and pour over apple mixture. Sprinkle remaining cinnamon-sugar on top. Bake for 15 minutes.

Calories per serving: 265

Fat per serving: 8 g

Calories from fat: 25%

Potassium per serving: 1,582 mg

Sodium per serving: 36.3 mg

K Factor: 44

Dill Pickles (6 PINTS)

Wash and sterilize 6 pint jars, lids, and bands. In *each* jar place:

1/4 teaspoon whole peppercorns
1 1/2 teaspoons onion flakes
1 small or 1/2 large clove garlic
1 teaspoon dill seed
1 pint scrubbed young cucumbers, cut into spears

Syrup

1 quart white vinegar
3 cups water
1/2 cup sugar
Cheesecloth bag containing 2 tablespoons pickling spice,
1 tablespoon whole allspice

Simmer syrup ingredients together for 15 minutes. Discard cheesecloth bag. Pour syrup into the jars over the cucumber spears and pepper, onion, garlic, and dill. Leave 1/2 inch of headroom over syrup. Use a wide-mouth funnel to keep jar rim clean. Place sterile lids and bands on jars, tighten moderately, and place jars in boiling water to cover. When water returns to a rolling boil, boil for 15 minutes. Remove jars with tongs and set in a draft-free place to cool. Allow to season for a few weeks before eating.

Calories per 100 g (2 medium-size pickles): 10

Fat per 2 pickles: 0 g

Calories from fat: 0%

Potassium per 2 pickles: 144 mg

Sodium per 2 pickles: 5 mg

K Factor: 29

George has been eating these for some time (for his blood pressure), but Dick, who loves dill pickles and is genetically resistant to hypertension, hadn't tasted them until recently. Dick's comment was that at first the pickles tasted very slightly different from the usual dills, but after the third pickle (he ate five the first time), he thought he actually liked them *better* than the usual dill pickle.

Lentil Casserole (SERVES FOUR GENEROUSLY)

   3 cups unsalted chicken or vegetable broth
   ¾ cup dry lentils
   ¾ cup chopped onion
   1 cup raw brown rice
   ¼ cup dry white wine
   ½ teaspoon crushed basil
   ½ teaspoon oregano
   ½ teaspoon thyme
   ⅛ teaspoon garlic powder
   ⅛ teaspoon black pepper
   1 cup shredded Swiss cheese

Combine all ingredients except ½ cup of cheese in an oiled three-quart casserole dish with a tight cover. Bake for 1½ to 2 hours at 350°F. Stir twice during baking. When lentils and rice are tender, sprinkle reserved ½ cup of cheese on top and bake uncovered until cheese melts.

   Calories per serving: 356

   Fat per serving: 8.8 g

   Calories from fat: 22%

   Potassium per serving: 1,166 mg

   Sodium per serving: 25 mg

   K Factor: 46

Luncheon Loaf (MAKES SIXTEEN SLICES)

   ¼ cup oats
   ¼ cup chopped onion
   2 tablespoons oil
   1 pound ground turkey
   1 tablespoon Bell's poultry seasoning
   1 teaspoon ground allspice
   1 packet unflavored gelatin
   2 cups cold water

Toast oats in a dry skillet, stirring frequently, until light brown. Sauté onion in oil; add turkey and brown. Remove from heat and add spices.

Soften gelatin in ½ cup of the water. Heat remaining water in medium saucepan. When boiling, add softened gelatin and dissolve. Add meat mixture and oats, stir, and heat all to boiling. Stir and pour into oiled loaf pan; cover with plastic wrap. Cool, then chill for several hours.

Before slicing for sandwiches, blot top of loaf with paper towel to remove any traces of fat. Cold cuts are the first to go when one begins a salt-free diet, and this is our savory answer to the challenge. Try it, you'll like it!

Calories per serving: 59

Fat per serving: 3.2 g

Calories from fat: 5.5%

Potassium per serving: 98 mg

Sodium per serving: 23 mg

K Factor: 4.2

Maple Bran Muffins (MAKES TWELVE MUFFINS)

1 egg, beaten
½ cup maple syrup
2 tablespoons oil
¾ cup water
1½ cups unprocessed wheat bran
1 cup whole wheat flour
¼ cup powdered milk
3 teaspoons sodium-free baking powder

Beat egg, maple syrup, oil, and water together. Mix bran with this mixture.

In a separate bowl, mix flour, powdered milk, and baking powder. At this point, the wet and dry ingredients can be set aside separately until morning and put together in a great rush in time for breakfast.

Preheat oven to 400°F. Mix wet and dry ingredients briefly, stir just until moistened, fill greased muffin pan, and bake for 15 minutes.

Calories per serving (2 muffins): 234

Fat per serving: 6.8 g

Calories from fat: 26%

Potassium per serving: 504 mg

Sodium per serving: 37.5 mg

K Factor: 13

Moore's Lumberjack Chili (SERVES 2 FORESTERS OR 6 PEOPLE)

¼ pound lean ground beef
2 cups chopped onions
15 ounces unsalted tomato juice
40 ounces (5 cups) canned kidney beans
1 teaspoon salt substitute
3 teaspoons chili powder (or to taste)

Break the ground beef into small pieces, brown, and drain on paper towels. Remove excess grease from pan. Add chopped onions and browned meat, cover, and cook on low heat, stirring frequently, until onions are tender and just starting to brown. During this time, puree half the kidney beans in a blender—this is the key to the success of this recipe!

After the onions are cooked, add the tomato juice and then add the pureed and the whole kidney beans. Add salt substitute and chili powder slowly while stirring over heat. Allow to simmer for at least 30 minutes. Consistency can be altered by changing the proportion of tomato juice.

The flavor is excellent, the amount of animal fat is very small, and the K/Na ratio is high. Dick developed this recipe while working his way through school as a cook in a forestry camp—it was a favorite with the foresters and with everyone since who has tried it. Enjoy it!

Calories per serving: 236

Fat per serving: 2.6 g

Calories from fat: 10%

Potassium per serving: 1,300 mg

Sodium per serving: 600 mg

K Factor: 2.2 (This *K Factor* is not very good because of the canned kidney beans, which are italicized in the table in Chapter 13. This illustrates that you can get away with an occasional italicized item if the rest of the day uses boldfaced items, as on day 28.) By using home-cooked kidney beans without salt for half of the beans, you can raise the *K Factor* to over 4.0 (but then save it for days when the *K Factor* for other meals is not as high as it is on day 18).

Oriental Meatballs with Rice (SERVES EIGHT)

1½ pounds lean ground beef
1 teaspoon minced garlic
1 teaspoon ground ginger
1 tablespoon cornstarch
1 cup canned pineapple chunks in natural juice (not heavy
 syrup), juice reserved
2 tablespoons cider vinegar
½ cup cranberry jelly
¾ cup carrot slices, cut diagonally
½ package (3 ounces) frozen Chinese pea pods or fresh
 edible-pod peas
2 cups brown rice cooked with 5 cups water

Mix ground beef, garlic, and ginger, and shape into small meatballs. Brown in nonstick pan, and drain well on paper towel. Make a paste of the cornstarch and a little of the pineapple juice. Pour the rest of the juice (about ¾ cup) into a saucepan with the vinegar and cranberry jelly. Add the cornstarch paste and cook, stirring, until transparent and thickened. Add carrot slices and cook until almost tender but not quite. Then add snow peas, pineapple, and meatballs. Cook until carrots and peas are crisp-tender. Serve with brown rice.

Calories per serving: 416

Fat per serving: 9.7 g

Calories from fat: 21%

Potassium per serving: 729 mg

Sodium per serving: 54 mg

K Factor: 13.5

Pineapple-Prune Compote (SERVES EIGHT)

1 pound dried prunes
20-ounce can crushed pineapple in unsweetened juice

Mix ingredients and refrigerate overnight.

Calories per serving: 190

Fat per serving: 0

Calories from fat: 0%

Potassium per serving: 557 mg

Sodium per serving: 10 mg

K Factor: 56

Pita (SERVES EIGHT)

¼ teaspoon sugar
1¼ cups warm water (115°F.)
1 envelope yeast
1½ tablespoons safflower oil
¾ cup white flour
2 cups whole wheat flour

Mix sugar into warm water and sprinkle yeast on top. Add safflower oil and white flour; beat well with a wire whisk. Mix in whole wheat flour and beat with a wooden spoon. Turn dough out onto floured board and knead well until smooth and elastic.

Place dough in an oiled bowl, turn once to oil top of dough, cover loosely with plastic wrap, and let rise an hour or until double in volume. Punch dough down; divide into eight balls. Flatten each into a 6-inch circle, using a rolling pin or your hand. Place on pan or foil, cover loosely with plastic wrap, and let rise again about ½ hour.

Preheat oven to 500°F.

Bake pita for 7 minutes on lowest rack of oven. Serve warm or cool. May be stored in plastic bag or frozen.

Calories per serving: 160

Fat per serving: 3.5 g

Calories from fat: 19%

Potassium per serving: 152.6

Sodium per serving: 1.24

K Factor: 123!

Potato Salad (SERVES FOUR)

4 cups cubed raw potatoes, unpeeled
2 tablespoons *Webb Dressing
½ cup chopped celery
1 medium onion, chopped
¼–½ teaspoon celery seeds
¼ cup unsalted mayonnaise
1 teaspoon unsalted mustard

Steam potato cubes in steamer basket until just barely tender— about 15 minutes—then sprinkle with Webb Dressing and place in covered refrigerator jar. Marinate overnight, stirring twice (or inverting jar to mix marinade twice). Next day, add remaining ingredients and mix well. Leave in refrigerator several hours for flavors to blend.

Of all the foods we modified for a salt-free diet, bread was the easiest and potato salad and cold cuts were the most difficult. The first potato salads we made were consistently unpalatable. Summon your courage and try this one. Part of its flavor actually comes from the noble potato itself, scrubbed but not peeled, and cooked in a way that retains its natural flavor contribution.

Calories per serving: 273

Fat per serving: 11.2 g

Calories from fat: 37%

Potassium per serving: 904 mg

Sodium per serving: 65.9 mg

K Factor: 12

Rye Bread (MAKES TWO LOAVES, TWENTY SLICES EACH)

2 *packages active dry yeast*
2 *teaspoons grated orange peel*
2 *teaspoons caraway seeds*
4 *tablespoons brown sugar*
2 *cups all-purpose flour*
2 *tablespoons butter-flavored soy oil*
2⅔ *cups hot water*
6 *cups rye flour (approximately)*

Mix together yeast, orange peel, caraway seeds, brown sugar, and all-purpose flour. Mix oil and hot water together, then add to dry ingredients and beat well with a wire whisk.

With a wooden spoon, beat in rye flour until dough becomes too stiff to beat. Turn out onto a floured board or cloth and knead well, adding rye flour, until dough is no longer sticky but plump and elastic (like a baby's bottom). Place in an oiled bowl, turn once to oil top of dough, cover loosely with plastic wrap, and let rise about an hour or until doubled in volume. Punch down, form into two loaves, place in greased pans, and cover loosely with plastic wrap.

Let dough rise again about ½ hour or until doubled.

Preheat oven to 400°F. Bake for 30 minutes.

Calories per slice: 98.3

Fat per slice: 1.1 g

Calories from fat: 9.8%

Potassium per slice: 16.2 mg

Sodium per slice: 0.9 mg

K Factor: 18

Sham Tonkatsu Sauce (SERVES SIX)

   $\frac{1}{2}$ *cup very hot water*
   2 tablespoons apricot jam
   1 tablespoon tomato paste
   1 teaspoon Worcestershire sauce

Mix all ingredients well. Refrigerate, and use on oriental-style dishes, especially to dress celery cabbage as a salad. Until some-one invents a really low sodium soy sauce, we offer this to assuage your craving for oriental foods. It is somewhat reminiscent of the famous Japanese sauce used on pork cutlets, but makes no claim to be an imitation.

   Calories per serving: 26

   Fat per serving: 0.02 g

   Calories from fat: 0.9%

   Potassium per serving: 44 mg

   Sodium per serving: 70 mg

   K Factor: 4

Sole with Mushrooms (SERVES SIX)

   4 tablespoons chopped scallions
   $\frac{1}{2}$ *cup sliced mushrooms*
   1 tablespoon butter-flavored oil
   $\frac{1}{2}$ *cup water*
   $\frac{1}{4}$ *cup lemon juice (white wine may be substituted for the water and lemon juice)*
   1 pound fillets of sole
   1 tablespoon cornstarch
   $\frac{1}{2}$ *cup water*
   $\frac{1}{2}$–*1 teaspoon tarragon*
   Black or white pepper to taste

Sauté scallions and mushrooms in oil very gently over medium heat. In this dish, all the flavors should be kept delicate, so the heat should never be too high. Add water and lemon juice or wine; adjust heat so that the broth is just simmering. Place fish gently on vegetables and simmer at low heat for a few minutes— just until fish is white and opaque. Transfer fish and vegetables to a platter and keep warm.

Make a paste of the cornstarch and a little water, then add water to make ½ cup. Add to the broth and cook, stirring, until it boils and thickens. Remove from heat and add tarragon; add pepper to taste. Pour sauce over fish and serve. Bon appetit!

Calories per serving: 93

Fat per serving: 3 g

Calories from fat: 28%

Potassium per serving: 308 mg

Sodium per serving: 61 mg

K Factor: 5

Tabouleh Salad (Serves eight)

First Mixture:
½ cup boiling water
½ cup bulgur (cracked wheat)
4 tablespoons chopped onion
2 tablespoons chopped parsley
1 tablespoon chopped mint
1 tablespoon lemon juice
1½ tablespoons safflower oil

Second Mixture:
1 pound tomatoes, chopped
½ cup chopped scallions
½ cup diced cucumber
½ cup diced celery
¼ cup diced green pepper
Dash of basil and oregano
2 tablespoons wine vinegar
2 tablespoons safflower oil
Greens

Pour boiling water over the bulgur. When cool, add chopped onion, parsley, mint, lemon juice, and 1½ tablespoons oil. Chill first mixture.

In a second bowl, mix tomatoes, scallions, cucumber, celery, green pepper, basil, oregano, wine vinegar, and 2 tablespoons oil.

Chill both mixtures for several hours. Toss together to serve.

Calories per serving: 135

Fat per serving: 33 g

Calories from fat: 41%

Potassium per serving: 264 mg

Sodium per serving: 21.8 mg

K Factor: 12

Tahini Sauce (SERVES SIX)

½ cup tahini (sesame paste)
Garlic to taste
¼ cup lemon juice
Water as necessary

Mix tahini, garlic, and lemon juice. Add water by the tablespoon while beating, until sauce is thick but still pourable.

Calories per serving: 95.6

Fat per serving: 8.2 g

Calories from fat: 77% (go light on this)

Potassium per serving: 132.5 mg

Sodium per serving: 10 mg

K Factor: 13

Turkey–Water Chestnut Casserole (SERVES EIGHT)

4 cups cooked turkey, cut into bite-size chunks
1 clove garlic, diced
1 medium onion, grated

    2 tablespoons butter-flavored oil
    Dash of cayenne pepper
    ¼ teaspoon freshly grated black pepper
    1 pound fresh mushrooms, sliced
    1 cup salt-free bouillon or meat juices with the chilled fat
      layer removed
    ⅛ teaspoon nutmeg
    1 8-ounce can water chestnuts, sliced and drained
    2 cups yogurt
    1 tablespoon chopped parsley

Brown turkey chunks, garlic, onion, and mushrooms in oil. Add pepper, nutmeg, water chestnuts, and bouillon. Use some of the bouillon to deglaze frying pan, then place cooked ingredients in an oven-proof dish, cover, and bake for 1 hour at 350°F.

Add yogurt and chopped parsley, cover, and return to oven for about 15 minutes.

Serve with brown rice.

Calories per serving: 233

Fat per serving: 8.7

Calories from fat: 34%

Potassium per serving: 822 mg

Sodium per serving: 120 mg

K Factor: 6.8

Webb Dressing (SERVES SIXTEEN)

    ½ cup wine vinegar
    ¼ cup water
    ½ teaspoon paprika
    1 teaspoon dry mustard
    2 teaspoons bitters
    ¼ teaspoon marjoram
    1 teaspoon grated lemon rind
    1 teaspoon sugar
    1 cup safflower oil

Mix all ingredients except oil in a jar and shake well. Add oil and shake again. Refrigerate. Use on tossed salads, and see our recipe for potato salad.

Calories per serving: 121

Fat per serving: 15 g

Calories from fat: 100% (go lightly when using)

Potassium per serving: 7.06 mg

Sodium per serving: 0.07 mg

K Factor: 101

Zero Cocktail (Serves one)

1 slice lemon (cross section)
2 dashes bitters
1 glass sodium-free seltzer water

Place a thick slice of lemon in a glass. Add three dashes of bitters. Then pour on the fizz water and sit back and enjoy.

Essentially zero calories

Zero fat

Zero sodium

Zero alcohol

Zero guilt, nirvana before dinner

Zucchini Relish

10 cups shredded zucchini (about 5 medium)
4 cups minced onion (about 4 large)
5 tablespoons potassium chloride (salt substitute)
2¼ cups vinegar
5 cups sugar
1 tablespoon dry mustard
1 teaspoon celery seeds
1 tablespoon turmeric

1 tablespoon cornstarch
1 tablespoon nutmeg

Mix zucchini, onion, and potassium chloride. Let stand over-night.

Drain and rinse twice. Add all other ingredients, heat, and cook until clear, stirring—about 30 minutes.

Place in hot sterile jars, seal, and process in boiling water bath for 15 minutes, following the directions given in the Dill Pickle recipe.

Calories per serving: 16

Fat per serving: 0

Calories from fat: 0%

Potassium per serving: 15 mg

Sodium per serving: 0.005 mg

K Factor: 3,000

CHAPTER 11

Step Three: Exercise

The finding that exercise lowers blood pressure significantly in a group of sedentary hypertensive patients suggests that "essential" (or primary) hypertension is a result primarily of life-style and can be prevented or treated effectively by reasonable physical activity.
—Robert Cade, M.D., et al., 1984[1]

The theme of this book is that high blood pressure is due to an imbalance of life-style, particularly nutrition and exercise. Therefore, the proper prevention and reversal of high blood pressure is to be found in life-style, not only in the *K Factor* approach to nutrition but, as Dr. Cade says, in "reasonable physical activity."

In this chapter, we discuss additional benefits of exercise, from helping you keep your weight down to maintaining a proper hormone balance in your body to enhancing your mood, and we answer the typical arguments against exercise. Then we provide some principles and guidelines for a comprehensive aerobic exercise program that you and your physician can tailor to your own personal situation.

Benefits of Regular Exercise

Regular aerobic exercise has many benefits, including that it:

○ Returns blood pressure toward "normal."
○ Decreases body fat.
○ Restores hormone balance.
○ Decreases blood lipids (fats), which cause heart attacks.
○ Increases blood levels of the "good" cholesterol (high density lipoprotein cholesterol, or HDL-C).
○ Increases stability of electrical activity of the heart.
○ Increases resistance to fatigue.
○ Decreases craving for smoking.
○ Adds life to your years.
○ Probably adds years to your life.

Return of Blood Pressure toward "Normal"

It is probably no surprise to you that exercise helps you lose weight (and thereby helps bring down your blood pressure). But several scientific studies (discussed in Chapter 7) have shown that regular exercise programs are effective in lowering blood pressure even if you're not overweight and even if you don't lose excess weight. We discussed the study of Dr. Cade and his co-workers, which demonstrated that aerobic exercise can be a remarkably effective way to enable your body to better regulate its blood pressure and can even produce a fall in blood pressure in patients with severe hypertension.

Several studies have shown that keeping fit by regular exercise also helps *prevent* the development of high blood pressure.[2] A study of six thousand women and men showed that people whose blood pressure was in the "high normal" range (130–139/85–89) and who had a low level of physical fitness were *ten* times more likely to develop hypertension than those with blood pressure in the normal range (120–129/81–84) and who were physically fit. Even when the blood pressure was less than 120/80, lack of physical fitness resulted in a 50 percent increased probability of getting hypertension.[3]

Decrease of Body Fat

As we discuss in the next chapter, losing excess weight may be essential for reducing your blood pressure. And exercise (at least three times a week) plays a very important—in many people a necessary—role in maintaining normal weight. In fact, any effective weight (and blood pressure) reduction program requires at least some aerobic exercise, especially in the long run (pun intended).

Restoration of Hormone Balance

Exercise makes muscles more responsive to insulin and decreases the blood level of this hormone,[4] allowing your kidneys to excrete more sodium and calming your sympathetic nervous system. And the effect of both lowers your blood pressure (remember Chapter 7). Lower levels of insulin also decrease any tendency of your body to convert calories to fat, and some studies suggest that lower insulin levels suppress feelings of hunger. The resulting weight loss also lowers your blood pressure.

Decrease of Blood Lipids

Blood cholesterol occurs primarily in two forms: low-density lipoprotein cholesterol (LDL-C), and high-density lipoprotein cholesterol (HDL-C).

It is the LDL, which contains a large amount of cholesterol and other fat, that is "bad," because it contributes to the formation of fat deposits in your arteries. Another type, very low density lipoprotein (VLDL), is also bad. VLDL contains more fat (mostly triglycerides) than protein and explains why high levels of blood triglycerides should be avoided.

Exercise can lower the level of blood triglycerides, VLDL cholesterol, and low-density lipoproteins (LDL cholesterol).[5]

Increasing Blood Levels of the "Good" Cholesterol (High Density Lipoprotein Cholesterol or HDL-C)

On the other hand, HDL (specifically HDL-2) carries the bad

cholesterol to your liver, where it can be converted into bile and excreted.

Several studies have shown that exercise can raise the amount of HDL in your blood while lowering the level of LDL. The ratio of total cholesterol to HDL should be less than 5.0 for men and less than 4.5 for women. There is some dispute as to what the total cholesterol level should be. Although it is generally considered normal if below 220 or 240 milligrams per 100 milliliters of blood (220 or 240 mg/dl), there is good reason to be more conservative and say that the total blood cholesterol should be no more than 200 milligrams per 100 milliliters of blood. In fact, life insurance statistics show that your chances of death rise once your total cholesterol count rises above 170 milligrams per 100 milliliters. On the other hand, in the 35 years of the scientific study of the people living in Framingham, Massachusetts, there evidently has not been even *one* death due to heart attack in a person whose blood cholesterol is below 150 milligrams per 100 milliliters.

Increased Stability of Electrical Activity of the Heart

Of course, the all-important muscle that can benefit from exercise is your heart. Evidence suggests that regular exercise increases your chances of surviving a heart attack. This may be because the electrical activity of your heart muscle is more stable if you exercise regularly.

In a study of animal death from sudden cardiac arrest, the chance of fibrillation (abnormal electrical activity) of the ventricles (the large chambers of the heart) was decreased in those animals that had experienced exercise training.[6]

Increased Resistance to Fatigue

Regular aerobic exercise increases the number of mitochondria, or "powerhouses of the cell" (tiny membrane "sacks" within the cell that contain special proteins that combine oxygen with food products to provide energy to the cell), which allows your body to increase the percent of energy you can get aerobically (*aerobic* means "using oxygen"). Therefore, your body needs to place *less* reliance on the less efficient anaerobic (without oxygen) metabolism and so is more resistant to fatigue.

Initially, as you get in shape, you may well need a bit more sleep than usual. But joggers who regularly cover at least 20 miles (or expend about 2,000 calories) a week frequently report that they require less sleep than before they took up regular exercise. In fact, you may find that once you've made it a habit, regular exercise may not decrease the number of hours you have for other activities. Regular aerobic exercise also increases your stamina for everyday work.

Decreased Smoking

A frequent observation is that many people who take up regular aerobic exercise either decrease the amount they smoke or stop altogether.

Adding Life to Your Years

People who exercise regularly also know that it makes them feel better and even changes their mood. Exercise stimulates the brain's production of opiatelike substances called beta-endorphins, which some think explain why exercise is often beneficial for mild depression. "Runner's high" describes a common experience in which euphoria or elation is felt during or immediately after a good aerobic workout.

The Bottom Line: Adding Years to Your Life

Although the medical profession is still debating this, the life insurance companies are already betting their money that exercise will make you live longer. Allstate Life Insurance Company is giving up to a 35 percent discount for those who exercise regularly. Most of the companies giving discounts on premiums for life insurance require a minimum of 30 minutes of aerobic exercise (such as running) at least three times each week.

Recently there has been controversy about the safety of exercise, and about whether or not exercise can extend your years. We think the discussion that follows will help you realize that with proper precautions, exercise can be safe and that it almost certainly can extend your life span.

The Controversy about Exercise

Exercise, especially jogging, has become almost a national obsession. The popular opinion is that exercise makes us more healthy, and many joggers believe it will make them live longer.

Is Aerobic Exercise Safe, or Is It Dangerous?

For several years, the view had even circulated that enough exercise could "immunize" you against a heart attack. It was claimed that no one who finished a marathon had ever died of a heart attack. But then it was found that marathoners like U.S. Congressman Goodloe Byron, age forty-nine, who had run six Boston marathons; New Zealander Dennis Stephenson, who held records for 100-mile runs; and forty-eight-year-old Frenchman Jacques Bussereau, who died of a heart attack during the 1984 New York City marathon, had died from their cholesterol-filled coronary arteries. And then in 1984 Jim Fixx, the well-known author of *The Complete Book of Running* and a finisher in twenty marathons, collapsed and died of a heart attack at the end of a jog on a Vermont road.

What About Jim Fixx?

When one of the main running gurus, a man who regularly put in about sixty miles per week, dropped dead at the end of a four-mile jog, the antiexercise group sallied forth, claiming that exercise not only doesn't make you live longer but it can kill you. So many uncertainties were triggered by Jim Fixx's death that some thought the exercise boom would begin to die. Certainly Fixx died while, or immediately after, exercising. But did exercise kill him? Or was it something else?

The autopsy of Jim Fixx revealed that of the three coronary arteries in his heart, one was almost completely plugged by fat deposits, one was 70 percent closed, and the other 80 percent closed. Not only that, but scar tissue was present on three regions of his heart, each a record of a previous myocardial infarction, or heart attack. One of these heart attacks had occurred about two weeks and another about four weeks before he died.[7]

These heart attacks had not felled him but probably had been associated with classic symptoms that were, unfortunately, not recognized. For example, during that last month, Jim Fixx had mentioned to his friends that at times he felt a tightness in his throat when he was at rest. In Kenneth Cooper's newsletter *Aerobics*, Jim's son, John, is quoted as saying, "It turns out that when he was running all that summer he would have to stop because of the tightness in his chest about five minutes into a run. He would walk a little and then he would be fine and go on and do his miles."

It's not unusual for people with coronary artery disease to experience chest or throat tightness or pain about six minutes after starting to run, only to have it get better if they continue for a while at a slower pace. This happens because it takes about six to ten minutes for the body to get "warmed up," and for blood vessels in the muscles to open, decreasing blood pressure and thus decreasing the load on the heart.

The two heart attacks before the fatal one were probably associated with symptoms. On one occasion, Fixx complained of pain in his jaw. The other nonfatal attack probably occurred when he was running with his son John, just two weeks before he died. Very early in the run, Jim remarked that he had to go to the bathroom. The two then walked to a nearby airplane hangar, where they stopped to talk with someone for about ten minutes before resuming their run. When the son questioned Jim's remark about going to the bathroom, Jim said he was all right now and did not have to go. It's possible that he was having a mild heart attack and the brief rest, plus the "warm up" effect, decreased the load on his heart enough to diminish any symptoms.

Not only had he had at least three previous heart attacks, not only were his coronary arteries almost completely plugged, but the autopsy showed that Jim Fixx had an enlarged heart—probably since birth. This type of enlarged heart, known as biventricular hypertrophy, is fairly rare and has been associated with sudden death in athletes, usually at a much younger age. Running didn't kill Jim Fixx, but heart disease and probably a congenital heart condition did.

But could this sudden death have been prevented? Or does

this mean that you shouldn't exercise because you might have heart disease? Let's take a look at the coronary artery disease and the three heart attacks that resulted. Jim Fixx had had several "risk factors" for heart attack. He had a family history of heart trouble (his father died at the age of forty-three of a second heart attack), and before Jim took up running at the age of thirty-six, he had smoked, worked in a high-stress environment, eaten a high-fat diet, been obese, and lived a sedentary life. In addition to these risk factors, Jim's blood cholesterol had been found to be elevated; it was 253 milligrams per 100 milliliters in 1980 and was 254 at autopsy. Although his ratio of total cholesterol to HDL was in the normal range—2.91 in 1980 and 3.48 at autopsy—his total cholesterol level was abnormally high.[8]

So before Jim Fixx died, there were plenty of indications that there might be something seriously wrong with his heart. These included:

- Recent unexplained fatigue.
- Recent chest pains while running.
- Family history of heart disease.
- Previous high-fat diet.
- History of overweight.
- Former high-stress life-style.
- History of smoking.
- Elevated blood cholesterol.

Putting Exercise-associated Death in Perspective

The examples of Jim Fixx, Goodloe Byron, Dennis Stephenson, Jacques Bussereau and others clearly show that exercise doesn't immunize you against heart attacks. Dr. L. E. Lamb, of the U.S. Air Force School of Aerospace Medicine, has emphasized that most American men over age forty have "silent" coronary artery disease—a condition that does not produce symptoms, may not show up in a stress test (treadmill electrocardiogram, or EKG), and may not even prevent completion of a marathon. Nonetheless, according to Lamb, a fatty cholesterol deposit in the coronary arteries of these men may eventually trigger a blood clot that clogs an artery, causing a heart attack, especially during or just after exercise. Dr. Lamb does not claim that exercise actually causes a heart attack; just that it can trigger one.

FREQUENCY OF SUDDEN DEATH DURING EXERCISE. In a six-year study of joggers in Rhode Island, only one death during jogging occurred per year for every 7,620 joggers.[9] Similarly, in King County, Washington, with a population of 1.25 million, only 9 cardiac arrests occurred during vigorous exercise during one fourteen-month period.[10] To put things in perspective, another Rhode Island study found that of 81 people who died during recreational exercise, the largest number of deaths (23% of the total) occurred during golf! Jogging was second (20%), and swimming third (11%).[11] In almost 90 percent of these deaths, the underlying cause was hardening of the arteries, or atherosclerosis, and 93 percent of those who died either had a medical history of heart disease or had recognized risk factors. Another way to keep this in perspective is to realize that of *all* sudden deaths that occur, very few occur during exercise. In a study of 2,606 sudden deaths studied in Finland, only 22 were associated with exercise.[12]

The statistical evidence suggests that among people, most of whom did not have a stress test, the chance of sudden death occurring *during* exercise is about seven times that of it occurring during sedentary activity. If you exercise 2 hours per week, you do accept a slightly higher incidence of sudden death during those 2 hours. But as we'll discuss, during the other 166 hours, you may be decreasing your chance of death. In any case, the overall chance is only about one jogger out of every 7,620 during a whole year.

Not only that, but with today's medical knowledge, it's possible to improve the odds a good deal more. As an example of the value of proper medical evaluation, at Dr. Kenneth Cooper's Aerobics Center in Dallas, over five thousand participants have been followed who have collectively run more than six million miles (an average of over 1,000 miles per person), with only two cardiac-related events and *no* fatalities. These people had all been screened with an exercise-tolerance stress test as well as complete physical and history.[13]

Can anything be done to identify whether exercise is dangerous for you? If anything, the running death of Jim Fixx demonstrates that sudden death during exercise rarely if ever happens unless there is underlying disease, usually heart disease. And usually there are previous symptoms and/or risk factors that can provide warning signals that heart disease is present. As cardiologist-runner George Sheehan says, "Nobody with a normal heart is going to drop over" while exercising.[14]

Most important, an adequate medical examination by your physician can catch many of these cardiac problems in time, especially if a proper stress test is done. Even as far back as 1973, a physical exam of Jim Fixx had picked up some signs of problems with his heart. That exam revealed abnormalities in his resting EKG (heart tracing) as well as an enlarged heart on X ray and a heart murmur. Today we have not only better techniques, such as echo cardiography, lithium angiography, and advanced types of EKG stress tests, but we also have more knowledge and more insight with which to detect and evaluate the existence of heart disease. Had physicians known then what is known today, or had Jim Fixx recently been tested with a modern treadmill stress test, the likelihood is high that his underlying heart disease would have been revealed before it was too late.

Shortly we will discuss the main things you and your doctor should check to decrease the odds of sudden death during exercise. Along with Nathan Pritikin,[15] Dr. L. E. Lamb[16] has pointed to several studies showing that major diet changes can reverse the effects of coronary artery disease. Lamb and Pritikin believe that exercise, if accompanied by a diet low in fat and cholesterol, actually helps prevent heart disease.

On the other hand, because of the high fat content typical of the Western diet that most of us have been eating, there is some risk of having a heart attack while exercising especially if you haven't had a medical workup before you start. But you can exercise without worry if you meet the following conditions:

- Your blood cholesterol is "normal" (see Chapter 9).
- Your doctor evaluates you for certain other risk factors (see Chapter 9 and page 196).

○ You can pass a properly conducted treadmill stress test (see Chapter 9), even if you're over 40, you have risk factors, or your diastolic pressure is above 95 mm Hg.
○ You have been eating a low-fat diet (see Chapters 10 and 12)
○ You follow our recommendations in the section Aerobic Exercise Guidelines on page 204.
○ You have a complete medical evaluation, and you start the exercise program *slowly*, as we describe.

Keep in mind that because high blood pressure is a major risk factor for heart attack and because some drugs interfere with exercise, the last item on the foregoing list is *especially* important.

Does Exercise Lengthen Your Life?
But how about the other 166 hours in your week? Does exercise influence your chance of death during the hours you are *not* exercising?

Although the interpretation is disputed, in 1978, the first study of 16,936 graduates of Harvard University—the Paffenbarger Study[17]—appeared and indicated that regular aerobic exercise equivalent to jogging at least 20 miles (about 2,000 calories) every week may significantly lower the risk of heart attacks.

THE ANTIEXERCISE ARGUMENTS. But in his book, *The Exercise Myth*, Dr. Henry Solomon, a New York cardiologist, disputes practically every claim ever made for exercise promoting longevity. He admits that exercise may make people feel better or make them stronger. But, scrutinizing the defects in the studies claiming that exercise prolongs life, he questions if exercise really does make people more healthy or live longer.

In the last analysis, however, Dr. Solomon seems to base his negative conclusions solely upon the claim that no large-scale controlled study has demonstrated conclusively that exercise increases life span, decreases the chance of heart attacks (he disputes the interpretations of the 1978 Paffenbarger Study), or otherwise improves those measures of health that show up in statistics. Large controlled studies with statistical analysis can, of course, be an important aid in deciding whether a given procedure works. But as we discuss in Chapter 19, they're not the only evidence that must be considered.

Studies sufficiently rigorous to satisfy Dr. Solomon are not only difficult to do, they can take as long as twenty years to complete. Worse, the interpretation of such clinical studies can be misleading if not supported by other lines of evidence (see Part V). In the meantime, we need to form judgments based upon currently available evidence. Let's look at some of that evidence.

THE PROEXERCISE ARGUMENTS. After Solomon's *The Exercise Myth,* Dr. Paffenbarger published an updated report of his study of those 16,936 Harvard alumni.[18] This recent report shows that men who expended over 2,000 kilocalories (kcals) per week on physical activity had about *half* the death rate from heart disease as did men who were sedentary (expending less than 500 calories per week), even though both groups of men were living similar life-styles in other respects. Expending 2,000 calories per week on exercise is roughly equivalent to jogging 20 miles per week.

Incidentally, this same report shows that having hypertension puts a man (the alumni were men) at greater risk for having a heart attack than does a sedentary life-style, cigarette smoking, being overweight, or having a family history of coronary artery disease.

This recent Paffenbarger report contained another unexpected—but pleasant—finding. The death rate *due to cancer* of those men expending more than 500 calories per week on physical activity was 25 percent lower than the cancer death rate of men expending less than 500 calories each week. This means that men who jogged even 5 miles each week apparently had less chance of dying of cancer. While this is not "proof" (see Chapter 19 if you confuse *proof* with *statistics*), it certainly is a promising clue.

There is other evidence that supports the view that regular aerobic exercise can help extend life. In a study published in late 1984, Dr. David Siscovick and co-workers compared the exercise history of 133 men who had cardiac arrest without prior known heart disease to a random sample of healthy men of the same age, marital status, and similar life-style. The overall risk of heart attack—during vigorous exercise as well as the rest of the time—was 60 percent lower in the men who exercised regularly than in those who didn't.[19]

Summary of the Controversy

Although one can argue the validity of the purely *statistical* evidence that exercise extends life (see Chapter 19 if you think statistics are the answer to everything), it is clear that exercise has several desirable effects, each of which reduces your chance of death. Exercise helps:

○ Decrease body fat.
○ Reduce blood pressure.
○ Reduce the "bad" (LDL) blood lipids.
○ Increase the "good" (HDL) blood lipids.
○ Stabilize electrical activity of the heart.
○ Normalize hormones that affect the body's ability to balance sodium and potassium.

So if you look at the whole picture, it's a pretty safe bet that with the proper precautions, exercise is on your side. As Dr. David Siscovick and his co-workers conclude, "Even though intense physical activity may be one of the factors that can precipitate primary cardiac arrest, habitual participation in such activity is associated with an overall reduction in the risk of primary cardiac arrest."

Dangers of Exercise

Sudden Death

We have just discussed the danger of sudden death while exercising. The chance of sudden death occurring is quite small—almost 1 in 7,600—but it is there. The problem for older people is that coronary artery disease can precipitate a heart attack.

Because of this, we believe that everyone over thirty should obtain a serum cholesterol level before embarking on an exercise program. If the serum cholesterol is above 200, a properly conducted exercise stress test EKG should also be done. With this information, your doctor can advise you as to your risk of having a heart attack and any special precautions you should take.

Injuries

Of course, exercise can cause such minor problems as "runner's heel" (achilles tendonitis), strained muscles, and sore feet. But as we mention in the next section, there are ways you can prevent these.

How about joints? Won't running for years wear your joints out? Some people, apparently considering bones and joints as just another machine, have maintained this, but the evidence doesn't bear it out—provided you don't have arthritis or other joint disease, are not greatly overweight, and take proper precautions. The body is not a machine. True, over a very short period (seconds or minutes), the body *acts* like a machine: after all, we can break a bone or wreck a knee. That "mechanistic" view is part of an old scientific paradigm (see Chapter 19) that is outdated. But in the new paradigm, we realize that over time—periods of days or weeks—the body is a dynamic self-renewing living organism with remarkable potential for self-repair. Recent basic research has shown that to an extent far greater than we previously thought, your body can actually rebuild itself (see Chapter 19).

The Tarahumara Indians in northern Mexico virtually make running a way of life. For fun, they play kickball games that go as far as 200 miles, and have been known to run 500 miles in five days *and* they run well into their sixties and seventies. No joints made of a nonrenewing substance could hold up to a lifetime of that sort of activity. And it's not just this group, or anything special about their inheritance. Early American Indians used running as a means of communication, and it was part of their ritual of relating to nature. In the last century, one Hopi Indian was asked by the local Indian agent to deliver a message 78 miles away. He set out at three in the morning, reached his destination at about noon, where he rested a half-hour and got rubbed down, and varying his gait, ran back home, covering the round trip of 156 miles in less than twenty-four hours. He was almost a hundred years old when he died.[20] Regular exercise helps strengthen your bones as well as your muscles. Thus, regular exercise can help prevent osteoporosis (weakening of the bones), which is especially frequent in older women.[21] Conversely, if you have been sedentary, your bones may be weak, and this emphasizes, once again, our recommendation that sedentary people begin their exercise program *gradually*, preferably with walking. Otherwise you're more likely to develop "stress" fractures or joint damage. But, since the body is a self-renewing organism, if you don't *over*stress it, and if you give it a chance to respond, moderate exercise will stimulate your body to renew itself, strengthening your bones, muscles, and, some evidence suggests, even the ligaments that stabilize your joints.

One of the authors (Dick) has a trick knee that was uncomfortable and would occasionally "lock." When he began jogging, he really had to take it easy and slow down every time the knee bothered him. Now, after several months of jogging four to six times a week, he tends to forget that the knee ever bothered him. The other author (George) used to get "tennis elbow" until he started doing pushups every day. Now it never bothers him.

The head of the ski patrol at Sugarbush, in Vermont, had badly damaged his knee with several severe sprains during bike racing, basketball, and tennis. The damage was so bad that he experienced pain walking and his knee would dislocate and buckle under him even when playing tennis. Then he began gradually to jog, slowly increasing his workouts. Today, he skis and runs footraces of over five miles without any pain in his knees.

Don't jump to the conclusion that we're saying exercise is good for all bone, ligament, and joint ailments. Some orthopedic conditions could be made worse by exercise, especially if it's too strenuous or the changes are too sudden. Remember, with *sudden* stress, the bones do act like a machine— and break. There's still a lot we don't understand about how the body maintains itself, but provided you take proper precautions, the evidence is that running not only won't hurt your joints, it may even be good for them.

Aerobic Exercise Guidelines

The key to increased physical endurance—and an aid to loss of weight and to achieving normal blood pressure—is aerobic exercise. Aerobic exercise refers to repetitive movements involving the large muscles of the legs or arms. These movements require more oxygen (hence, aerobics) and thus make us breathe more heavily.

Because only 1/5th of all the energy released actually moves your muscles, the remaining 4/5ths appears as heat, causing you to get warm and sweat a lot. In aerobic exercise, motion is the name of the game, but not motion so strenuous that it prevents you from doing it continuously for a period of many minutes.

In contrast to aerobic exercise, power weight lifting (pumping iron) or progressive resistance exercise may require comparatively little continuous motion of the large muscle groups and so may use relatively few calories. It therefore may not increase your breathing or heart rate very much. In addition, during power weight lifting, the blood pressure may rise to extreme levels. In five young body builders, even a one-arm curl raised the blood pressure to an average of about 255/190 mm Hg, and during maximum exercises, such as the double-leg press, the pressure rose to an average of 320/250 mm Hg![22] Even in those who aren't body builders, lifting as little as 50 percent of their maximum weight can raise blood pressure from normal resting values to about 170/108 mm Hg.[23] If you recall chapters 5 and 6, there is pretty good reason to believe that the blood vessels in people with hypertension are weakened. Therefore, since power weight lifting is not aerobic and since at present there isn't sufficient information about its dangers in people with hypertension, it would seem the wiser course for people with hypertension to restrain from this activity until further information becomes available.

However, if you do repetitive resistance exercises involving high numbers of repetitions with small weights with little rest in between, you can raise your heart rate sufficiently and for a long enough time to obtain the benefits of aerobic exercise.[24] Also, as we will mention under *preventing injuries,* for some sports, such as jogging or running, you may need to work with very small weights in order to maintain balance between opposing groups of muscles.

Outdoor forms of aerobic exercise include bicycling, jogging, running, cross-country skiing, swimming, rowing, active skating, singles tennis, and fast walking. The exercise that burns the most calories per hour is cross-country skiing, followed by rowing, and then by running.[25] Indoor aerobic exercises include aerobic dancing, riding a stationary bicycle, using a rowing machine, a cross country ski simulator, or an exercise treadmill. Tennis or racquetball may qualify if performed vigorously enough over a sufficient period of time. Jumping rope is another option.

There is now evidence[26] that aerobic dance can cause as large an increase in the capacity for aerobic exercise and endurance as jogging. A note of caution: Be sure to wear proper shoes and to exercise on a resilient surface rather than on something hard like concrete. Also remember that in any exercise, you should progress slowly under the supervision of a well-trained instructor who will be sure not to place you in a class with "young turks" ahead of your fitness level. (The "young turks" could be young ladies.) Dick got into a women's advanced aerobics class ("Sure, I'm in shape," he told the instructor) and had all he could do to keep up. You can do aerobic dancing at home, either to your own music or to videotapes. Videotapes can be a good motivator, providing discipline and some instruction. But since they can't be tailored to your particular degree of fitness, be careful not to let yourself be overworked by them, especially if you're just starting. Also be certain to avoid those videotapes that have a lot of stretches that involve bobbing. *Slow,* constant stretching is not only much more effective for flexibility but much safer.

For those who are significantly overweight (20 pounds) or

who have orthopedic problems, you should start by riding a bike, swimming, or walking leisurely followed by faster walking. These are good ways to get aerobic exercise without overstraining joints and ligaments.

If you are interested in starting to jog, take a look at any of several good introductory books for advice on how to prevent injuries. Especially good are *The Complete Book of Running*, by James Fixx (Random House, 1977) (don't do what he did—skip an exercise EKG; do what he said—and take one), and *Dr. Sheehan on Running* (Mountain View, California: World Publications, 1975).

Here are seven basic points to keep in mind as you begin your exercise program:

1. Begin with a proper medical examination.
2. Start your program slowly.
3. Never overexert yourself.
4. Listen to your body.
5. Exercise frequently.
6. Warm up and cool down.
7. Take steps to prevent injuries.

Begin with a Proper Medical Examination

The very first thing is to check with your doctor, who will want to do a physical examination as well as take some blood tests, including a blood cholesterol. This is Step One of our program. (See Chapter 9 for details.)

SEE YOUR DOCTOR!
This step is extremely important!

Start Slowly

As with most things dealing with your health and body, it's important not to make sudden changes. Begin your exercise program only after you have had a medical evaluation, and begin it slowly.

To emphasize the importance of increasing the intensity of exercise gradually, consider the following: In a study of 2,606 sudden deaths, Vuori and co-workers found that the chance of death being triggered by strenuous physical exercise was highest if the exercise had been intensified without a gradual increase in training.[27] If you have high blood pressure, the importance of *gradually* increasing the level of training is even greater. So don't start off by taking an all-out fitness test. Begin gradually.

Especially if you have a diastolic blood pressure of 100 mm Hg or above, or are taking antihypertensive drugs, begin very slowly, walking at a pace that allows you to carry on a conversation at the same time. If you can carry on a conversation, that means your metabolism is still "aerobic"; that is, your body is getting enough oxygen to use more fat and less carbohydrate for energy.

Your doctor may need to consider the drugs you're on before you begin your exercise program. For example, if you are on a beta blocker, this drug will prevent your heart rate from rising as much as normal and so would be expected to limit your exercise capacity. This is borne out in the studies done so far that conclude that taking a beta blocker for hypertension will probably decrease your ability to exercise easily, especially if it's endurance exercise lasting more than 30 minutes.[28] It is essential to discuss this with your doctor: he or she may want to replace your present drug with one that has less effect on your exercise capacity. If you do exercise while taking a beta blocker, keep in mind that it may make you tire more easily, so be very careful to not overdo it and keep the sessions under 30 minutes, but at least five times per week. Finally, a slow warm-up may help reduce the effect of the beta blocker and a longer, slower cooldown will prevent you from feeling lightheaded, a symptom often experienced by exercisers on beta blockers.

In summary, although more research is being done, we would recommend that you be *very* careful not to overexert if you are on a beta blocker. If you stick to the *K Factor* program, your physician may be able to take you off these drugs eventually. But *never* stop any drugs, except under your physician's supervision: suddenly stopping some drugs can cause rebound hypertension and can be lethal.

If you have an elevated blood cholesterol level, we believe you should be in a supervised program and should have an exercise stress test before you start the program. However, so that you can reach your maximum heart rate during the test (which we consider important in order to perform the stress test properly), some exercise physiologists point out that it may be necessary for you to do a few weeks of very gentle exercise first. This is important not only to improve muscle tone but to get you used to detecting the symptoms of normal fatigue.

The exercise stress test has been underrated in our opinion, and it is not a bad idea for *anyone* who is out of shape to take one before beginning an exercise program. We especially recommend this for those with hypertension, certainly if the diastolic pressure is 95 mm Hg or above and if coronary risk factors are present.

Dr. Lamb recommends that until the blood cholesterol has been down to normal levels for at least three months, the only unsupervised exercise that you should do is walking at a conversational pace and light calisthenics.

If you haven't been exercising regularly or are overweight, start out by taking walks—even if your diastolic pressure is less than 100 mm Hg. This will help strengthen your bones and muscles before you start fast walking or jogging. Your muscles, joints, ligaments, and cardiovascular system need time to toughen up a bit before you take on anything more vigorous. This is especially important if you're overweight. It's surprising how a few extra pounds put extra strain on your joints and can increase the chance of injuries to the knees or ankles.

The American College of Sports Medicine points out that beginning joggers tended to have "increased foot, leg, and knee injuries when training was performed more than 3 days per week and longer than 30 minutes duration per exercise session."[29] Also, keep in mind that elderly people apparently need longer to get the benefits of training.[30]

Dr. Rachel Yeater of West Virginia University recommends walking at a leisurely pace for 10 minutes each day if you are out of shape. Increase your daily walk by 5 minutes each week. Keep increasing the duration until you walk 30 to 60 minutes each day. Don't be in a hurry; this will take at least six weeks.

Don't start jogging until you can walk at a 4-mile-per-hour pace, that is, cover 2 miles in your half-hour walk. Then, if your blood cholesterol level is normal and your resting diastolic blood pressure is not above 95 mm Hg, you can begin jogging a few paces every couple of minutes during your walk. Slowly increase the amount of the distance covered by your short jogging periods. Play it by ear. As you proceed, you'll automatically jog more and walk less, until you can do the whole 2 miles at a slow jog. It should now take you about 20 to 25 minutes—not much faster than a brisk walk. During these early stages, you may need a little more sleep; listen to your body. Later on, you'll probably actually need less sleep!

For older persons, walking may be enough exercise. If you are jogging, just keep up an easy pace, and over a period of time, as your conditioning improves, you will find you gradually speed up automatically, thereby covering more miles in the same time. Take it easy; don't rush; be patient. Don't force it. It may seem slow at first, but progress is inevitable with this approach. You'll be surprised how much progress you've made after three or four months. We emphasize that you *must* not overdo it initially or you will risk becoming discouraged from unnecessary soreness or injuries and not continue your regular exercise program long enough to see those satisfying results.

Intensity and Duration

INTENSITY: NEVER OVEREXERT YOURSELF. Overexertion is dangerous—and completely unnecessary. In fact, during overexertion, the systolic blood pressure can rise to levels that might present danger to a person with hypertension. And too great an intensity of exercise can make hypertension worse.[31] Fortunately you need never strain or work to exhaustion to get in shape and lower your blood pressure.

Patience is the name of the game. If you are a beginner, during the first few months, you should never push yourself. Even when you get into better shape, we don't think you should push yourself until you have been evaluated with a properly conducted treadmill stress test. If you feel muscle pain, or if afterward your muscles are more than slightly sore or your resting pulse upon awakening is elevated, you are pushing yourself. Don't push yourself into injuries.

Don't ignore any unusual sensations during or after exercise. Pain caused by a heart attack isn't felt in the heart; it's carried by nerves, or "referred" to other parts of the chest, arm, throat, neck, jaw, or stomach. And it may not cause pain at all—just a feeling of tightness, discomfort, nausea, severe dizziness, extreme breathlessness, or fatigue. Therefore, if you have pain in either the front or the back of the chest, a choking sensation, or a tightness in your chest or throat—as Jim Fixx did about a week before he died—don't ignore the warning: *Stop exercising and see your doctor.*

If you have orthopedic or other health problems, your physician may advise that you would be better off limiting your exercise to brisk walking, which is still very beneficial but much less stressful on the joints.

How do you determine the intensity of your exercise? There are three indicators:

1. How you feel.
2. Whether you can carry on a conversation.
3. Your heart rate.

How you feel, whether you are relaxed or straining—in other words, "listening to your body" is a constant indicator to you about your level of exercise.

An excellent indicator is whether you can carry on a conversation. If you can, you are going at a pace that will help burn off fat but not unduly strain your heart.

Your heart rate is an objective measure of your pace, and we discuss this further.

Use all three of these signs. Work out at a pace that allows you to feel comfortable, carry on a conversation, and keep your pulse at about 50 to 60 percent of its maximum value.

If you are just beginning to get in shape, most exercise experts would say that your intermediate goal should be maintaining a heart rate of 60 to 70 percent of its maximum for about 20 minutes. But if you keep your heart rate to between 50 and 60 percent of its maximum predicted rate, it will help you lose weight just as well and perhaps better than a faster rate. The reason is that at a rate greater than 60 percent of the predicted maximum, you may experience an increased appetite, after the first meal, for up to thirty-six hours after your workout. If you really want to get in shape, aim for 70 percent of the maximum rate for over 20 (preferably over 30) minutes—once you have your weight at a good level (percent of body fat preferably below 15%).

There are two methods of estimating your predicted maximum heart rate (PMHR). According to Dr. Kenneth Cooper,[32] who started the aerobics movement in the 1960s, if you are a male and have been exercising regularly, simply subtract one-half your age from 205. For a fifty-two-year-old, that gives 179 beats per minute. Sixty percent of that is about 107. So the target range for that person would be a pulse of 107 while exercising.

If you are a woman, your predicted maximum heart rate is determined by subtracting your age from 205. This formula also applies if you're an out-of-shape male. If our fifty-two-year-old were a woman or a man who was out of shape, that would give a predicted maximum pulse rate of 153. So if that person were just beginning to get in shape, her or his pulse should be raised to between 76 and 92 while exercising (50 to 60 percent of the maximum). After a few weeks, he or she could move into the higher range.

Many exercise physiologists prefer a more conservative formula for calculating your maximum heart rate: 220 minus your age for males and 215 minus your age for females.[33] For a fifty-year-old male, this gives a predicted maximum pulse of 170, as compared to 180, which is arrived at using Cooper's formula. This difference emphasizes that the "predicted maximum pulse" is an *estimate* only.

If you have been steadily active in athletics, your actual maximum pulse may be higher. For example, cardiologist-runner Dr. George Sheehan is sixty-six years old and his *actual* (not predicted) maximum heart rate determined during a treadmill stress test is 179. One of the exercise physiologists who critiqued this chapter, a former member of the Canadian Olympic Team, Dr. Robert Kochan, is thirty-six and has a treadmill-determined *actual* maximum pulse of 209.

On the other hand, keep in mind that if you are taking a beta blocker, your actual maximum heart rate will be much *lower* than the predicted maximum.

For a quick and easy way to measure your heart rate while exercising, count the pulse on the inside of your wrist for 6 seconds, then multiply by 10 (just add a zero). Checking your pulse while exercising will help keep you from overdoing. If you overdo it, you will fall back and risk quitting because of discouragement. Haste makes waste when you are getting your body back in the condition it was meant to have.

And even if you do feel comfortable with longer workouts, don't go to 85 percent of your maximum heart rate, especially if you are over forty or have been obese, *unless* you have been told that your EKG is normal at at least that heart rate while doing a stress test, your resting diastolic blood pressure is below 90 mm Hg, and you do not have other coronary risk factors, such as:

○ A blood cholesterol level above 200 mg/100 ml blood (200 mg per dl).
○ A history of cigarette smoking.
○ Family history of heart attacks.
○ High-stress life-style.
○ Diabetes.
○ High-fat diet.
○ Obesity.

Don't *ever* go above 85 percent of your maximum heart rate without a coach and special medical evaluation. World-class athletes can do it, but most of us would be playing Russian roulette. We cannot overemphasize this enough: *Don't force it!* Sudden changes in intensity can trigger what had been silent heart disease into becoming a heart attack. So—**make no sudden changes in intensity** and **never change intensity and duration at the same time**.

DURATION: TIME IS THE IMPORTANT THING. At least initially, don't set goals of distance in your exercising—particularly if you're jogging, swimming, or cycling. It is more important to increase the time you spend exercising than it is to achieve a distance goal. By emphasizing time spent exercising rather than competitive goals, you reduce the chances of overdoing it and injuring yourself. You don't need to be competitive to get into really good shape.

Apparently there are two important time thresholds for aerobic exercise. The minimum amount of time you should spend exercising depends on the intensity of the exercise. To get a good "training effect" if you're walking, 30 minutes is the minimum and 45 to 60 minutes is better. If you're jogging or running, 20 minutes is the minimum and 30 to 45 minutes is better.

If you find you can't spare at least 20 minutes one day, even a 5- or 10-minute walk, especially when you're starting your program, is better than nothing. But try for the 20-minute minimum if you're jogging or the 30 minutes if you're walking. If you feel lazy and don't want to go for a 20-minute jog, remember: the real trick is to get out the door and take those first steps. Once you have gone 10 minutes, it's easy to say, well, let's do another 5, and at 15, well, this feels good, so 5 more minutes isn't much time out of the day. And there you are—you did your 20 minutes even though you hadn't felt in the mood.

Whatever the form of exercise, the same guidelines apply: Just start off slowly, and gradually work up to 30 or more minutes of walking or 20 or more minutes of jogging, running, or other more active forms of aerobic activity.

Exercising at your target heart rate for 20 to 30 minutes (enough to expend 300 kilocalories of energy) at least three times a week (1.5 hours per week) is the minimum to help reduce body fat.[34] This is also enough to produce a significant increase in your body's ability to use oxygen (maximum oxygen uptake or Vo_2 max). However, depending upon the fat "set point" of your own body (see the next chapter), you may well need to spend more than 1.5 hours per week to get a significant weight reduction effect. Some people (like Dick) need to do aerobic exercise for at least 3 hours per week to maintain a normal weight, and some people (who have a lot of fat cells) are going to have to do 3 or 4 hours per week and also cut down on calories. You will just have to find out for yourself by doing it.

To get the optimum effect on your blood pressure, you also may need to exercise more than 1.5 hours (90 minutes) per week, although the total amount required is well within reason. It is documented that three 55-minute sessions of aerobic exercise (including jogging, dancing, and light gymnastics) per week (a total of 165 minutes per week) can produce a significant lowering of blood pressure.[35] The study by Dr. Cade and co-workers showed that once people had been jogging 2 miles per day, seven days per week (a total of about 140 minutes per week) for three months, half of those being treated with drugs for *primary* hypertension achieved normal blood pressure and were able to stop taking their medicine without changing any other factor such as diet.[36] And 96 percent of the 105 patients in the exercise program achieved a significant reduction in blood pressure.

Thus, the evidence so far is that to get your blood pressure down, you need to spend a *total* of about 2¼ to 2¾ hours per week doing aerobic exercise. This must be done at least three— and we believe preferably five or six—times a week. This probably is enough to help you maintain both normal weight and normal blood pressure.

We agree with the American College of Sports Medicine that because of the greater chance of discouragement or of injuries associated with high-intensity activities, "lower to moderate intensity activity *of longer duration* is recommended for the non-athletic adult," especially older people.[37]

If you want to go beyond this level for other reasons, for example, to help lose weight, do it gradually. After a few weeks or so, start increasing your daily jog by about 5 minutes each week until you can comfortably jog for 45 minutes. After several months, as you really begin to get in shape, you may have a few 45-minute and eventually 60-minute workouts.

But remember, as we discussed in Chapter 7, Dr. Cade and his co-workers showed that better than 70 percent of their younger patients achieved blood pressure in the "normal range" within three months of when they were able to run only 2 miles every day.

Listen to Your Body

To get the most benefit while avoiding overdoing it, you'll need to keep track of your heart rate—your pulse. Keeping track of your pulse while exercising is one of the best ways of monitoring whether you are overdoing it, underdoing it, or doing it right.

Your heart rate at rest is important, too. One of the best indicators of progress is your resting heart rate upon awakening in the morning. As you achieve better cardiovascular fitness, the resting morning pulse will decrease. As you really get fit, it should come down to about 60 and may approach 50. If one morning you notice your resting pulse is higher than usual, especially if you feel tired, you probably have been overdoing it and need to take it easy for a couple of days or even skip a day to give your body some extra rest.

Other signs of overdoing it include lack of energy for other things, trouble sleeping, and the development of aches and pains that don't go away. As time goes by, you will become better "tuned in" to your body and find it easier to notice small aches or signs of tiredness before they become serious. You will develop the ability to judge your exercise level by "listening to your body."

Frequency

We have already stressed the importance of regular exercise. This is the main thing: at least three or four times a week, do some active, or aerobic, exercise such as jogging or swimming. If you're only walking, try to make it more often than that; there's nothing wrong with a walk every day.

Remember:

○ The most dangerous exercise is infrequent, sporadic exercise.
○ Never increase frequency at the same time as intensity or duration.

Warm Up and Cool Down

Warm up slowly during the first 10 minutes of each exercise session. Even world-class Olympic athletes start their warmups jogging at a pace not much faster than walking. It's the amateurs who want to get off to a flying start.

The warm-up is especially important for those who have high blood pressure or heart disease. When you first start exercising, both your systolic and your diastolic blood pressure increase. However, later, as your body begins to warm up, the tiny blood vessels, or arterioles, in your muscles open, or dilate, allowing easier flow of blood. As a result of this vasodilation, your diastolic blood pressure then begins to drop, placing less strain on your heart. It is very important that you go slowly until this decrease in peripheral resistance occurs. That way you will be placing a smaller load on your heart while you exercise.

The cool-down (or "warm-down") period is also important. It allows the blood in the muscles you've been using to get back into your main circulation. (This point can be underscored by the experience of a man who ran in a park and then drove home without a cool-down and fainted at the wheel.) So at the end of your exercise, slow down for the last 3 to 5 minutes.

Dr. George Sheehan, cardiologist and noted runner, doesn't think cooling down is so important.[38] He says at the end of a run he just sits—and watches the others cool down. Dr. Kenneth Cooper, the aerobics expert, disagrees.[39] He believes that a warm-down is *very* important. Cooper points out that at the end of a run, blood tends to pool in your legs, slowing its return to the heart. This can decrease the amount of blood delivered to your coronary arteries and, if they are narrowed with cholesterol plaques, could trigger a heart attack. Cooper points out that the first marathon runner, the runner who brought Athens the news of the Greek victory on the Plain of Marathon, didn't die until *after* he stopped. He died during the "cool-down" and not the run. Cooper points out that we still don't fully understand the importance of the cool-down period and suggests that this may be what happened when Jim Fixx died right at the end of his run. So Cooper recommends that you continue brisk movement for a few minutes, slowing to a walk before stopping.

Dr. Sheehan does point out that lying down right after a run allows blood from your legs to return to your heart faster than normal and so can place an extra load on your heart. In addition, the increased output of the heart, plus the fact that it doesn't have to push the blood against gravity to your head, would increase the blood pressure within your head. If you already have high blood pressure, this could be very dangerous. *So don't lie down* right after a run. Wait five or ten minutes for your system to readjust.

OUR COMMENT. Slowing down during the last three to five minutes of your exercise can't hurt. Look at it this way: even though you're slowing to a walk, that last three to five minutes of cooldown is still exercise. It counts. So it seems wise just to make sure that the last few minutes of your exercise are done at a progressively slower pace. If you want to put out some hard effort, do it before the last five minutes of the workout.

Preventing Injuries

Perhaps one of the most common reasons that people stop exercising is because they get hurt. So take steps to prevent injuries. If you're jogging, proper running shoes are essential. Tennis shoes or sneakers won't provide adequate support or cushioning for your foot, and if you jog in these shoes, you'll likely end up with painful foot problems. Running on dirt roads or on grass (beware of hidden stones and holes) is better than running on harder surfaces, such as asphalt and concrete. This is especially important when you are beginning. If you do aerobic exercise, stay off floors without resilience, such as concrete. If you jog or run, try to stay off concrete.

Jogging and running tend to result in an imbalance between major muscle groups. For example, the gastrocnemius, or calf muscle, becomes much stronger than the small muscles in the front of your shin. This muscle imbalance can cause a continuous pull on your achilles tendon (the strong tendon you can feel at the back of your ankle), which can result in achilles tendonitis. Since this tendon attaches to bone on the *bottom* of your heel, achilles tendonitis causes pain on the bottom of the rear of your foot, so you may confuse it with a bruise and not recognize the cause.

Of course, the best medicine is to prevent injury; fortunately, you can take simple steps to prevent the bad effects of muscle imbalance. Light weight training and stretching are necessary to prevent this type of muscle imbalance. For example, stretching will increase blood flow to the shin muscles and help prevent shin splints. Perhaps the most important stretching is to prepare the calf muscle by slowly leaning into a wall for 1 minute, as illustrated in Figure 17.

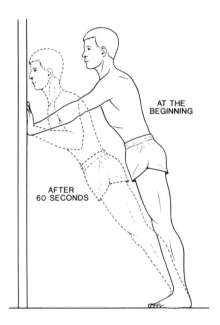

FIGURE 17. *This exercise can prevent, or reverse, "runner's heel," a painful condition that occurs when the achilles tendon pulls on the back of the heel.* A stretching exercise, simply stand a distance equal to one-half to two-thirds of your height away from a wall, leaning forward with your arms outstretched, and then, over a 60-second period, slowly pulling in your arms so that your head approaches the wall. Keep your body straight and your feet flat on the ground. This exercise slowly pulls on the achilles tendon, lengthening the gastrocnemius to counter the shortening effect of running. Take it easy: Stretching exercises should never cause pain, just a sense of tension in the muscles being stretched.

Do this stretching exercise both before *and* after your walk, jog, or aerobic dancing. Stretching not only helps preserve muscle balance and prevent injuries, it helps your workouts. Stretching is especially effective when done at the end of your exercise period. It not only helps prevent muscle cramps, but because your muscles are warm, you can stretch them further and help keep them from shortening. So after cooling down, do some stretching exercises for at least 2 to 5 minutes.

Light weight training, to strengthen arm, shoulder, and back muscles and the muscles in the front of your thighs, also helps maintain a proper balance among your muscles. See *Running and Being* (Simon and Schuster, 1978), by Dr. George Sheehan for his "magic six" stretching and weight exercises. Dr. Sheehan has since modified the "magic six" by changing the "backover" (or yoga plow) to the "knee clasp" and has added two extension exercises for the low back. As Dr. Sheehan emphasizes, stretch slowly and only to the point of tension, not pain.

An excellent book on stretching exercises for any sport is Bob Anderson's *Stretching* (1980, Shelter Publication, Bolinas, California 94924). Yoga is another way you can increase body flexibility.

Learn to listen to your body. If you feel tired, and if your resting heart rate is higher than usual, take it easy for a day or two. (On the other hand, be sure to do something, such as walk.)

Motivation

We hope this chapter itself helps motivate you. George Sheehan's books and seminars are *excellent* motivators, making you wonder how you ever could have lived (maybe you really haven't) without regular exercise; running is his particular game.

Keeping in mind that regular aerobic exercise not only benefits your health but is virtually a necessity for proper weight and blood pressure should help you use the discipline necessary to get started—and keep going. After two to four months, you will probably begin to look forward to most sessions.

Realize that regular aerobic exercise is as important to your health as sleeping or eating. So it is not an indulgence or something to try to work in when you can. Reserve a regular time slot for it each week, and don't feel guilty if this requires some people to readjust their schedules (lunch, for example) to fit yours. To the contrary, announce to your boss, your spouse, close colleagues, and friends that you are committed to a regular exercise program and it *must* be scheduled. Most of them will understand, especially when they realize how important it is to your blood pressure and overall health.

Try to pick pleasant surroundings. If you walk, jog, or run, vary your route to give variety, but keep in mind that it's best to avoid hard surfaces if you can. Another way to get variety is to change the type of exercise you do occasionally. For example, if you are a jogger, try riding your bike, an aerobics dance class, or swimming as an occasional alternative.

Another motivator for many people is to get involved with a group—an exercise class, a running club, a friend. An Irish setter named Charley got one of the authors back into running. Exercise videotapes may also help motivate you, but remember the precautions we mentioned.

If you like music (ever meet anyone who said he or she didn't?), you may find that a portable tape player is a big help in making it especially enjoyable. Just one word of warning: Don't listen to songs such as Laura Branigan's "Gloria" while you run unless you're in almost competitive shape. If music gets to you, songs like that can put you into overdrive and you may wind up really overdoing it without realizing it—until the aches and pains set in afterward.

If you stay with it during those first slow weeks, you will feel encouraged as your body begins to remember what it is to feel young.

Finally, following your progress will help as you see your resting heart rate drop and the distance you cover in a given time go up (see Chapter 14). Seeing that progress charted out will help encourage you. But be patient—you can't reverse the effects of a lifetime of sedentary living in a couple of weeks or months.

Summary

Regardless of what the antiexercise groups say, several points appear well established:

- Exercise decreases your blood pressure.
- Exercise helps decrease obesity.
- Exercise can be safe if proper precautions are taken.
- Exercise increases the quality of life and helps keep you out of hospitals.
- We believe that the total evidence suggests that exercise also increases your chance of having a longer life. Besides the fact that some statistical studies indicate this, it's hard to see how something that helps normalize both your blood pressure and your weight, helps balance your body's hormones, and helps relieve psychological stress can do anything other than that.

To the point of this book, regular aerobic exercise almost certainly can help lower your blood pressure toward normal.

CHAPTER 12

Step Four: Help Your Body Find Its Proper Weight

The fourth step in the program for lowering your blood pressure and increasing your well-being is to shed excess body fat.

Of course, observing Step Two (eating right) and Step Three (exercise) overlaps considerably with this step. Nonetheless, since overweight people have particular problems not shared by people with normal weight, we feel losing excess weight deserves a discrete focus.

We hardly need to tell you that losing weight is not easy, and keeping it off is even more difficult. But hypertension occurs twice as often among obese people as it does in people with normal weight. In its 1984 recommendations for dealing with hypertension, the Joint National Committee warned obese people with high blood pressure to shed some of those excess pounds.

In an obese person, some of the blood hormones do not work properly; they do not maintain a correct balance between sodium and potassium in the cells, thus contributing to hypertension. Getting rid of excess fat helps return the blood hormones to normal levels, allowing the body to maintain a more normal balance between sodium and potassium. For example, shedding extra pounds lowers blood insulin, and in many people, this helps the kidneys excrete more sodium, thereby lowering blood pressure.[1]

Losing excess weight alone, without doing anything else, can sometimes bring blood pressure back to normal. In clinical studies, loss of one-third to one-half of excess body weight has reduced blood pressure significantly.[2] On the other hand, if you *don't* get rid of the extra fat, your abnormal blood hormone levels may prevent the *K Factor* or even drugs from reducing your blood pressure. So if you have hypertension and are overweight, it is *very* important that you reduce your weight.

Getting your weight toward normal has other benefits, too. There is a good deal of evidence that maintaining normal weight decreases your chances of having a heart attack, and it is a major factor in preventing you from developing adult onset (Type II) diabetes. Normal weight, along with good physical fitness, increases your energy. You just plain feel better.

Are You Overweight?

How do you know if you are "obese" or have "normal" weight? Actually it's not weight but the amount of *fat* in your body that counts. You can have normal weight and be too fat! If you haven't put on any weight since high school, when you weighed in at 195 and were "all muscle," don't brag too much. Unless you work out a lot, there is a good chance that a lot of that muscle has wasted away, or atrophied, from lack of use. You may have gained several pounds of fat even though your weight is the same.

The most accurate way to tell if you're obese is to determine, with the underwater immersion test, the percent of your body weight that is fat. This involves some special equipment that measures your naked weight when you are completely submerged in a water tank. This weight is compared with your naked weight in air. Since the fat part of your body is lighter than water and the rest of your body is heavier, the percent of your body that is fat can be calculated from the difference between your weight in air and your weight in water.

There is also a more advanced way to determine your body fat, based on an electrical property (called conductivity) of your body,[3] using the principle that the electrical conductivity of lean tissue (such as muscle) is far lower than that of fat, but this method is not yet widely used.

Once you know the percentage of your weight that is fat, you can compare that with the "average" to determine whether you are overweight. For men, the national average is about 15 to 20 percent; about 22 to 23 percent is considered healthy for a woman. Some people who exercise a lot have only about 9 percent body fat. The lowest value is found in some world-class male athletes: about 5 percent body fat. For women, the figures are somewhat higher.

Tables for ideal body weight are of limited help for many people because they cannot take into account the wide variations in amounts of bone and muscle. As an example, Dick had his body fat measured scientifically in the water tank. After subtracting his body fat from his total weight, the resulting lean weight was still 3 pounds over his "ideal" total body weight as listed in one table! Even if he removed all fat from his body (which is impossible), he would still be 3 pounds "overweight."

Of course, there is a much easier guide to determine if you are too fat: skin fold thickness, which you can estimate right in your own home. Pinch the skin of your abdomen. If, while sitting, you can pinch more than 1 inch, your body has too much fat. By using calipers, you can estimate your percentage of body fat more accurately. This requires determining the skin fold thickness in several body locations and then using a table to estimate the percentage of fat in your body. Some of the fancy calipers have a built-in microchip that contains the information of the table and does the calculation for you. You need to determine the thickness in several locations, because body fat tends to go to different places on different people. In fact, although we don't yet understand why, recent studies indicate that if your body fat tends to accumulate in the abdomen, your chances of having a heart attack are increased.

Finally, just looking at yourself nude is not only one of the simplest but one of the best ways to determine if you are overfat. If you can see folds of fat sagging, you are too heavy. If you look nice and trim, you probably aren't.

What Determines Your Body Fat?

We used to be convinced that if you were overweight, you ate too much—period. That's all there was to it. Dick remembers a physician friend of his examining a very obese teenager whose mother insisted, "Doctor, she eats just like a bird," to which the young physician wryly replied, "Yeah, a giant Condor." Neither he nor Dick could believe anyone could be that overweight without overeating. Why? Because the First Law of Thermodynamics, or the Conservation of Energy Law, says that energy can neither be created nor destroyed. This law, which was discovered in the 1840s, is well established and has appropriately influenced not only physics and medical thinking but the thinking of society at large. The obvious solution for losing weight was simple: Don't eat so much. But decreasing your calorie intake does not necessarily decrease your weight. It's just not that simple. Some obese people really do eat like birds, yet they stay fat. In fact, many overweight people actually eat fewer calories than do thin people.

How could this be? Well, the Conservation of Energy Law does hold true; none of us, the obese included, can create energy out of nothing. But the situation is a bit more complicated. We need to follow the newer scientific approach (see Chapter 19) and look at the whole picture.

Perhaps we can most easily see the true situation by looking at the way energy enters and leaves the human body. Figure 18 shows what happens to the calories you eat:

- As much as 80 percent are "burned off": they are turned into heat (#1) (that's what keeps your body warm).
- Some are burned off by doing work (#2).

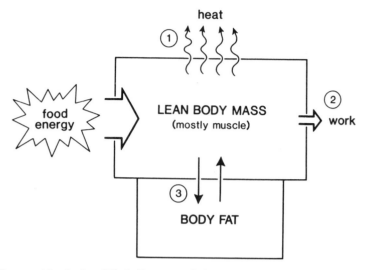

FIGURE 18. *A simplified diagram of the energy input and output of the body.* (Not shown is the normally small amount of calories lost through feces and urine, although with people in disease states, such as diabetics losing sugar through the urine, or those with diarrhea, this can become considerable.)

○ Some are turned into proteins and other structural components of your body (this is less than 1% in an adult).
○ Some are lost in the stool.
○ The rest are stored as fat (#3).

You want to eliminate the last possibility; you want to avoid having "the rest" left over for fat. In fact, if you don't take in enough calories to provide for the other possibilities adequately, the fat you already have will be burned off and you will lose weight.

Let's look at this in more detail.

Almost all your energy comes into your body in the form of food. The two main ways we lose energy are by the body giving off heat and by the body performing work on the environment (exercise). Any energy left over must, according to the Energy

Law, be used to increase body protein (such as muscle) *or* must be stored as fat (#3).

So far, so good. Eating more should make you gain weight, and vice versa, right? Not necessarily; if we look closer, we see that there are other possibilities.

Inside your body are several mechanisms that determine the balance between the energy stored as fat (#3) and that given off as heat (#1) or work (#2). To oversimplify a bit, these mechanisms can be divided into those that primarily regulate the amount of energy that goes into fat and those that primarily regulate the amount of energy given off as heat.

FACTORS THAT INCREASE ENERGY GOING INTO FAT	FACTORS THAT INCREASE ENERGY LOST AS HEAT
Insulin	Thyroid hormone
White fat cells	Brown fat cells
	Sodium-potassium pumps

Insulin prevents fat from being used up; thyroid hormone increases heat production; sodium-potassium pumps also produce heat directly and especially indirectly. Brown fat cells tend to burn fat more than store it. On the other hand, white fat cells tend to store fat.

These mechanisms all work together to regulate the amount of fat in your body. The balance among these mechanisms determines if you will be "fat" or not. No one can "control" your amount of fat; your body itself does that. But we will see that within fairly wide limits, you can help your body reset the fat level.

To look at this, scientists borrowed a concept from modern control systems theory (which deals with the way complex systems, such as airplanes, computers—or human beings—are regulated) called the *set point*. Just as the thermostat in your home establishes a set point, or target temperature, mechanisms inside your body that determine the balance between energy stored as fat versus that given off as heat tend to keep the amount of body fat constant at a "target" amount *even if you cut back on the calories you eat.* That is why in the long run, dieting alone won't and can't work!

Since the extent to which we can change the set point depends upon our genetics and upon the number and type of fat cells in our body, part of this regulation is beyond our ability to influence. Fortunately, however, a large part of this fat set point *can* be influenced.

All this means we've got some good news and some bad news. The good news is that you *can* change the amount of fat in each of your white fat cells: you can change your body's set point for body fat. If you have a lot of white fat cells you'll just have to change the "set point" further. But you *can* do it—naturally. How?

It should be obvious from Figure 18 that doing more work— exercising—is one way to get rid of excess calories. Some people used to downplay this, saying that the amount of energy lost through exercise isn't enough to make a difference. But for each mile you walk or jog, you lose at least 100 calories—and each pound of fat contains 3,500 calories. So walking or jogging just nine miles each week would be enough to burn off about a pound of fat a month. Maybe that doesn't sound dramatic, but that's twelve pounds in a year.

But exercise also changes the set point that determines the balance between energy going into heat or into fat. We not only lose more heat during exercise than we do during rest (the body temperature actually increases a degree or two, and we sweat), but regular exercise produces changes in blood hormones, involving insulin, adrenaline, and thyroid hormones, which cause the body to lose more heat *even between exercise sessions*. So the effect of exercise is actually more than just the amount of energy it takes for each mile, or hour, of aerobic exercise.

Now merely decreasing caloric intake changes the levels of some of your blood hormones, such as thyroid hormone and insulin, which signals your body to waste fewer calories in heat and hold onto its fat. The purpose of this is to prevent your body from using up spare fuel (fat) and thus to help you survive longer if you are faced with starvation. (Of course, this is a great advantage if the possibility of actual starvation is imminent, but for most of us, surrounded by plenty of food, it's a catch-22.) To make matters worse, the fatter you are, the fewer calories you need to eat just to maintain the same weight. And as you become older, the problem gets more acute. Fat cells of obese people have a defect that makes them give off less heat than the fat cells of thin people.

A major part of the calories you eat—perhaps a quarter to a third—goes into running the "pumps" that move sodium out of your cells and potassium into them.[4] Most of the energy used by these pumps eventually winds up as heat. Some overweight people apparently have fewer of these sodium-potassium pumps than do people with normal weight.[5] This means that obese people expend fewer calories as heat than do thin people; their calorie needs are therefore a few hundred less per day. (The altered sodium-potassium balance might also help explain the fact that obese people are twice as likely to have high blood pressure as people with normal weight.)

Interestingly, a potassium deficiency has been shown to decrease the number of sodium-potassium pumps in skeletal muscles (which make up most of your lean body mass).[6] So it's possible that restoring the proper *K Factor* in your diet may provide some assistance in resetting your body fat set point.

Another problem is that being overweight tends to increase your blood levels of insulin, a hormone that works to promote the storage of fat (and may also make you feel hungrier).

Unfortunately, you can't decrease the *number* of your fat cells.[7] Worse, you can *increase* the number of fat cells by gaining and losing weight—which is common in obese people, who try one diet after another. Most of the diets work temporarily; few work permanently. Also, white fat cells just store fat, but brown fat cells actually help turn energy into heat—they can actually help keep body weight down. Recently, there has been a lot of talk about brown fat cells. But only a few lucky people have enough brown fat cells to keep them from gaining weight. But the rest of us have mostly white fat cells—so we have a harder time losing weight than those who have more brown fat cells. Well, you win some and lose some.

Fortunately, by changing the set point, you change the

amount of fat in each fat cell. A person who has more fat cells will have more body fat at a given set point than one who has fewer fat cells. Thus to lose weight, a person with more fat cells will have to change his or her set point more than a person with fewer fat cells will have to change his or hers.

The Vicious Cycle

So the more overweight you are, the tougher it can be. Being obese is a vicious cycle. The more obese you are, the more your body hormones and metabolism change to make you even more obese from the calories you eat. Not only that, but since the fat surrounding your body is a good insulator, just having more body fat tends to decrease the energy you lose as heat. And being obese makes it more difficult to work off calories during exercise.

In addition, some people have so many fat cells, or have predisposing genetic factors, that it's extremely difficult to achieve healthy weight even using the principles outlined here. Those people especially need the help of a physician-nutritionist in order to handle their problem.

But fortunately the "new" paradigm, with the systems approach and its set point concept, shows that by working *with* nature, most of us can influence our body's fat storage—we can break out of the vicious cycle.

How to Lose Weight

In order to lose weight, you must:

○ Pay attention to your diet and restrict calories.
○ Increase the number of calories you use doing work.
○ Change your body's fat set point to increase the amount of calories you burn.

Pay Attention to Your Diet

So what else is new? Are we just telling you to eat less—as though you hadn't heard that already countless times? Not exactly. It's important not just to eat less but also to manage the kinds of foods you do eat. If you are following our recommendations from Chapter 10 (Step Two: Eat Right), you're probably doing the right thing. However, here we want to make a significant—and simple—distinction between kinds of foods: between high-energy-density foods, which have a high ratio of calories to bulk, and low-energy-density foods, which have a low ratio of calories to bulk. We want you to avoid the first kind (in spite of its nice-sounding name) and concentrate on the second kind. The high-energy-density foods tend to make you obese.

HIGH-ENERGY DENSITY FOODS	LOW-ENERGY DENSITY FOODS
Fat foods: butter, margarine, nuts, gravies, marbled beef, etc.	*Low- or nonfat foods*: low-fat yogurt, skim milk, nonfat dry milk, etc.
Simple carbohydrates:* refined sugars, foods with added sugar, white bread, etc.	*Complex carbohydrates** and foods containing fiber*: fresh vegetables (potatoes are great), fruits, whole grains (including rice), pasta
Alcohol	*Protein foods*: skinned chicken, fish

Some nutritionists say simple carbohydrates are absorbed rapidly into the bloodstream. This raises your blood levels of insulin, a hormone that, among its many actions, causes storage of fat. Alcohol is also absorbed fast; it is readily metabolized by

*Simple carbohydrates include table sugar (sucrose), milk sugar (lactose), and dextrose (glucose). Honey contains sucrose predigested by the bee into a mixture of glucose and fructose. Sucrose is composed of one molecule of glucose joined with one of fructose. Lactose is composed of one molecule of glucose joined with another sugar called galactose. Some people don't have the enzyme to break lactose into these two sugars.

**Complex carbohydrates include starch and cellulose, both of which are made of hundreds or thousands of glucose molecules bonded together. In starch, these glucose molecules are bonded in a single chain which our digestive system breaks down into glucose molecules; but in cellulose, the glucose molecules are bonded in a way that can't be digested by people. So cellulose, which is one type of fiber, doesn't give us calories even though it helps satisfy hunger.

the body for quick use, *or* its energy can be converted into fat. Fat is absorbed more slowly than either simple carbohydrates or alcohol but has about twice as many calories as the same weight of carbohydrate or protein. Simply put, fat is fattening. In contrast, the low-energy-density foods release their energy slowly and gradually, over a sustained period and in a form your body can use.

There is evidence that high-energy-density foods increase your hunger. One study showed that people who ate high-energy-density foods, containing lots of fat and refined sugar, required almost twice as many calories to satisfy their hunger as did a group who ate low-energy-density foods. The high-energy foods tend to stimulate your appetite, whereas the fiber in low-energy-density foods produces bulk to help satisfy your hunger.

When you eat high-energy-density foods, the level of insulin in your blood increases far more than it does when you eat low-energy-density foods. This insulin stimulates your hunger, according to some researchers. And the extra insulin raises your blood pressure by causing the kidneys to retain sodium and by stimulating activity of the sympathetic nerves.

In contrast, low-energy-density foods are high in *K Factor* and fiber and low in fat. Eating them will not only help you avoid overeating, it will provide you with the nutrition you need to keep your blood pressure down as well as decrease your chances of getting coronary artery disease or cancer.

EAT LOW-FAT FOODS. Avoid butter, margarine, sour cream, nuts, gravies, cream, and other fats.

Since dietary fat contains about twice as many calories per gram as does dietary protein or carbohydrate, cutting dietary fat intake is the most effective way to cut calories. Besides, eating fat stimulates your appetite and thus encourages you to overeat.

Fat may be even more "fattening" than we thought. A study published in 1984 reported that laboratory animals eating a diet containing 42 to 60 percent of the calories as fat became obese (51% body fat), whereas the control group which ate a low-fat diet containing the *same number of calories* ended up with normal (30%) body fat.[8] This thought-provoking study indicates that it's not only the extra calories in fat and the fact that fat may stimulate hunger that makes fat especially fattening, but the way the body processes fat. From what we know of basic biochemistry, this isn't too surprising. When food is turned into body fat, some of the energy is wasted in the conversion process: when protein is converted to fat, 25 percent of the calories are lost as heat; with carbohydrate the figure is 20 percent; but when dietary fat is converted to fat, only 4 percent of the calories are lost as heat—the rest going into fat.[9]

So the next time you're tempted to pour on the butter, sour cream, or add whole cream to your coffee, go ahead if you must—it's your choice. But in your mind's eye, visualize that almost all of that pad of butter going straight into those unsightly bulges on your abdomen or legs.

In 1984, Americans consumed, on the average, 44 percent of their calories from fat. This may well be part of the explanation that today Americans are more obese than in 1910 when they obtained only 27 percent of their calories from fat.[10] And the evidence indicates that you need even less fat than that.

Your body manufactures most of the fat it needs: several fatty acids (both saturated and unsaturated), cholesterol, and other steroids. (There is one fat, though, that the body cannot manufacture: an unsaturated fat called linoleic acid, which, incidentally, helps to keep your blood pressure normal. If you are an active adult, you need about 30 to 60 calories—7 grams, or about ½ tablespoon—of linoleic acid every day. In addition, you need some fat in order to absorb vitamins A, D, E, and K, which are all fat soluble. If you were to cut your dietary fat to below 10 percent, you might not get enough of these essential vitamins.)

We agree with the 1984 American Heart Association recommendation that you cut your fat consumption down to 30 percent of your total caloric intake—and if you have a cardiac "risk factor," to 20 percent. In fact, we recommend everyone cut it to 20 percent. (Keep in mind, however, that you couldn't eat a totally fat-free diet even if you wanted to. Everything we eat, whether animal or vegetable, is made of cells, and all cells have membranes that contain fat. Therefore, even crisp iceberg let-

tuce has 7 percent fat (by calories), and loose leaf lettuce has almost 15 percent of its calories in fat! Hardly anything—except such starchy foods as potatoes, rice, and beans—has less fat than lettuce.)
Our menu plan in Chapter 10 helps you do just that: cut your fat intake to 20 percent.

EAT FOODS CONTAINING COMPLEX CARBOHYDRATES. If you avoid simple sugars and processed carbohydrates (candy, sugar cookies, white bread, cakes, etc.), you can eat a fair amount of complex carbohydrates (carrots, cucumbers, broccoli, green beans, fresh fruits, cornstarch, brown rice, potatoes, beans, whole grain breads and cereals, etc.) and still lose weight. Remember, carbohydrate doesn't promote obesity as much as does dietary fat.

RESTRICT THE TOTAL CALORIES YOU EAT. Exercise and changing your set point can do a lot, but if you want to lose excess fat, keep a "cap" on your calories—don't *over*eat.
Listen to your body—not to the situation or the environment. Avoid temptation. Don't keep fattening foods in the house. If everyone else is going to indulge at dessert, explain that you must leave the table—and then do it! Use vegetables such as celery or carrots as a substitute for fattening desserts or snacks. If you find it helpful, join a weight-reduction group or class.

Increase the Amount of Calories You Use Doing Work

Decreasing the amount of calories you take in is not enough. Remember, when you diet without exercise, your body actually wastes *fewer* calories as heat. This slows the loss of body fat. Worse than that, some of the weight you lose may be muscle.
In order to lose weight, you also need to increase the amount of calories your body burns. Unfortunately, as we've already pointed out, even at rest, overweight people tend to give off less heat than do people of normal weight. And studies have shown that obese people automatically learn to do tasks with the smallest amount of body movement. For example, they actually expend *less* work making a bed than thin people do. Therefore, it's

down to work: You must burn off calories by doing work—that is, by exercising.

In the previous chapter, we discussed exercise in detail. Here we want to present some ideas specifically for those of you who are overweight. Obesity and lack of exercise are closely related. Obesity makes it more difficult to exercise, and without exercise, many of us have difficulty keeping our weight down. This can become another vicious cycle, as illustrated in Figure 19. By the same token, exercise does help you lose weight, and losing weight makes it easier to exercise, especially if you jog or run.

In a slow jog for one hour, a 110-pound woman would burn up about 500 calories. For a 150-pound man, the figure would be 650 calories, and a 200-pounder would burn about 800 calories. Aerobic exercises, such as cross-country skiing or swimming, can burn off as many calories per hour as jogging.

If you are very overweight, instead of jogging, you can walk, ride a bike, or swim. If the 110-pound woman were to walk briskly for one hour, she would burn off 230 calories; the 150-pound man would burn off 300 calories, and the 200-pounder would burn off 360 calories. For a one-hour leisurely walk, the figures are 150, 180, and 220.

As an example of the value of walking, one group of women who had a sedentary life-style and had repeatedly failed to lose weight were instructed to walk for a half-hour each day. After one year, they had all lost at least ten pounds. Those who walked more lost still more weight.

Try to get in the habit of taking advantage of everyday oppor-

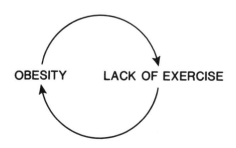

OBESITY   LACK OF EXERCISE

tunities. For example, use the stairs instead of the elevator; if you have to take things to the basement, make two or three trips instead of one; if you are walking, do it at a brisk pace and don't take the shortcut. Use your imagination.

The bottom line is: you must have patience. Regular exercise may take fat off slowly, but it will *stay* off as long as you continue exercising.

Change Your Body's Fat Set Point to Increase the Amount of Calories You Burn

Exercise not only uses more calories while you are working out, it also helps reset your set point to cause your body to "waste" more energy, in the form of heat, during the whole rest of the day—even when you sleep. Exercise builds up your muscles and at the same time actually increases the activity of the fat-burning enzymes in your body.

Even moderate regular physical activity helps elevate the level of hormones such as adrenaline that promote fat breakdown and decrease the blood level of the hormone insulin, which prevents fat breakdown.[11] Thus exercise tends to prevent the calories you eat from being turned into fat (since, again, a high level of insulin tends to shift calories into making more fat) and allows fat to be released from the fat cells so the muscles can burn it up. The lower levels of blood insulin may also be the reason exercise helps match your appetite to your body's needs.

CUT BACK ON FOODS CONTAINING SIMPLE CARBOHYDRATES (SUGAR). Besides exercise, *how* and *what* you eat can influence your body's set point. For example, carbohydrate in the form of sugar causes your blood insulin level to rapidly increase, or to "spike," more than complex carbohydrate. The increased level of blood sugar promotes the production of fat and the retention of sodium by the kidneys, and the combination of elevated blood sugar and elevated blood insulin tends to stimulate the sympathetic nervous system, thus raising your blood pressure[12] (remember Chapter 7?). One study showed that in people on low-calorie ("reducing") diets with lots of simple sugar, blood pressure did not drop, whereas people whose diets had the same number of calories but very little sugar did obtain a reduction in blood pressure.[13]

TIMING. Timing is important: It helps if you coordinate your eating with your physical activity. As you recall, a high blood level of insulin tends to shift calories into making more fat. From this, you can correctly conclude that eating just before going to sleep will spike your blood insulin and maximize the storage of the calories in fat at a time when you are going to do *no* exercise to burn calories or to lower the insulin. So midnight snacking may be one of the worst things you can do. Taking in more of your food in the early part of the day can decrease the number of calories used to make fat.

A few minutes of mild exercise, such as a leisurely walk or a bike ride after a meal, will help keep the blood insulin level from rising and will thus decrease the number of calories in the meal that are converted into body fat. Taking a fifteen-minute walk after supper, for example, can burn off about 50 calories. That amounts to about five pounds of fat per year! Walking after meals seems to be especially effective for those who have trouble losing weight.

Finally, remember that if you not only want to lose weight but want to keep the weight off, you will need to do regular aerobic exercise.

STRESS. Stress can contribute to obesity in at least two ways. From your own experience, you may already know that stress tends to promote overeating and binge eating. But stress also causes the release of certain hormones, such as adrenaline, that stimulate insulin release, thus decreasing fat breakdown. In this way, stress tends to increase the fat set point.

If you know stress is a problem, make an effort to learn what you can do about it; there is a lot of literature on the subject. For starters, though, you might try listening to music or taking a short walk as a substitute for binge eating when you feel stress driving you to the icebox. You might also consider various relaxation techniques, including yoga or meditation, to counter the effect of chronic stress on your fat set point. A swim, a long walk, or a jog outdoors is also good for relieving stress.

Precautions

Do not begin a new exercise regimen—or substantially change the one you are currently on—without first consulting your doctor. If you are dieting (decreasing your caloric intake), do not exercise as strenuously as you would if you were not dieting; balance the two activities. Never exercise strenuously after a meal because more blood is flowing to the stomach and intestines then and less to the muscles.

Group and Professional Support

Many people can adjust their life on their own so that their body seeks its healthy weight. But many others, especially those with too many fat cells or the wrong genes, will have difficulty achieving a healthy weight. Most overweight people have already tried to lose weight and are now discouraged.

In that case, you really have to consider getting into an organized program. It helps to realize that for most of the obese, there *is* a way to lose weight. But many of us can't do it on our own but must participate with others. If you insist on doing it on your own, you will probably get very discouraged. On the other hand, a program can give you structure, support, and guidance, such as do *this* this week and *that* next week. Although you can monitor your progress, a program can help monitor you and provide reinforcement.

Finally, there are a few who are going to have a very difficult time achieving a healthy weight, and they should not feel guilty but should realize that they *especially* can't do it on their own and need to participate with others and receive professional help.

Summary

Actually this is a simple illustration of the change in the way scientists think about things, an illustration of the "paradigm shift" (the working scientific philosophy or viewpoint) we discuss in Chapter 19. The Conservation of Energy Law (from the "old" paradigm) is not only still true but necessary for us to understand fat regulation. But it's not enough. Alone, it is misleading. Thinking in terms of the old paradigm, which emphasized only the Conservation of Energy Law, led us to "blame overeating as the major cause of obesity and has stimulated the development of hundreds of diets and other techniques [including pills] to 'control' how much we eat."[14]

We need more than the Energy Law. We need to look at the whole system and focus on the *relationships* (or feedback loops, as they are called) inside the system.

You can participate with your physician—and with nature—to achieve a more healthy weight in the following ways:

1. Change the set point by:
   a. Exercising more.
   b. Watching what you eat, especially your sugar intake.
   c. Relieving stress.
2. Restrict calories by:
   a. Decreasing the percentage of calories in your food that is obtained from fat.
   b. Cutting back on alcohol.
   c. Eating fiber-containing foods, such as fruits and vegetables (which fill you up more quickly and also have a high *K Factor*).
   d. Regulating the amount you eat (some may need to restrict calories).

PART FOUR
The Tally Sheet

The next breakthrough in medicine is the patient taking responsibility for his own health.

—Dr. John Knoll, 1950

In the early months of adopting our program, it is important that you keep records of your progress. Otherwise it will be too easy for you to slack off on some days or make a major mistake (such as eating commercial pickles or several olives for lunch) and thus sabotage your possibility for success.

At the end of this part, we will provide you with a sample chart on which you can record your progress. Other copies are in the Appendix.

Remember that earlier in the book, we made the point that lowering your blood pressure is not enough. You must give your body the care it needs to restore the normal balance between potassium and sodium in your body's cells. So in contrast to the past, where only a symptom (actually a sign) was treated—blood pressure—we want you to record other signals that reflect the actual condition of your body.

241

The most important things for you to do for your blood pressure are the following:

- Keep track of your *K Factor*.
- Keep track of your exercise.
- Keep track of your weight.
- Keep track of your blood pressure.

There is a small chapter in this part devoted to each of these. In addition, for your general health, you should:

- Keep track of your dietary fat intake.

Again, you need to record your progress on the chart provided at the end of this part.

CHAPTER 13
Keep Track of Your *K Factor*

One of the most important things you can do is to monitor your progress on our program by keeping track of the *K Factor* in your body. You can do this by monitoring your diet, your urine, and your blood.

Monitoring Your Diet

While you follow our sample menu plan in Chapter 10, you can look up your daily *K Factor*, which is given at the end of each day's menus.

However, you will no doubt want to plan some of your own menus as well as alter some of ours. In this case, you can determine your *K Factor* by using the table we have provided starting on page 245. Or, if you use one of our recipes, you can look up the values given at the end of each recipe.

After a while, you'll get familiar with the potassium and sodium contents of various foods, and you won't have to do any calculations. But in the beginning, you may find it reassuring to double check the values of what you are eating. You can get a quick idea of how good or bad some common foods are by looking over the table.

Potassium and Sodium Content of Foods

The items printed in boldface are very good in terms of sodium (Na) and potassium (K) balance and were selected because their sodium content is less than 65 milligrams (mg) and their potassium-to-sodium ratio is greater than 5, or their sodium content is less than 40 mg and their potassium-to-sodium ratio is greater than 3. The italicized foods should be avoided because their sodium content is greater than 200 mg and their potassium-to-sodium ratio is less than 1.0, or their sodium content is greater than 20 mg and their potassium-to-sodium ratio is less than 0.5, or their sodium content is greater than 400 mg. Even though beer and wine are in boldface, they are not recommended (except in moderation), because chronic alcohol consumption has been shown to cause hypertension. Although nuts are in boldface, they are not recommended in large quantities because their fat content is high.

The usual portion size for some foods is close to 100 grams (g). Many of the portion sizes were rounded to exactly 100 g to simplify comparisons. For your computations, it helps to know that 100 grams weigh 3.5 ounces, 100 grams of water have a volume of 3.4 fluid ounces, and 1 ounce weighs 28 grams. Beverage ounces are given in fluid ounces; all other ounces are avoirdupois weights. Remember that a K/Na ratio of less than 1 means that the food has more sodium than potassium, whereas when it's greater than 1, there's more potassium than sodium.

Go for the **boldfaced items**, avoid the *items in italics*, and normal print items are okay.

TABLE 4.

Food	Portion Size	Calories/ Portion	K Content (mg)	Na Content (mg)	K/Na (mg/mg)
Beverages					
Apple juice	6 oz. (182 g)	86	184	1	180.00
Beer (Pabst)	12 oz. (351 g)	147	128	6	22.00
Beer (Natural Lite)	12 oz. (353 g)	96	105	7	15.00
Club soda (Seagram)	12 oz. (358 g)	0	1.4	93	0.02
Coffee	3.4 oz. (100 g)	1	36	1	36.00
Coke	12 oz. (373 g)	146	2.5	16	0.16
Cranberry juice*	8 oz. (253 g)	147	61	6	10.00
Dr. Pepper	12 oz. (370 g)	144	1.4	31	0.05
Ginger ale (Schweppe's)	12 oz. (370 g)	115	0.7	26	0.03
Grapefruit juice	6 oz. (184 g)	72	298	2	140.00
Milk, skim	12 oz. (368 g)	132	532	190	2.80
Orange juice	8 oz. (250 g)	112	500	2	250.00
Orange pop (Sunkist)	12 oz. (370 g)	170	1.8	38	0.05
Root beer (Hires)	12 oz. (370 g)	152	1.8	66	0.03
7-Up	12 oz. (370 g)	160	1.4	39	0.04
Tap water (Burlington, VT)	12 oz. (355 g)	0	0.7	2.8	0.25
Tomato juice	6 oz. (182 g)	35	413	364	1.10
unsalted	6 oz. (182 g)	35	413	5	83.00
*V-8 juice**	8 oz. (242 g)	53	527	715	0.74
unsalted*	8 oz. (242 g)	53	527	47	11.00
Wine, red	3.5 oz. (102 g)	87	94	5	19.00
Wine, sherry	2 oz. (59 g)	81	44	2	22.00
Wine, white	12 oz. (345 g)	293	248	3.9	64.00
Breads/Cereals					
Bagel	1 bagel (55 g)	163	41	198	0.21
Barley, dry	½ cup (100 g)	349	160	3	53.00
Biscuit	1 (35 g)	92	29	156	0.19
Blueberry muffin	1 (40 g)	112	46	253	0.18

Food	Portion Size	Calories/ Portion	K Content (mg)	Na Content (mg)	K/Na (mg/mg)
Bread, corn	1 piece (78 g)	161	122	490	0.25
Bread, cracked wheat	1 slice (25 g)	66	34	132	0.26
Bread, Italian	1 slice (30 g)	83	22	490	0.12
Bread, raisin	1 slice (30 g)	79	70	110	0.64
Bread, rye	1 slice (25 g)	61	36	139	0.26
Bread, white	1 slice (27 g)	74	33	134	0.25
Bread, whole wheat	1 slice (25 g)	61	68	132	0.52
*English muffin**	1 (57 g)	135	319	364	0.88
*Grapenuts flakes**	1 oz. (28 g)	102	99	218	0.45
Noodles, egg cooked, no salt	1 cup (160 g)	200	70	3	23.00
Oatmeal	1 oz. (28 g)	109	98	0.7	140.00
Puffed wheat	1 cup (14 g)	50	35	1	35.00
Quaker 100% Natural	¼ cup (28 g)	130	120	15	8.00
*Raisin bran (Post)**	2 oz. (57 g)	174	350	370	0.95
Rice, brown, dry	¼ cup (46 g)	166	99	4	23.00
Rice, white, dry	¼ cup (46 g)	168	42	2	19.00
Roll, white hard	1 (50 g)	156	49	313	0.16
Spaghetti, dry	2 oz. (57 g)	209	112	1	110.00
*Sugar pops**	1 oz. (28 g)	109	20	63	0.32
Crackers					
Cheese nips	100 g	479	109	1039	0.10
Graham	100 g	384	384	670	0.57
Ritz	100 g	458	113	1092	0.10
Ry-krisp	100 g	344	600	882	0.68
Saltines	100 g	433	120	1100	0.11
Desserts					
Angel food cake	100 g	269	88	283	0.31
Animal crackers	100 g	429	95	303	0.31
Apple pie	100 g	256	80	301	0.27
Applesauce (unsweetened)	100 g	41	78	2	39.00

Food	Portion Size	Calories/ Portion	K Content (mg)	Na Content (mg)	K/Na (mg/mg)
Apricots (canned)	100 g	66	239	1	240.00
Banana custard pie	100 g	221	203	194	1.00
Brownies	100 g	485	190	251	0.76
Cherry pie	100 g	261	105	304	0.34
Chocolate cake	100 g	369	154	235	0.66
Coffee cake	100 g	322	109	431	0.25
Custard, chocolate*	½ cup (112 g)	142	186	153	1.22
Donut, plain	3 (100 g)	391	90	501	0.18
Fig newtons	5½ (100 g)	358	198	252	0.79
Fruitcake, dark	100 g	379	496	158	3.10
Fruitcake, light	100 g	389	233	193	1.20
Lemon meringue pie	100 g	255	50	282	0.18
Orange sherbet	100 g	134	22	10	2.20
Peach pie	100 g	255	149	268	0.56
Pecan pie	100 g	418	123	221	0.56
Pumpkin pie	100 g	211	160	214	0.75
Raisin pie	100 g	270	192	285	0.67
Vanilla pudding (instant)*	½ cup (148 g)	147	207	422	0.49
Vanilla tapioca	100 g	134	135	156	0.86
Vanilla wafers	100 g	462	72	252	0.29
Fats/Oils					
Butter, salted	1 Tbsp. (14.2 g)	102	3	140	0.02
Cooking oil	1 Tbsp. (13.6 g)	120	0	0	—
French dressing	1 Tbsp. (16 g)	66	13	219	0.06
Margarine	1 Tbsp. (14.2 g)	102	8	140	0.06
Mayonnaise	1 Tbsp. (14 g)	101	5	84	0.06
Fish/Seafood					
Catfish	100 g	103	330	60	5.50
Clams, cherrystone	6–7 (100 g)	80	311	205	1.50
Clams, soft	100 g	82	235	36	6.50

Food	Portion Size	Calories/ Portion	K Content (mg)	Na Content (mg)	K/Na (mg/mg)
Cod, fillet	100 g	170	407	110	3.70
Flounder, or sole	100 g	202	587	237	2.50
Haddock	100 g	165	348	177	2.00
Halibut, steak	100 g	171	525	134	3.90
Lobster, cooked	100 g	95	180	210	0.86
Oysters, fried	100 g	239	203	206	0.98
Oysters, raw	100 g	66	121	73	1.70
Pike, walleye, raw	100 g	93	319	51	6.30
Salmon, canned	100 g	141	361	387	0.93
Salmon, steak	100 g	182	443	116	3.80
Sardines, Atlantic, canned, oil	100 g	311	560	510	1.10
Scallops	100 g	81	396	255	1.60
Shrimp	100 g	91	220	140	1.60
Tuna, canned, oil	½ can (100 g)	288	301	800	0.38
Whitefish	100 g	155	299	52	5.80

Fruits

Apple	1 med. (150 g)	80	152	1	150.00
Apricots	3 (114 g)	55	301	1	300.00
Avocado	100 g	167	604	4	150.00
Banana	1 med. (175 g)	101	440	1	440.00
Blueberries	1 cup (145 g)	90	117	1	120.00
Cantaloupe	½ (477 g)	82	682	33	21.00
Cherries	100 g	70	191	2	96.00
Coconut	100 g	346	256	23	11.00
Cranberries	100 g	46	82	2	41.00
Dates	10 pieces (80 g)	219	518	1	520.00
Grapefruit	1 med. (400 g)	80	265	2	130.00
Grapes	10 pieces (40 g)	18	42	1	42.00
Olives, green	100 g	116	55	2400	0.02
Orange	1 med. (180 g)	64	263	1	260.00
Peach	1 (175 g)	58	308	2	150.00
Pear	1 (180 g)	100	213	3	71.00
Pineapple	1 slice (84 g)	44	123	1	120.00
Plantain	1 med. (365 g)	313	1012	13	77.00
Plums	10 med. (110 g)	66	299	2	150.00

Food	Portion Size	Calories/ Portion	K Content (mg)	Na Content (mg)	K/Na (mg/mg)
Raisins	1 Tbsp. (9 g)	26	69	2	34.00
Strawberries	1 cup (149 g)	55	244	1	240.00
Watermelon	100 g	26	100	1	100.00

Meats/Poultry

Bacon	1 slice (15 g)	86	35	153	0.23
Beef, ground	3.5 oz. (100 g)	287	270	60	4.50
Beef, rib roast	1 piece (85 g)	374	189	41	4.60
*Bologna (beef)**	1 slice (23 g)	72	36	230	0.16
Chicken	2 pieces (50 g)	83	206	32	6.40
Egg	1 med. (50 g)	72	57	54	1.10
Ham	2 pieces (85 g)	318	220	48	4.60
Hot dog	1 (45 g)	139	99	495	0.20
Lamb chop	3.4 oz. (95 g)	341	234	51	4.60
Liver, beef, cooked	100 g	229	380	184	2.10
Liver, chicken, cooked	100 g	165	151	61	2.50
Pork chop	3 oz. (85 g)	308	233	51	4.60
Pork sausage	1 patty (27 g)	129	73	259	0.28
Steak, sirloin	8 oz. (226 g)	876	583	127	4.60
Veal cutlet	3 oz. (85 g)	184	258	56	4.60
Veal breast	8 oz. (226 g)	684	471	103	4.60

Milk Products

Cheese, American	1 slice (14 g)	52	11	159	0.07
Cheese, cheddar	1 slice (24 g)	96	20	168	0.12
Cheese, cottage	1 oz. (28 g)	30	24	65	0.37
Cheese, cream	1 Tbsp. (14 g)	52	10	35	0.29
Cheese, Swiss	1 slice (14 g)	52	15	99	0.15
unsalted	1 slice (14 g)	52	15	6	2.50
Cream, light	1 Tbsp. (15 g)	32	18	6	3.00
Cream, heavy	1 Tbsp. (15 g)	53	13	5	2.60
Ice cream	1 cup (133 g)	257	241	84	2.90
Milk, skim	1 cup (245 g)	88	355	127	2.80
Milk, whole	1 cup (244 g)	161	342	122	2.80
Yogurt, skim milk	1 cup (245 g)	123	350	125	2.80
Goat milk	1 cup (244 g)	163	439	83	5.30
Human milk	1 cup (244 g)	188	124	39	3.20

Food	Portion Size	Calories/ Portion	K Content (mg)	Na Content (mg)	K/Na (mg/mg)
Miscellaneous					
Almonds	100 g	598	773	4	190.00
Honey	100 g	304	51	5	10.00
Maple syrup*	5 Tbsp. (100 g)	252	176	10	17.60
Peanut butter	100 g	589	627	605	1.00
Peanuts, unsalted	100 g	582	701	5	140.00
Pecans	100 g	687	603	trace	600.00
Walnuts, English	100 g	651	450	2	225.00
Prepared Food					
*Burrito, beef (Taco Bell)**	184 g	466	320	327	0.98
Chicken chow mein, canned	100 g	38	167	290	0.58
*Chicken chow mein, frzn. din. (Banquet)**	12 oz. (340 g)	282	241	2268	0.11
*Chicken, drumstick (Kentucky Fried Chicken)**	47 g	117	122	207	0.59
Corned beef hash	100 g	181	200	540	0.37
*Fried shrimp (Arthur Treacher)**	115 g	381	99	537	0.18
*Hamburger (Burger King)**	110 g	290	240	525	0.46
*Hamburger (McDonald's)**	102 g	255	142	520	0.27
*Lasagna, cheese, frzn. (Stouffers)**	10 + oz. (298 g)	385	580	1200	0.48
Pizza, sausage	100 g	245	114	647	0.18
*Salisbury steak, 3 course frzn. din. (Swanson)**	16 oz. (45 g)	490	545	1680	0.32
Turkey pot pie	100 g	197	114	369	0.31
Vegetables (fresh when not specified)					
Asparagus	4 spears (100 g)	26	278	2	140.00

Food	Portion Size	Calories/ Portion	K Content (mg)	Na Content (mg)	K/Na (mg/mg)
(cooked, no salt)	100 g	20	183	1	180.00
Beans, green	100 g	25	151	4	38.00
(canned)	100 g	18	95	236	0.40
Beans, kidney	100 g	118	340	3	110.00
(cooked from dry)					
*(canned)**	⅖ cup (100 g)	90	264	300	.88
Beans, lima	100 g	111	422	1	420.00
Beans, navy (dry)	100 g	340	1196	19	63.00
Beans, pinto (dry)	100 g	349	984	10	98.00
Beans, yellow wax	100 g	22	151	3	50.00
Beets	100 g	32	208	43	4.80
(canned)	100 g	34	167	236	0.71
Broccoli	100 g	32	382	15	25.00
Brussels sprouts	100 g	45	390	14	28.00
Cabbage	100 g	24	233	20	12.00
(cooked)	100 g	20	163	14	12.00
Carrots	100 g	31	222	33	6.70
Cauliflower	100 g	27	295	13	23.00
(cooked)	100 g	22	206	9	23.00
Celery	100 g	17	341	126	2.70
Corn, sweet	1 ear (140 g)	70	151	1	151.00
(canned)	100 g	83	97	230	0.42
Cucumber	100 g	15	160	6	27.00
Eggplant	100 g	19	150	1	150.00
Green pepper	100 g	22	213	13	16.00
Lentils (dry)	100 g	340	790	30	26.00
Lettuce, iceberg	100 g	13	175	9	19.00
Lettuce, leaf	100 g	18	264	9	29.00
Mushrooms	100 g	28	414	15	28.00
(canned)	100 g	17	197	400	0.49
Onions, cooked	100 g	29	110	7	16.00
Peas, cooked	1 cup (160 g)	114	314	2	160.00
Peas, canned	100 g	77	96	236	0.41
Pickles, dill	100 g	11	200	1428	0.14
Potato, baked	1 med. (202 g)	145	782	6	130.00
Sauerkraut	100 g	18	140	747	0.19
(canned)					

Food	Portion Size	Calories/ Portion	K Content (mg)	Na Content (mg)	K/Na (mg/mg)
Soy beans (dry)	100 g	403	1677	5	340.00
Spinach	100 g	26	470	71	6.60
Squash, acorn	100 g	55	480	1	480.00
Squash, zucchini	100 g	12	141	1	140.00
Sweet potato, baked	100 g	114	243	10	24.00
Tomato	1 med. (135 g)	27	300	4	75.00
(canned)	100 g	21	217	130	1.67

Table information adapted from: Watt, B. K., and A. L. Merrill, *Composition of Foods*, Agriculture Handbook No. 8, U.S. Department of Agriculture, U.S. Printing Office, Washington, D.C., 1975; Adams, C. F., *Nutritive Value of American Foods in Common Units*, Agriculture Handbook No. 456, U.S. Department of Agriculture, U.S. Government Printing Office, Washington, D.C., 1975; and J. A. T. Pennington and H. Nichols Church, *Food Values of Portions Commonly Used*, 14th ed., New York: Harper & Row, 1985. The values for the food items with a * came from this third reference. We recommend this book for readers who wish additional information on food values. We thank Harper & Row and the authors, J. Pennington and H. Nichols Church, for allowing us to use their copyrighted material.

If you are eating mainly foods that are boldfaced in the table, you probably don't need to calculate your *K Factor*. But if you eat some major regular type or italicized items, your *K Factor* could drop below 3.

We will give you two examples of calculating your *K Factor*. First let's consider a cheese sandwich lunch. We can calculate the *K Factor* of this lunch by making a table of the ingredients (remember, K = potassium, Na = sodium):

Notice that in the version of this lunch with a dill pickle made with our recipe, the *K Factor* is 2.1, even though commercial salted bread was used. If unsalted whole wheat bread had been used, dropping the two-slice amount of sodium from 264 to about 2 mg, the lunch's *K Factor* would have been 5.7. However, 2.1 isn't bad, as the *K Factor* for the day could still be kept above 3 by eating a healthy breakfast and dinner.

But suppose you were to sneak in a commercial dill pickle

TABLE 5.

Item	K (mg)	Na (mg)	*K Factor* (K/Na)
2 slices commercial whole-wheat bread	136	264	0.52
1 slice unsalted Swiss cheese	15	6	2.5
1 tablespoon unsalted eggless mayonnaise (data from label)	34	13	2.6
2 leaves lettuce (10 g)	18	1	18
1 glass skim milk (8 oz)	355	127	2.8
1 apple	152	1	150
1 large dill pickle, our recipe	180	6	30
Totals	890	418	
K Factor			2.1

instead of the pickle from our recipe. After all, every ingredient but the bread has a *K Factor* well above 2. The commercial dill pickle should do little harm, right? Let's take a look:

TABLE 6.

Item	K (mg)	Na (mg)	*K Factor* (K/Na)
2 slices commercial whole-wheat bread	136	264	0.52
1 slice unsalted Swiss cheese	15	6	2.5
1 tablespoon unsalted eggless mayonnaise	34	13	2.6
2 leaves lettuce (10 g)	18	1	18
1 glass skim milk (8 oz)	355	127	2.8
1 apple	152	1	150
1 large commercial dill pickle	*200*	*1428*	*0.14*
Totals	910	1840	
K Factor			0.49

Quite a bit of harm was done just by that pickle! The huge amount of sodium in the pickle shot the sodium total so high that the *K Factor* for the whole lunch is now only 0.49. You sabotage the entire meal just by eating one pickle. Now it would be extremely difficult to bring the day's *K Factor* above 3 even with a very good breakfast and dinner.

The important point here is that you cannot just estimate the overall *K Factor* by averaging the individual *K Factor(s)*. You have to divide the *total* potassium by the *total* sodium in order to determine the overall *K Factor*.

Now let's consider an entire day. Suppose it looks like this:

TABLE 7.

Item	K (mg)	Na (mg)	*K Factor* (K/Na)
Breakfast	1572	204	7.7
Lunch	1065	1016	1.0
Snack	159	1	159.0
Dinner	3137	156	20.1
Totals	5933	1377	
K Factor			4.3

Notice that the overall *K Factor* for the day is a healthy 4.3.

But suppose it's Friday and you decide to celebrate by having a commercial pizza for dinner instead of the lentil casserole and squash dinner you had originally planned. Table 8 shows what happens to the *K Factor* for the day.

In this example, the beer-and-pizza dinner, considered by itself, had a very unhealthy *K Factor* of 0.37:

Item	K (mg)	Na (mg)	*K Factor* (K/Na)
1/2 sausage pizza (200 g)	228	1294	0.18
Two 12-oz. beers	256	12	21.3
Totals	484	1306	
K Factor			0.37

The pizza-beer fling brought the *K Factor* for the entire day down to 1.3, from the menu plan value of 4.3. By changing canned chunky chicken soup for lunch to a low-salt soup, you could bring the *K Factor* up to 1.8. Since 1.8 is a much healthier *K Factor* than most people eat, you might allow yourself a pizza once in a rare while if your other meals for the day are very healthy ones. (A better alternative, though, is to make your own

TABLE 8.

Item	K (mg)	Na (mg)	K Factor (K/Na)
Breakfast	1572	204	7.7
Lunch	1065	1016	1.0
Snack	159	1	159.0
1/2 sausage pizza (200 g)	*228*	*1294*	*0.18*
Two 12-oz. beers	*256*	*12*	*21.3*
Totals	3280	2527	
K Factor			1.3

pizza, without adding salt, using less cheese, and putting on green peppers, onions, and/or mushrooms instead of sausage. Use unsalted tomato paste and spice it up!)

Estimating Your K Factor from Urine Samples

We have provided space on your progress sheet for recording your *K Factor*. But even if the *K Factor* in your food is high enough, you might blow it by getting sodium from another source, such as by drinking water from a water softener or from some over-the-counter drug. Or perhaps you are eating lots of foods that aren't in the table and you're not sure about the *K Factor*.

Well, there is another way to keep track of your *K Factor*, although it's somewhat inconvenient. You can collect your urine for a twenty-four-hour period and take it to your doctor or medical laboratory for a potassium and sodium analysis.

To collect a twenty-four-hour urine sample, you'll need a clean, 1-gallon plastic bottle. In it you must collect every drop of urine you produce over a twenty-four-hour period. Here's how to do it.

When you get up in the morning, completely empty your bladder into the toilet as usual. This way you get rid of the previous day's urine and start fresh for the new day. From then on, you need to collect *all* your urine in the bottle. It will be hard to remember. If you're at home, place the bottle on the toilet seat to remind yourself. If it's a workday, keep the bottle (in a bag if you wish) somewhere where it will remind you, and tie a string on your finger.

Continue to collect every drop of urine through the evening and night. When you get up the next morning, completely empty your bladder *into the bottle*. You now have a twenty-four-hour urine sample.

Take this to your doctor or medical lab to have it analyzed to determine how much sodium and potassium you excrete in your urine over a twenty-four-hour period. This will be approximately equal to the amount you are eating per day. (Actually it's a little less, since small amounts are lost in the stool and in sweat. If you sweated a *lot* during the twenty-four-hour period, make a note of it, as the lab may want to correct for the estimated loss of sodium and potassium in your sweat (see Chapter 21).

Since your eating habits are likely to be different on weekdays than they are on weekends, we recommend you collect samples for analysis from each of these periods.

Monitoring Potassium

One simple step that can sometimes indicate if your body is deficient in potassium is to ask your physician to have your blood potassium level measured.

Unfortunately, however, this doesn't always give you the information you need. If the level is between 4 and 5 milliequivalents per liter (the upper limit of normal), you still may or may not have enough potassium in your body. Why can't you be certain? What you need to know is the level of potassium in your cells, not your blood, and it is possible to have sufficient amounts in the blood but not in the cells.

On the other hand, if the blood level is low (below 4 milliequivalents per liter), you may have a problem. The level of potassium in the blood seldom drops unless your body cells are deficient. If it is below the accepted "normal" limit of 3.5 milliequivalents per liter, you can be sure the cell level is low as well.

Thus a blood test cannot assure you that your *K Factor* is high enough, but it can indicate a problem.

CHAPTER 14

Keep Track of Your Exercise

On the progress chart, we have provided space for you to enter the number of times each week you have vigorously (and continuously) exercised for at least 20 minutes, for 20 to 30 minutes, and for over 30 minutes.

Your pulse rate, taken upon awakening, is an easy measure of your progress in the exercise program. Take your pulse before sitting up or getting out of bed. Count the pulses in your wrist or neck for 30 seconds and multiply by 2.

Please review Chapter 11 for our recommendations about exercise.

CHAPTER 15

Keep Track of Your Weight

Because of variations in the amount of water in your body during the day, it is best to check your weight at the same time each day, without clothes. Be sure the scale is accurate.

If your weight is normal, a weekly check will ensure that you don't start to gain. But if you use the principles we have outlined for choosing and preparing your food (see Chapter 10) and get at least some regular exercise (see Chapter 11), you shouldn't have any trouble maintaining normal weight.

If you are overweight, our program should help you reduce gradually. If it doesn't, cut your calories by a quarter and be especially careful to eat as little fat as possible (see Chapter 12). A loss of about one or at most two pounds per week is realistic *and* better than the more rapid loss that you could get by severe calorie restriction. If it seems you need to make a conscious effort to reduce calories in ways other than by reducing your dietary fat intake, get the advice of your doctor or a nutritionist before restricting your calories to less than 1,200 per day.

CHAPTER 16
Keep Track of Your Blood Pressure

Measuring your own blood pressure at home is easy, and you really should do it if you want to make sure your blood pressure is getting—and staying—down within the "normal" range. Furthermore, keeping track of your own progress is an excellent way to stay motivated to cure your hypertension. The feedback you get will encourage you to get or keep your *K Factor* high, your dietary fat low, your weight normal, and your exercise patterns regular.

In this chapter, we'll discuss the equipment you will need as well as explain how to check its reliability and how to use it.

Here is a diagram of the circulatory system, showing how a blood pressure cuff is used to measure the blood pressure inside the artery in your arm.

The small diameter arterioles the blood has to pass through before reaching the capillaries should remind you of the "nozzle" in our "hose" drawing in Chapter 6.

.

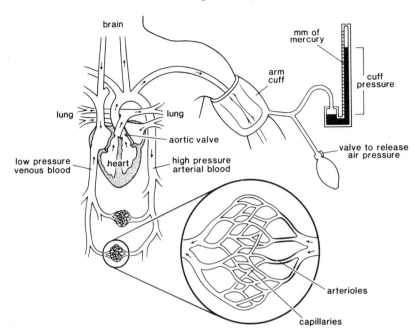

FIGURE 20. *The circulatory system and a blood pressure cuff.*

Getting the Right Equipment

First you need to get the right equipment for measuring your own blood pressure. You need some kind of *blood pressure cuff* and, if the cuff does not have a built-in listening device, a *stethoscope.* You can obtain both devices in a "blood pressure kit," or you may buy them separately.

The Blood Pressure Cuff

The blood pressure cuff is made of cloth with a rubber bladder sewn inside. This bladder is attached by rubber tubing to (1) a rubber bulb with a one-way valve (like the heart, so that repeatedly squeezing the bulb pumps air into the bladder), (2) an adjustable release valve for letting the air out of the bladder, and

(3) a device for measuring the air pressure inside the bladder. The measuring device itself can be one of the following:

○ A mechanical dial.
○ A column of mercury in a calibrated glass tube.
○ An electronic pressure sensor with a digital display.

The most inexpensive cuffs are the dial type (you can buy a reasonably good one for under $30).

If you buy the dial type, you will need to check its accuracy by comparing it with your doctor's cuff (see the next section). The mercury type, more expensive and more likely to break, is more reliably accurate; it is probably the type your doctor has.

The new electronic automatic type has a built-in microphone, eliminating the need for a stethoscope. The systolic and diastolic blood pressure appear on a digital display. Some cost under $100. George recently purchased an electronic digital blood pressure monitor by mail order for $49.95 and has found it to be very accurate and reliable. It not only displays systolic and diastolic pressures, but it also displays pulse rate. The air pressure release valve has two positions: a slow release (which you adjust with a screwdriver to 2 or 3 mm Hg per second) and a rapid release.

Cuffs come in three sizes. Before you rush out to the medical supply store, use a tape measure to determine the circumference of (the distance around) the midsection of your upper arm. This is the only way you can decide which size to get.

ARM CIRCUMFERENCE	CUFF SIZE
6.5–10 inches	small adult cuff
9.5–12.5 inches	standard adult cuff
12.5–16.5 inches	large adult cuff

It is important to get the right size cuff, since the wrong one will give you incorrect readings. Since it's a nuisance to keep more than one size cuff on hand, even doctors sometimes make the mistake of using the wrong size. For example, suppose you have a large muscular (or fat) arm, measuring fifteen inches around. A standard cuff is not wide enough to transfer the full amount of pressure that is inside the cuff to the tissues surrounding the artery in your arm. You would need to pump in more air to collapse the artery, so that the reading you get will be too high. It could be as much as 30 mm Hg too high! Thus there are some people who are being treated for high blood pressure who don't really have it; they just have big arms!

The Stethoscope

The stethoscope brings the sounds of blood pulsing through your arm's artery to your ears through rubber or plastic tubing. A stethoscope costs only about $5, and some blood pressure kits come with one. There are two types: one has a bell-shape end for collecting the sound; the other has a thin plastic diaphragm. Either type will work, but we prefer the bell-shape type.

Checking the Accuracy of Your Equipment

Considering that there are all kinds of cuffs, it is important that you make sure you are getting the same readings your doctor is getting. Check its accuracy against your doctor's mercury type, especially if you have the dial type. You can connect the two with a Y-shape tubing connector. Sometimes the two cuffs can have a discrepancy of as much as 5 percent. You can correct for this if you know about it. Your readings will be misleading if you don't.

If you have the electronic type, there is the possibility of error from variations in the position of the microphone. When the microphone is not over the artery, you usually get diastolic pressure readings that are too high (or you may get an error signal). Again, you should compare your instrument's reading with the reading your doctor obtains. George compared his electronic cuff system with a mercury type and was pleased to find almost perfect agreement.

Taking the Measurement

You should be completely relaxed, both mentally and physically, before your blood pressure is measured. You should be in a warm, quiet room, seated in a comfortable chair beside a table of some kind. All your muscles should be as relaxed as possible, and you should not talk. (You may be pleasantly surprised to find that your blood pressure measured at home is lower than the reading obtained in your doctor's office. If you know that your equipment measures the same as your doctor's, or if you have corrected for any discrepancy, your lower home reading is probably because you aren't nervous or worried, as you may have been in the doctor's office. Chapter 6 explains how your sympathetic nervous system, activated by being nervous or worried, constricts your arterioles [small arteries], thus raising your blood pressure.) In the less likely event that your home readings are higher than your doctor's, you should schedule an appointment with the doctor and take in your cuff to figure out why.

Getting back to your home measurement, rest your arm on the table that is beside the chair you are sitting in (so that the middle of the cuff will be even with the level of your heart, thus eliminating "hydrostatic" pressure). Your palm should face up. Wrap the cuff around your bare arm and fasten it so that it is snug but not tight. The lower edge should be about one inch above the bend of your elbow (to allow room for the stethoscope over the artery). The arrow on the cuff should be pointing approximately to where your artery is—aimed slightly toward your torso from the middle of the upward surface of your arm, just above the bend at your elbow. Find out exactly where it is by feeling the pulse with your fingers. If you have an electronic cuff, place the circle showing the location of the microphone directly over the artery where you feel your pulse.

If you do not have an electronic cuff, place the end of your stethoscope on your skin over the artery just below the cuff. Apply very light pressure on the head of the stethoscope, just barely firm enough to make even contact with your skin.

By squeezing the bulb, inflate the cuff to a pressure about 40 mm Hg higher than your last systolic reading in order to collapse the artery completely. You will not hear any sound through the stethoscope at this time because all blood flow to your lower arm has been cut off.

Now gradually (at a rate of 2 or 3 mm Hg per second) let the air out of the bladder by turning the screw at the end of the bulb to open the pressure release valve. Or, if you have a "two-position" air release valve, make sure it is in the slow release position before you pump up the cuff. When you can hear a beating sound (as little spurts of blood begin to open the artery again), take a reading of the pressure. This is your systolic blood pressure. (The electronic cuff gives you this reading automatically.)

As the air pressure in the cuff continues to drop, you will continue to hear rhythmic beating sounds in the stethoscope. (Some electronic types make a beeping sound.) The artery is now open when the heart beats, but it is still collapsing between beats because the cuff pressure is greater than the diastolic blood pressure.

As soon as the beating sounds first disappear (the artery is open continuously), take your second pressure reading: this is the diastolic blood pressure. (Again, the electronic cuff gives you this reading automatically.) After diastolic pressure is reached, you may switch to rapid air release to relieve the pressure on your arm. You have now measured your blood pressure.

Repeat the measurement after five minutes. Take your blood pressure on at least two different days a week and record the lowest of the readings on the progress chart.

CHAPTER 17
Keep Track of Your Dietary Fat

In addition to keeping track of your *K Factor*, you will also need to watch the amount of fat you eat. As we discussed in Part III, this will help you lose weight as well as reduce atherosclerosis and decrease your chances of having a heart attack or of developing cancer.

Since fat has about 9 calories per gram, you can calculate what percentage of your calories is from fat with the following formula:

$$\frac{9 \times \text{fat}}{\text{calories}} \times 100$$

For example, if the label on a package of ice cream says there are 9 grams of fat and 160 calories per serving, you would do the following calculation:

$$\frac{9 \times 9}{160} \times 100 \text{ or } \frac{81}{160} \times 100 \text{ or } 0.51 \times 100$$

or 51 percent. You now know that 51 percent of the calories in the ice cream come from fat. Try this calculation on some dairy product substitutes. You may be surprised to find that most nondairy creamers and some nondairy ice cream substitutes are loaded with fat.

As we have said, you should keep your daily fat consumption down to less than 20 percent of your calories. The rest of your calories should come from carbohydrates and protein.

The currently recommended minimum protein consumption is 56 grams per day. You will stay healthy and keep your kidneys happy if most of your calories come from complex carbohydrates.

Using the Progress Chart

On page 269 is a sample progress chart; a blank chart for your use has been included as an appendix (see pages 408 and 409).

The first line of the chart is for recording your blood pressure. We suggest that you measure it twice each day on at least two days each week, and measure it at least twice in a row. On the chart, record the lowest of all the readings.

When you enter your *K Factor*, you will usually have to estimate your average for the week from your diet. This will be easy while you are following our menu plan. During the transition week, the *K Factor* averages 1.9, during the first week of the permanent plan (days 8–14) the average is 4.9, during the next week (days 15–22) the average is 5.6, and during the last week of the menu plan the *K Factor* averages 6.6. If you have a determination of the *K Factor* in your urine, then during a particular week use that value and indicate with a "U" on the chart. Where the chart says drugs, write the names of prescription drugs you're taking, and use a horizontal arrow to indicate the time span.

A central theme of this book is participation with your doctor and, of course, we have already participated by writing the book. But to close the circle, we are offering *you* the chance to participate also.

We would appreciate your help in building a data base on the results of the *K Factor* program. If you wish to participate, after completing 14 weeks and recording the results on the chart, photocopy it and mail it along with any shopping tips or other suggestions you may have. If you miss a week here and there, leave those weeks blank. In order to help us verify the reports, have your physician sign it and include his printed name and address. Then mail the form to:

K Factor
P.O. Box 253
Warren, VT 05674

If you have a micro-computer with a modem (either 300, 1200, or 2400 baud) you can enter your results directly in to our computer, which will be on-line 24 hours a day, by having your micro-computer dial (802) 496-4862

You are also encouraged to send in, either typewritten or through your micro-computer, any suggestions or recipes you may want to share. The best ones, in our judgment, will be maintained, along with recognition to you, in our computer's memory. Then those of you who choose to can use your micro-computer to obtain—free of charge—shopping tips, recipes, ideas, suggestions, or other results from other readers of *The K Factor*.

By communicating with us in either of these two ways, you will not only be helping yourself, but others. By working together, we can hasten the day when high blood pressure will no longer be the problem it is today.

As a sample, two weeks are filled out on the facing page. Again, please see the Appendix for a blank chart you can use.

Progress Chart

Age __50__   Initial weight __168__   Height __6'0"__   Sex __male__

Week	1	2	3	4	5	6	7	8	9	10	11	12
Blood Pressure Systolic		138								127		
Diastolic		87								82		
Pulse upon awakening		64								58		
Weight (lbs.)		166								163		
Number of workouts (aerobic exercise)												
less than 20 minutes		2								2		
20 to 30 minutes												
greater than 30 minutes		1								2		
K Factor (K/Na ratio)		0.5(u)								4.4		
Serum K (mEq./liter)		3.8								4.1		
Drugs							Diuril					

PART FIVE
Why Drugs?

One of the most highly developed skills in contemporary Western civilization is dissection: the split-up of problems into their smallest possible components. We are good at it. So good, we often forget to put the pieces back together again.

—Alvin Toffler[1]

271

CHAPTER 18

The Emphasis on Drugs

We often miss the forest for the trees. Antihypertensive drugs usually do get high blood pressure down, and in moderate and severe hypertension, they do protect against death. But the drugs don't improve the death rate in mild cases of hypertension, and they appear to do harm in borderline cases. In addition, the drugs make almost everyone feel bad and cost the country billions of dollars each year. Thus the drug approach to treating high blood pressure can hardly be called a howling success. Given what we now know, this isn't too surprising. As long as we didn't have much insight into the mechanism of hypertension, drugs could only be developed to treat the blood pressure rather than the underlying problem.

Now it's time to put the pieces together again. But first let's ask how a whole society, professionals and laypersons alike, could have gone so far down a path that missed the mark so badly.

In the 1950s, the decade of the "miracle drugs," the time was ripe for acceptance of drugs as the answer to any condition for which the cause wasn't known. And we really didn't understand what was going on in primary hypertension. This is revealed in the term itself: Health professionals use the term *primary* to describe a condition for which they don't know the cause; if they know its cause, they call it *secondary*.

A personal example illustrates this almost automatic reliance upon drugs. In 1957, Dick worked with a group doing research on a drug that inhibited cholesterol in food from being absorbed from the intestine into the blood, thereby helping to prevent heart attacks. At the time, the thought entered his mind that it might be easier simply to eat foods that didn't contain cholesterol. Had he known that only animal products (meat, milk, and egg yolks), not fruits or vegetables, contain cholesterol, this thought might have been more than a passing one, but he had been told that diet just wasn't a practical way to treat people, since they wouldn't follow it. So, like so many others, he fell back in line and returned to research on a drug to treat a nutritional problem. The moral: When everyone is marching in a given direction, it's hard to go the other way.

But can the explanation for the almost unquestioning belief in drugs simply be our enthusiasm for "miracle" drugs? We think the reason lies deeper, in the basic assumptions of Western—especially American—culture. As Pogo used to say, the problem is not them (the medical establishment and drug companies), but us—all of us.

The Technology Myth

Like other people, doctors and scientists are products of their culture. Since American society values pragmatism so much, even in the highly theoretical science of physics, American scientists are more pragmatic and somewhat less inclined toward theoretical approaches than are their European counterparts. Furthermore, the American culture has also emphasized activism, optimism, and a belief we inherited from the seventeenth-century thinker Francis Bacon: that nature can be, and should be, dominated. This cultural background, this Baconian view, has until recently reinforced our notion that technology can solve all our problems.

Our society has been mesmerized by technology, which we often confuse (even in our schools) with science. The overuse of the phrase *science and technology* has led, in the minds of many, to the confusion that the two are the same. We have forgotten that science is the discovery of *insight* into nature, whereas technology is only an *application* of science. Unless we keep our focus upon the *insight* that science can give into the whole system (as emphasized in the "new" scientific paradigm discussed in the next chapter), the application of science—technology—could produce an effect opposite to what we desire. Examples abound, ranging from the use of lead in paint and gasoline and the widespread application of DDT to the use of drugs to treat everyone with high blood pressure.

In our view, the excessive dependence on drugs in the treatment of hypertension, especially borderline cases, is not based upon basic scientific understanding. It does not take into account the whole picture. It results in part from blind faith in technology and from our belief that the purpose of science is to bend nature to our will, to dominate it rather than to understand it, cooperate with it, and find ways to live in harmony with it.

Consistent with the Baconian view that total control over nature is possible was the development, around the turn of the century, of the chemist Paul Ehrlich's "magic bullet" concept. Ehrlich, sometimes called the father of the pharmaceutical industry, sold the notion that we could have drugs that not only would find their way, as if by magic, to the desired site in the body, but, like bullets, would not affect anything other than the desired target. We could thus control not only the rest of nature but ourselves also—the ultimate in better living through chemistry!

In an article on the ethics of hypertension, scholars at Columbia University have commented on this cultural bias toward technology and the resultant use of drugs to treat borderline cases of hypertension.[2]

It is, we believe, an instance in the medical domain of the more general phenomenon of technological optimism—the disposition to employ technologies in the belief that the benefits that flow from them will outweigh whatever unforeseen and undesirable effects ensue, and that these effects will themselves be manageable by existing or potential technological means. . . . Among physicians, technological optimism is conjoined with and bolsters a disposition toward therapeutic activism. When making decisions under conditions of uncertainty (whether [blood] pressure will rise or fall without treatment), physicians prefer to take the risk of treating when intervention may not be called for to the potential error of not treating when treatment is needed.

Whether or not they are magic, drugs are certainly high tech. So in a culture mesmerized by technology, reliance upon drugs was a natural first reaction.

As an example of "the belief that . . . whatever unforeseen and undesirable effects ensue . . . these effects will themselves be manageable by existing or potential technological means," we now have drugs to treat the side effects of antihypertensive drugs. When we find ourselves using drugs to treat the effects of drugs, maybe we've gone too far. Maybe we should reexamine the game plan.

Sue-Happy, Pill-Happy Americans

Once incorporated not only into the education but into the culture in which doctors find themselves, the tendency toward technological activism is bolstered by legal considerations. A lot of doctors in private practice are skeptical about using these drugs to treat hypertension, but they're often afraid *not* to give them. Regardless of the treatment—or lack of treatment—used for any condition, it is still possible for patients to get worse or even die. Life is never certain. But it's a good bet that many physicians have had nightmares of a lawyer saying, "You mean, doctor, that the deceased had hypertension and you didn't even prescribe medicine?"

In our present culture, the best way for a doctor to protect himself or herself against unjustified malpractice suits is to follow conventional, accepted methods of treatment—even if the doctor has reason to believe that other alternatives may be better. Americans are so "sue happy" that doctors are often afraid to try anything new or different.

And patients *demand* drugs. If they have the flu, many of them demand a shot or a pill even if they've been told it won't do any good. In this busy world, Americans who don't feel well tend to say, "Give me a pill to make me feel better." The poor doc is bombarded not only by salespeople from drug companies but by patients demanding pills.

Pogo was right! We *all* created the drug culture. And the drug culture, together with a distorted view of the true meaning of *science*, created the drug-treatment approach to hypertension. So it is understandable that the dramatic ability that thiazide diuretics sometimes have in lowering blood pressure, as well as their apparent relative safety, led rapidly to the incorporation of these drugs as a foundation of the treatment of high blood pressure. After the thiazide diuretics were introduced in 1957, dietary approaches seldom received much attention. The pill had won—but we didn't.

The Dietary Approach—High Science but Low Tech

But what about the dietary approaches up to that time? Why hadn't they caught on? It frequently happens that the early pioneers of a new idea are ignored. Nowhere is this more striking than in the use of a dietary approach for high blood pressure treatment.

By 1957, when the first potent drugs for hypertension were introduced, the ability of dietary changes to lower elevated blood pressure had been demonstrated time and again. Such early pioneers as Ambard and Beaujard in France and Allen, Addison, and Priddle in the United States had demonstrated that either decreasing sodium or increasing potassium in the diet can cure high blood pressure. And Dr. Walter Kempner of Duke University had shown hundreds of times that his rice-fruit diet could return blood pressure to normal. These pioneering investigators—and more recently Dahl, Page, Tobian, and others—had the right idea, but they couldn't get anyone to listen. Reflecting their frustration, in 1972, Dr. Lewis Dahl, discussing Kempner's rice-fruit diet and his own studies of a high–*K Factor* diet, stated:

For reasons that are difficult to fathom, there appeared a great deal of antipathy to Kempner's reports as well as irrational disbelief in the effectiveness of the diet. . . . I have often felt that we became heirs to the antipathies originally directed at Allen and later at Kempner. We decided, nonetheless, to try to detect the dietary factor that made this diet effective. For those of you who are unfamiliar with the diet, let me define it as a low sodium, or a high potassium, or a high carbohydrate, or a low protein, or a low fat, or a high fluid diet. In its pristine form it is made up mostly of rice and fruit including juices, but certainly with no added salt (NaCl).[3]

Why were these successful dietary approaches so widely rejected? Dr. Dahl has pointed out that until the thiazide diuretics were introduced, very few physicians thought sodium had much to do with hypertension. Dahl had suggested that one reason for the skepticism about the importance of sodium is that even when they were urged to do so, very few patients had succeeded in reducing their sodium intake to a low enough level to obtain an antihypertensive effect. He suggested the following reasons for this failure:

(1) To palates accustomed since infancy to saltiness, the absence of salt is at first distressing. Substitution of herbs and seasonings other than salt requires a modicum of intelligence, imagination, and determination. (2) Most low sodium diets are prescribed haphazardly and unenthusiastically. (3) Even when prescribed by authoritative sources like the American Heart Association, these diets are so complex as to discourage all but the most persistent. (4) Most patients are unaware of . . . the added NaCl in most processed foods.

With the introduction of the diuretic chlorothiazide in 1957, both patients and physicians found its antihypertensive effects more convenient than dietary approaches. Skepticism about the role of dietary sodium persists today. But Dr. Lou Tobian has pointed out that every time these physicians use a diuretic, they "cast a vote for sodium" as a cause of hypertension, since these drugs act by causing the body to lose sodium through the kidneys.

But why were dietary changes prescribed "haphazardly and unenthusiastically"? Most physicians have neither the time, the inclination, nor the background to educate their patients about nutrition and exercise. As far back as 1963, the American Medical Association's Council on Foods and Nutrition stated that "medical education and medical practice have not kept abreast of advances in nutrition." In spite of the fact that nutrition is involved in both the cause and the treatment of diabetes and cancer as well as hypertension, the majority of medical schools still do not require a course dealing specifically with nutrition. Since nutrition is not usually part of their education, future physicians tend to ignore dietary approaches and view them as suspect and "unscientific." Accordingly they aren't prepared to believe in the importance of nutrition in hypertension, let alone to realize that the necessary changes are *not*, in fact, "so complex as to discourage all but the most persistent." Instead, they are trained to believe in drugs and they learn how to get patients to use them.

But why did even most nutritionists miss the importance of the *K Factor*? We suggest that even more important than the lack of emphasis upon nutrition in training doctors was the fact that until recently, there was no "model," or concept, to explain how raising the ratio of potassium to sodium in the diet could reduce blood pressure.

Thomas Kuhn, a leading historian of science, has emphasized the essential importance of a concept, or paradigm, in the perception and evaluation of familiar information. Without a concept—some idea of how things work that enables us to believe they *can* work—we often do not "see" the reality behind the facts.

A good example is provided by Semmelweiss's discovery that death rates dropped when doctors who worked in the morgue washed their hands before examining women in the lying-in hospital. Although such washing greatly reduced mortality in the lying-in hospital, the procedure was not widely accepted. Only with the birth of the science of bacteriology and the recognition that germs, or bacteria, can "carry" disease did the logic of Semmelweiss's recommendation become apparent. When this was recognized, the practice urged by Semmelweiss rapidly became the standard.

So probably the reason that the dietary changes discovered by Allen, Addison, Kempner, and others (see chapters 4 and 20) were ignored is that in their time, there was no clearly accepted concept of how sodium and potassium work in the body. If you don't understand something, it's natural to ignore it. So sodium and potassium seemed unimportant; one seemed the same as the other, and their relation to blood pressure must have seemed as relevant as the tooth fairy.

The importance of nutrition and exercise has finally dawned on us. But now the situation has changed. Not only has the drug approach failed to help approximately half of those with primary hypertension, but due to years of basic biomedical research, we finally have a model for understanding the role of potassium, sodium, calcium, and magnesium in the cell (see Chapter 6).

It was this model, with its prediction that added potassium could help lower blood pressure, that led us into the study of hypertension. Moreover, the model provides us with some good leads as to how weight loss and exercise can help restore blood pressure to normal. Finally, and perhaps most important, the model indicates that elevated blood pressure is not the primary problem but is instead a consequence of an imbalance at the level of the living cell. Fortunately, in many people, this imbalance can be corrected by the natural means of proper nutrition, exercise, and weight loss.

Summary

The nutritional approach to primary hypertension was ignored not only because future doctors were not educated about nutrition but even more because of the lack of a concept that made it seem realistic. And the bias toward drugs was inevitable in a society that believed that technology could fix anything.

But now we realize that drugs affect only some of the *consequences* of this imbalance, such as retention of sodium or increased activity of the sympathetic nervous system, without correcting the imbalance itself.

Drugs may be "magic bullets," but in the case of primary hypertension, they miss the mark.

CHAPTER 19

How Science Works: Scientific Paradigm and Scientific "Proof"

There's a great deal of intimidation by intellectuals in this country of less intellectual people. It comes in the form of pompous studies and pompous words to describe ideas that are fairly simple or have very little content.
—Richard Feynman, *Surely You're Joking, Mr. Feynman*

We have tried to avoid pompous words in our explanation of the *K Factor* and the way it works. You have seen that the scientific ideas that led to the *K Factor* program are, at least in outline, fairly simple. And we are hopeful that you understood the evidence without too much trouble and that you realize it doesn't take an advanced degree to form a sound opinion for yourself.

But if the ideas are basically simple and if there is now so much evidence that nutritional changes coupled with moderate exercise can restore normal blood pressure in most people with primary hypertension, why hasn't this become standard treatment? Why are so many specialists in medicine still skeptical and unwilling to accept the approach as "proved"?

As we discussed in the last chapter, there are several reasons

281

the evidence for the nutritional approach has been ignored. This was partly due to our cultural biases, including a fascination with high tech (our "technology block") and our belief that through science, we can dominate nature.

And it has also been due, until recently, to the lack of a paradigm, or concept, about hypertension. But the reason the new view did not catch on was also connected to blocks that were inherited from a nineteenth-century scientific paradigm and accordingly to an oversimplified view of how science really works and what constitutes adequate scientific proof. To understand this further, we need to consider briefly how science works, including three related questions:

Exactly what is a paradigm and what is its importance?

What is the scientific "method"?

What is scientific "proof"?

How Science Really Works

Science is not done simply by the schoolbook recipe of making an observation, forming a hypothesis, and testing the hypothesis. True, these are involved, but only *after* a paradigm has been developed and accepted. In fact, the method and the criteria for "truth" depend upon the scientific paradigm of the time.

People of each new age like to think they are up to date, or modern. So we may chuckle, but we shouldn't be surprised or too complacent when we learn that a paper written in 1898 began with: "In the modern way of doing things. . . ." In order to focus upon the day-to-day practicalities, people in each age begin to take its paradigm for granted. They become unaware of this unquestioning acceptance; the assumptions of the age seem self-evident. But we should remember that in science, we never quite have the final answer. Rather, we proceed by a series of successive approximations. And every couple of centuries, science outgrows its existing overall paradigm, and a major *paradigm shift* occurs.

Until the beginning of this century, the only overall paradigm in science was that provided by what is called classical physics, the physics governed by laws described by Isaac Newton. But discoveries in physics during the early 1900s have caused science to begin to modify its overall paradigm to include views and concepts undreamt of by physicists of the last century. As we will show, these changes affect not only what is considered by science and how science is done, but also how people in general think about their world, themselves, and ultimately about their responsibilities.

What Is a Paradigm?

We've already pointed out that a paradigm is a concept, or a set of related concepts, that gives a framework within which we have some idea of how things work—and enables us to believe they can work. But let's consider this further. As David Edge of Edinburgh University points out, a paradigm influences the *way* science is done:

The notion of paradigm refers to conceptual frameworks *and often (tacit) rules of procedure. . . . Scientists perceive problems in terms of common concepts; they are agreed on their relative importance and difficulty, on* what techniques *are relevant to their solution, and on* what will count as a "solution" [or "proof"]. . . . *Within the paradigm, an expanding programme of research topics is defined, on which scientists can embark with reasonable expectation of success. A paradigm is then like an empty crossword puzzle. In a mature specialty, "normal science" consists of the ever more exact specification of the shape of the puzzle and its clues, and the steady infilling of its blank spaces.*[1]

The overall paradigm, then, is like a game. The scientific paradigm determines the rules by which science is done and by which scientific "truth" is evaluated. The paradigm influences where we focus our attention. It determines the *style* of our approach.

The Old Scientific Paradigm

In the old Copernican, or Newtonian, paradigm, the universe and everything in it—including living beings—is built of atoms that interact in a mechanical way. Unlike the parts of a living system, however, none of these atoms depends upon the others for their existence. Rather, in the old paradigm, the atoms were visualized as behaving like hard billiard balls, which exist independent of each other and interact in a totally predictable fashion. In other words, the universe was viewed as being composed of parts that interact in a completely deterministic manner. This is the image of a machine, with gears and levers leading to perfectly predictable behavior. As Johannes Kepler said in the seventeenth century, "The Universe is similar to a clock."

This mechanistic paradigm is not to be totally disregarded: in its day, it was very productive. Indeed, it works well, and always will, for explaining things such as the orbits of the planets and the trajectory of satellites and nuclear warheads.

By the 1600s, thinkers such as Descartes realized that the subtle, unpredictable aspects of life, including free will, could not fit into this paradigm. Therefore Descartes suggested that there are actually *two* aspects to reality: the realm of consciousness or spirit, and the realm of matter.

In this dualistic view of reality, it was easy to accept Bacon's assertion that man (spirit) should dominate nature (matter). Why not? A machine certainly can be dominated, controlled, or managed, and, in fact, most of us would agree that we should control machines; after all, we don't want to let machines get out of control. If nature is a machine, then dominating it is the only logical thing to do.

So the old classical paradigm, based upon the success of classical, or Newtonian, physics, paves the way to the Western emphasis upon technology as the answer to most questions. Given enough technique—enough sophisticated machines—we can bend nature to our will and build a better world. "Better living through chemistry"—and thus through drugs and through mechanical hearts.

For reasons that will be explained shortly, this classical paradigm has dominated medical education since 1910—even though we now know that it is insufficient and in some major ways misleading.

The New Scientific Paradigm

We are now well into a period in which the old paradigm is giving way to a newer view of how the universe works that is at once more sophisticated and more tested. At the deepest levels of science, the working philosophy has begun to shift to a more "modern" view, in which the universe is seen less as a machine and more as an interconnected web of events. Physicists now realize that the Copernican or Newtonian world view was only a first approximation of the workings of the universe. Nature may in some ways be *similar* to a machine, but in many other ways, it is something quite unlike a machine. And at the cutting edges of physics, this new paradigm is being extended and deepened to include not only the nonliving, or physical part of the universe, but the problems of consciousness and of life.

This shift in the main paradigm, or world view, of Western science began at the turn of the century with two scientific discoveries. One was the introduction by Einstein of the theory of relativity, which shows that two measurable "things," distance and time, which were previously thought to be quite separate, are in reality inseparably tied together. The other was the discovery in 1900 by Max Planck and then by Einstein in 1905 that energy cannot be endlessly divided but comes in tiny, indivisible "packets," or quanta, which, unlike waves, have the ability to cross the entire universe without being diminished in any way.

The discovery of these energy packets or quanta eventually led to a new physical theory called quantum mechanics. In contrast to the mechanical paradigm of Newtonian physics, this new theory has been able to explain the structure of small objects such as atoms and molecules, thus providing the foundation for modern chemistry, and has led to technological marvels such as transistors. But while it was accomplishing these practical tasks, quantum mechanics has also demolished our old ideas of hard, immutable matter. Physicists have been forced to shift their attention from "matter" (things) to "fields" (interactions between things).

The development of quantum mechanics by physicists has led to a whole new scientific view, or paradigm, in which interactions are emphasized more than "things." Under this paradigm, iron-clad determinism, for example, gives way to a notion of limited causality involving some uncertainty or freedom. In Newton's physics, every cause produced a specific effect—if we could only know the exact position and velocity of every atom,

we could predict *exactly* the entire future of the universe. Everything would be predetermined. But the new paradigm of physics, which rests upon the quantum principle, clearly shows that
nature is much more flexible, subtle, and pregnant with possibilities. While nature does not work in an arbitrary fashion,
each event has a certain freedom—the link between cause and
effect is *not* iron-clad: we are not trapped by our history, as the
Newtonian paradigm suggested.

Along with this abandonment of the idea of absolute determinism has come the realization that absolute objectivity must
also be abandoned. The old absolute distinction between "subject" and "object" has disappeared.

Perhaps John Archibald Wheeler, head of the Center for Theoretical Physics at the University of Texas in Austin, says this
best:

*The quantum principle has demolished the view we once had that
the universe exists safely "out there," that we can observe what goes
on in it from behind a foot thick slab of plate glass without ourselves being involved in what goes on. We have learned that to
observe even so minuscule an object as an electron we have to
shatter that slab of glass. We have to reach out and insert a measuring device. We can put a device to measure position or we can insert
a device to measure momentum, but the installation of the one
prevents the insertion of the other. We ourselves have to decide
which it is that we will do. Whichever it is, it has an unpredictable
effect on the future of that electron. To that degree, the future of the
universe is changed. We changed it. We have to cross out that old
word "observer" and replace it by the new word "participator." In
some strange sense, the quantum principle tells us that we are
dealing with a participatory universe.*[2]

Physicists have realized that other ideas of the old paradigm
also have to be abandoned, namely, the idea of "things" existing
completely independent of each other, the idea of a rigid determinism, and the idea that nature is like a machine. In Wheeler's
words:

*On the one hand there is the view that the universe is a gigantic
machine with imperishable particles that goes on its way willy-
nilly with man a small actor in a very small corner in the whole*

thing—a view which is carrying what we call the Copernican view to its extreme. On the other hand, there is a point of view that has been put forward—that the tie between man and the universe is very much closer indeed—that in some sense the physical constants and even the scale of the universe itself is such a scale and such a set of constants without which life and mind could not have come into being.[3]

Since the early 1970s, when Wheeler made these comments, additional advances in physics have furthered the change to a new scientific world view. The new scientific world view has an underlying message that all is connected; nothing really has a separate existence. Even an indirect observation affects the observed. In the new paradigm, we see that nature is not a machine. Rather, everything is viewed as a process, or an evolving system, in which decisions people make actually may play a decisive role in the long-term outcome of at least this part of our universe. We probably are not "a small actor in a very small corner of the whole thing." We are participators in the whole thing.

In the new paradigm, the future is not locked in by the past. Rather, the universe offers us the opportunity to participate in creating the future.

In the normal course of science, when everything is done within one paradigm, the "squares" of the crossword puzzle are filled in and sometimes even the rules are modified—just like any other activity such as business or football. But in a paradigm shift, it's not just the rules that are changed but the game itself.

To illustrate the change, we can list some implications of the new paradigm as opposed to those of the old.

OLD (NEWTONIAN) PARADIGM	NEW ("MODERN") PARADIGM
SCIENTIFIC IMPLICATIONS	
Atomic (molecular) approach.	Systemic approach.
Focus on parts.	Focus on the whole.
Focus on one variable.	Focus on many variables.

Reductionist.	Synthesist.
Separate parts (machinelike).	Interconnected parts (organismlike).
Deterministic (inevitability).	Probabilistic (freedom).
Absolute objectivity.	Observer interacts with the observed.
Analytic.	Analytic *and* synthesistic.
Emphasizes "things."	Emphasizes relationships.

SOCIAL IMPLICATIONS

Nature can be dominated.	We must harmonize with nature.
Power and control in society.	Cooperation, symbiosis.
Supports centralized control.	Control must be more decentralized.
Supports emphasis upon competition.	Supports emphasis upon cooperation.
Economic "engine."	Economic systems.

MEDICAL IMPLICATIONS

Reinforces specialization.	Requires generalization and application of broad view.
Supports technical intervention in medicine.	Supports preventive medicine.
Emphasizes "managing" or "controlling": dualistic (authoritarian).	Emphasizes working with, being in partnership with "authorities."
Supports patient being bossed.	Supports patient and doctor working together.
Doctor is seen as an authoritarian "boss."	Doctor is seen as coach.

This paradigm shift originated primarily in science, most obviously in physics, but has also emerged in ecology and in psychology, especially in the writings of Jung. But although Jung's ideas originated independent of the revolution in physics, he was not unaware of the connection. In fact, Jung wrote a book with the physicist Wolfgang Pauli,[4] who played a leading role in the development of the physics of the "new" paradigm.

More recently this ferment in the leading edges of physics has bubbled to the surface, beyond the realm of science per se. Several popular books[5] and at least one excellent magazine article[6] have been written for the layman.

Art and ritual play important roles in paradigm shifts. Images of the new paradigm can be seen in representations of the planetary consciousness—for example, some of Picasso's paintings, and especially that beautiful picture, taken from the moon, of our lovely planet "suspended" against the dark, cold backdrop of space. Thinkers in other fields have pointed toward aspects of the new paradigm, including Margaret Mead with her concept of the global village and R. Buckminster Fuller with his "spaceship earth." More than fifty years ago, the Jesuit scientist-philosopher Teilhard de Chardin[7] envisioned an interconnected planetary information network. Recently the paradigm shift has begun to affect all levels of social and economic thinking—witness the phenomenal popularity of John Naisbitt's *Megatrends*[8] or Marylyn Ferguson's *Aquarian Conspiracy*.[9]

No human activity is escaping the influence of the paradigm shift. That includes medical education. In fact, a growing number of medical educators recognize that medical education is in a state of crisis.[10] But they haven't yet connected this to the fact that medical education is based on the paradigm of 1910, the "old" paradigm, which has given way to the "new."

THE PARADIGM OF MEDICINE. The paradigm for medical education was set by the publication, in 1910, of the Flexner Report.[11] The Flexner study was authorized by the Carnegie Foundation in 1908 and was considered a hallmark in that it emphasized that medical education should be thoroughly grounded in science. In particular, Flexner emphasized "the essential dependence of modern medicine on the physical and biological sciences. . . ." The Flexner report also rightly emphasized using the latest technology to extend the physician's ability to observe. The physician should rely not only upon the "senses with which nature endowed him, but with those senses made infinitely more acute, more accurate, and more helpful by the processes and the instruments which the last half-century's progress had placed at his disposal. . . . The self-registering thermometer, the stethoscope, the microscope, the correlation of observed symptoms with the outgivings of chemical analysis and biological experimentation, enormously extend the physician's range."

Flexner proposed a curriculum, used essentially to this day, for the first two years of medical school and suggested that it require "for admission at least a competent knowledge of physics, chemistry, and biology. . . ." The result was a major updating in the standards of medical education. But since the study was done between 1908 and 1910, the Flexner Report was cast in the terms of the "old" scientific paradigm. The work of Planck, Einstein, Bohr, and others had only begun in the decade from 1900 to 1910. It was not until the mid-1920s that the new concepts in physics consolidated into the coherent quantum theory that made inevitable a "new" scientific paradigm. Flexner could not have known that physics was on the verge of changing the paradigm; indeed, in 1910, only a handful of those in physics realized this. As a result, the pattern for present-day medical education was set in a scientific world view that was just on the verge of becoming outdated and that we now know to be misleading in many respects.

True, Flexner emphasized that the "main intellectual tool of the investigator is the working hypothesis . . . and of taking all of the facts. . . . He constructs a hypothesis . . . and the practical outcome of his procedure refutes, confirms, or modifies his theory." But Flexner equated *theory* with a working hypothesis or educated guess, whereas physicists not only emphasize the importance of theoretical frameworks, as opposed to hypotheses, but were on the verge of rethinking the whole basis of science, the very *style*, as opposed to the rote method of science.

At about the same time the Flexner Report was issued, the study of electricity was being deemphasized in medicine and medical education, in part because it smacked of quackery and of "vitalism," the idea that the body is a machine requiring some "vital force" to drive it. The importance of electricity to living beings was first suggested in 1786, when Galvani discovered that an electrical spark caused the muscles of a frog to contract. In 1868, Julius Bernstein proposed the "Bernstein hypothesis"—an explanation of the conduction of signals along nerves in terms of physical theory. This hypothesis has since been confirmed and is now presented in standard textbooks. Bernstein suggested that his hypothesis was related not only to nerve conduction but was involved in the fundamental activities of all cells, for example, the healing of wounds. Robert Becker, who discovered that electrical fields play an essential role in the healing of broken bones, has pointed out, however, that "Bernstein's hypothesis came at a time when the scientific establishment was most eager to rid biology of electricity, the last vestige of vitalism."[12]

In addition, the medical establishment was trying to protect the public from electrotherapy, most of which involved charlatans. So it came to be out of fashion to think of electricity as being relevant to medicine. As a result, in biomedical research the molecular approach has until very recently received more support and attention than have biophysical studies about the role of ions, such as sodium and potassium, and electrochemical events within the cell. As an example, for several years an enormous effort was made to isolate in the test tube the molecular intermediate which carried energy during the formation of ATP, the "energy currency" of the cell. The final outcome, which won Peter Mitchell the Nobel Prize, is that this molecular intermediate doesn't exist. Rather the energy is carried in an electrochemical or "battery" form due in part to a voltage. Since voltages are a property only of intact *systems*, such as mitochondria, chloroplasts, or other systems within the cell, the minute the cell is ground up in a test tube to look for a molecular intermediate, the energy is no longer there. This again illustrates the limitations of a purely reductionist approach and highlights the necessity of also using a systems approach. To find the truth, both the molecular and the systems approach must be used. And if you recall our discussion in Chapter 6 about voltages and the "sodium battery" in the cell, you will realize that it was the study of bioelectric phenomena which led us to the realization that primary hypertension can be avoided.

The late thirties and early forties saw the early successes of antimicrobials—"wonder drugs" such as the sulfa drugs and antibiotics. Today it's easy to forget their impact; we forget that they virtually eliminated many infectious diseases such as pneumococcal pneumonia, which had been a leading killer of young adults. The success of these drugs helped consolidate medical thinking into the atomistic or molecular Newtonian paradigm. From that point on, drugs were an almost automatic answer to every problem, and any considerations of systems approaches, especially if they involved electrical events, were shoved to the back shelf. Becker has commented on this:

During the period another area of industry was also rapidly expanding, the manufacture of chemical drugs. It would seem likely that the biochemical view of life then being promoted by scientific medicine would be most attractive to these companies and indeed, they actively contributed to the campaign to discredit the electrotherapeutic techniques. Only within the past few years has it become possible to raise questions about the Flexner Report.[13]

Reinforcing the persistence of the old paradigm in medical education is the fact that premedical students take courses that essentially cover the discoveries of physics only through about 1900. This is because the Flexner Report recommendation that students at the premedical level have a grounding in physics was followed by requiring these students take a one-year introductory physics course. In 1910, such a course could only deal with the "classic" physics and with the old physics paradigm. Indeed, only in the 1930s was the first course in "modern" physics added to the curriculum.

Because modern physics rests historically and epistemologically upon Newton's physics, physics departments have continued to teach essentially the same one-year course in classical physics. But this is no longer a true "introductory" physics course. To get a true introduction, it is necessary to take a subsequent course, usually called modern physics, which introduces the student to the developments in physics since 1900.

Many people point out that doctors don't need to use physics equations to make their calculations, so it doesn't matter whether they know the equations of the new, or quantum, physics. Other people, who know that the old physics is adequate for objects much larger than atoms, argue that the study of classical physics is relevant for medicine because people are very large in comparison to atoms. In fact, it is true that the principles of classical physics do enable us to explain many things that happen in people—or, for that matter, in other complex things such as computers.

But both these objections miss the point. It's true that beyond perhaps some applications in radiology, physicians do not need to make calculations using the equations of "modern" physics (or, for that matter, "classical" physics). But whether or not they think nature behaves like a machine, whether or not they think something must be inevitably determined, whether or not they think they can be "observers" rather than "participators" lie at the very core of any model, or paradigm, for healing and for preventing illness.

Besides, while classical physics has served well for the questions addressed by biomedical research thus far, research physicians may well soon run into areas in which quantum calculations *are* required. For example, some aspects of molecular interaction simply cannot be understood without using the newer means of calculation. We now realize that some of the events within the cell happen at the level at which the old physics becomes inadequate. And these events can be amplified into the large scale. For example, the old physics cannot account for the mutation of a gene, but the new physics can. And that mutation in turn can cause the entire organism to change, or even die. Events at the very small level of even one atom can be amplified into changes of the large system.

Computers provide another example. In computers, the basic functional element, the transistor or the microchip, cannot be understood purely in terms of the old mechanical paradigm. In fact, it was the *new* physics of Planck, Einstein, Bohr, and others that led directly to the development of the transistor and then the microchip. In the final analysis, the modern computer depends upon the operations of nature at the level of the atom and of the electron. Consequently the computer cannot be understood without the new physics and its new paradigm.

Since the first year physics course does not include the new physics, premedical (and many biology) students are exposed only to that part of physics that leads to the old, mechanical paradigm. Hearing nothing else reinforces their view of nature as a "machine" that can be "conquered," "controlled," or "bent to man's will." It's understandable that these students tend to become reductionists, believing that the important thing to focus upon is the *parts* of a system. It's also inevitable that they see little connection between physics and the study of complex living systems.

Partly because of the reinforcement of the old paradigm and partly because of the complexity of the living being, medicine has remained a science built on facts and descriptions of phenomena as opposed to theoretical frameworks that provide understanding as well as predictability. The emphasis in teaching medical students remains on providing facts. For example, except for its applications to nerves, little (if anything) in the education of future doctors deals with the theory of electricity and ions in regulation of the living cell—a key consideration in our research, which led to our development of the *K Factor* theory.

The parts of medical education that are very good are those that are consistent with the old paradigm: namely, the emphasis upon technical intervention. But while this applies to crises, it is less appropriate to prevention. American medicine is superb at crisis intervention, such as treating accident victims and bacterial infections. It is much less successful at prevention.

In this connection, it's important to emphasize that our national medical bill is huge not because of advances in basic science. Rather, it is due to the fact that our life-style is out of synch with the natural laws governing the human body and to our overreliance on high-tech approaches. Until we shift from these aspects of the old paradigm to the lessons of the new paradigm, our national medical bill will continue to spiral.

A successful paradigm shift does not mean we should throw out the baby with the bathwater. It should, and we hope will, take what was valid from the old paradigm and add the value from the new. This has already happened in physics, where "modern" physics still includes Newton's physics—but extends and deepens the concepts.

But medical education has yet to fully join the paradigm shift. True, there has been a growing development of concepts in several areas of basic biomedical science, and medicine has moved from pure empiricism to include the formation of hypotheses. But medical education continues to be based on the reductionist, mechanical world view that existed at the time of Flexner. By and large, medical schools still educate future doctors primarily in the empirical, or factual, aspects of science. The underlying emphasis is upon reductionism, with its corollaries of overspecialization, overreliance on statistical analysis of facts, and overemphasis on technology to control, or manage, nature. So the vast majority of medical students have never been exposed to the new scientific world view or to such "theoretical" questions as How do we decide scientific truth? or What is scientific proof? And as a result, they naturally develop a knee-jerk tendency to look to statistics to answer every question.

The Tyranny of Statistical Analysis

Along with the simplistic view that scientific truth is decided only with statistics, this mechanical world view has inhibited doctors' use of intuition, judgment, and what some would call common sense in evaluating scientific questions. It has led to the tyranny of statistics: Nothing is believed unless statistics show it to be true.

Since a purely empirical and phenomenological science—one that describes phenomena but has no reliable theory—is severely limited in making predictions, the only test of "truth" can be statistics. So it's understandable that in the past half-century, the medical establishment on the whole has adopted the position that nothing is to be believed unless it has been "proved" in a large-scale clinical study with adequate controls to enable a proper statistical analysis. In other words, in the minds of most doctors, the criterion of whether something is true or false lies in statistical analysis of a large number of facts. The myth is that proof can come only from statistics.

True enough, statistics are an essential tool in science. As John Wheeler[14] points out, "When one gives a number for an answer to any question, it is agreed in science today, one is not doing enough. One must specify in addition the limits of error of that answer." The use of statistics sets the limits of error and thus is necessary to evaluate the reliability of data, or facts, and is necessary to compare data to theory. But by itself, statistics can't do more than suggest clues.

The influence of a paradigm is both subtle and powerful—especially if we don't discuss it. For example, Dick didn't really appreciate the extent to which doctors are conditioned to accept only statistical analysis until he explained the *K Factor* approach to two friends who are physicians.

Before he had finished outlining the approach, both of them asked, "Have there been any large, controlled, double-blind clinical trials with statistical analysis?" (See Chapter 8 for a discussion of double-blind studies). This standard, automatic challenge surprised Dick; after all, these guys were not only smart but one of them, now a specialist in internal medicine, had obtained part of his education in modern physics and had gotten a doctorate in biophysics. In response to the standard challenge, Dick pointed out that there were other ways to decide "truth" in science. The internist immediately recalled these, and after a moment's pause, said, "Come to think of it, you probably can't do a large-scale well-controlled double-blind study on this." (For the first time, Dick himself began to realize fully the truth of this. How can experimenters hide from their "subjects" whether they are eating more fruits and vegetables? And how can it be hidden from people whether or not they are exercising regularly? It's impossible. And it's almost impossible to totally "control" what people eat and how much they exercise.)

The controlled double-blind study is almost entirely limited to drug testing, in which a fake pill (a placebo) can be made to look like the real thing. Only when the only variable is identical-appearing pills can the study be totally controlled as well as double blind. So the prescription for doing these studies is very hard to fill unless pills are used. Double-blind studies *require* drugs! Once again the cards had been stacked in favor of using drugs in treatment—this time in biasing the selection of what kinds of treatments can be studied. The outdated world view that is the basis for educating medical students had struck again.

THE LIMITS OF STATISTICS. The bias toward empiricism, reinforced by a Copernican-Newtonian world view, has led to an overemphasis on controlled statistical studies.

With that in mind, let's examine some "facts" about hypertension based upon statistics. Four different statistical studies, each analyzing the same data base from a large number of people, have been published on the relation between hypertension and nutrition. The results of these studies are summarized in the following table.

TABLE 9.

	Effect upon Blood Pressure of:		
Study	Increasing Sodium	Increasing Potassium	Increasing Calcium
#1[15]	none	down	up (in men) down (in women and in blacks)
#2[16]	none	down	down
#3[17]	down	down	down
#4[18]	up	down	down in nonwhite males only, no effect in others

You will notice that no two of the studies agree. This is all the more remarkable when you consider that each of these four studies used *the same data base* (the HANES I study). These data are provided on computer tape from the National Institutes of Health. The data were collected from 13,671 persons eighteen years of age or older in the United States during the years 1971 to 1975. The only point on which the studies agree is that potassium seems to lower blood pressure. Why the differences? Well, statistical evidence isn't really straightforward; it's easy to make serious mistakes. Analyzing data is much more difficult than just pouring it into a computer and seeing the answer come out. In fact, one of the studies used a "canned" statistical program, the SPSS (a program developed for the social sciences) to analyze the data.

The analysis of complex sets of data is extremely difficult; some professional statisticians maintain that it can only be done with confidence by developing a model for each case—a very tedious, difficult, and time-consuming task. In contrast to study 3, in study 4, the authors developed much of their own equations of statistical analysis based upon models they constructed for this specific study, which is the way it should be done.

But there are other reasons for error. For example, no information about whether sodium was used at the table or in cooking food was collected for the original HANES I data base.

As the authors of study 1 pointed out, there were other important variables besides those analyzed and listed in Table 9. For example, older adults used less salt than did young adults. Yet we know that hypertension tends to get worse with age. So if this variable of age was not considered *at the same time* as sodium, one could conclude—erroneously—that lowering sodium intake increases blood pressure, which is, in fact, the conclusion of study 3. The authors of study 1 pointed out that since we know that some people's blood pressure is genetically resistant to sodium, the failure of the data base to evaluate genetic differences in sensitivity to salt confuses the results. Confusion also results if one ignores the fact that the response to sodium depends upon the amount of potassium in the diet and that there is a "threshold effect" to the effect of sodium.

There are real dangers to studying only one variable, as the authors of study 4, who developed their own statistical models, found. When analyzed alone, increased calcium intake seemed to decrease blood pressure. But when age was considered, calcium intake was no longer related to blood pressure. On the other hand, when they simultaneously considered not only the effect of sodium but also the age, body mass, and race of the subjects, increased sodium intake was still associated with higher blood pressure.

As you can see, an empirical paradigm was not sufficient. It was not possible to understand what was really going on by simply analyzing the data, or "facts." And physicians are naturally wary of trying something that isn't understood scientifically.

The population studies, described in Chapter 2, of the effect of drug treatment provide another example of the limits of statistics. Remember, the MRFIT study[19] found that in people with mild hypertension, intensive drug treatment had no apparent effect on mortality and in borderline hypertension apparently *increased* mortality. Another study from Australia,[20] of the use of thiazide diuretics, showed similar findings. On the other hand, there are three other studies (HDFP,[21] the VA Study,[22] and the Australian Therapeutic Trial[23]) which indicate that drug treatment does decrease mortality in mild hypertension. One reason for the different conclusions is that these studies used different categories of mild hypertension, whereas the MRFIT study was more discriminating. For example, the other studies did not do a separate analysis of the groups in the 90 to 94 mm Hg nor in the 95 to 99 mm Hg range. Also, in some of the studies, the control groups received placebos but in other studies received various types of antihypertensive treatment. For example, in the MRFIT and in the HDFP studies, although they did not receive intensive drug treatment, the "control" groups received the usual medical treatment.

Still another example of this is the fact that in spite of an abundance of evidence, many specialists still doubt the conclusion that aerobic exercise can lower blood pressure toward normal. Why? Because none of the studies thus far published has been "controlled" (though one has been reported as an abstract at the 1985 Meeting of the American Heart Association; see Chapter 11). This insistence upon a controlled study for determining the effects of exercise again oversimplifies the matter since it is impossible to be confident the two groups of people (exercised and non-exercised) with hypertension will in other respects be the same. In fact, because of differences in heredity, life-style, and environment, we know they won't be *exactly* the same. The only way we could really have an adequate control group would be to have a group of identical twins, each of which was eating exactly the same food, under the same stress, etc. except for one exercising and the other not exercising. But there is a way to do almost as well. By using each individual as his or her own control, it is possible to eliminate the effects of heredity and minimize other effects such as life-style. In fact, the study by Dr. Cade[24] and co-workers used just this means of comparison in fifteen of the people they studied, yet their study is considered "uncontrolled."

Whereas many doctors have been led to believe that controlled studies are the *sine qua non*, or hallmark, of a scientific approach, it's interesting that such studies are seldom, if ever, done in physics. Why? Physics long ago advanced to the point that the *relationships* between the variables can be clearly stated (with mathematics): in other words, reliable theories have been established. Therefore, the relationships can be tested by studying even one system. On the other hand, in living systems there are not only so many variables, many unknown, but until recently there were no theories which could state with mathematical precision the relationships between these variables. In such cases, one can only attempt to keep constant—or "control"—all variables except the one being tested. Until recent times, the only way medical issues could be established was to base them on impressions gained over a life-time or upon reports of usually a few isolated cases. Controlled studies do represent an advance over that. But as we have seen, such controlled studies are difficult if not impossible to really accomplish.

To understand high blood pressure, we must use both empiricism (statistical analysis of "facts" from observations) *and* theory.

What Is Scientific "Proof"?

Now we are prepared to discuss how science determines what is "true" and what is not. The first thing to realize is that in science, we can't *prove* anything. Science can only *dis*prove ideas stated as hypotheses, "models," or theories of how things work. In the final analysis, science can only state the *probability* that something is true and at best this probability can only approach 100%. In other words, whereas science can often state that something is true beyond any *reasonable* doubt, it can never state that something is true beyond *any* doubt.

In order to evaluate scientific "proof" or scientific "truth," we need a paradigm, or concept. In other words, we have to think about *theory*. And although we scientists may not like to admit it, the values of the culture in which we live affect the way we study science. As Stephan J. Gould of Harvard University points out, "Science is no inexorable march to truth, mediated by a collection of objective information and the destruction of ancient superstition. Scientists, as ordinary human beings, unconsciously reflect in their theories the social and political constraints of their time. As privileged members of society, more often than not they end up defending existing social arrangements as biologically fore-ordained."[25]

The Role of Theory

As we illustrated, both the old and the new scientific paradigms are the outgrowth of scientific theories. In the newest theories of physics, even atoms do not have a totally independent existence but are connected in a web of interactions. These interactions make up a system that cannot be understood merely by studying its parts and applying statistics. Rather, a systems approach, based upon modern physical theory, is required to understand any complex system—*especially involving life*.

(Only theory can deal with the "whole picture," and not just the "facts." We need a sense of the whole picture to sniff out leads and to make judgments. Narrow specialization works against this and paves the way for overreliance on statistics. While theory isn't everything, its importance cannot be ignored if genuine insight into and understanding of a given question are to develop. In the final analysis, the aim of science is to understand—to find some explanation or *theory* to account for—what really goes on. In the original Greek, the word *theory* means "vision." That's what good science is after: vision and insight. Unfortunately, in the American culture, with its empiricist bias, *theory* has become a synonym for *hypothesis* or, worse yet, *speculation*. This is not what *theory* means in an established science such as physics, in which experience and analysis show that theory is to be trusted fully as much as "facts.")

Even a partially developed theory is a powerful help in deciding scientific "truth." Physicists have long realized that in any
field, "facts" cannot be identified, judged, or even measured
without at least some theory (remember what we said about
paradigms). When you think about it, measuring a simple fact
such as the number of sodium atoms in our body requires the
theory that underlies the periodic table of the chemists. We
could not even measure blood pressure were it not for "theoretical" developments in the seventeenth century that clarified
the concept of "pressure," or Isaac Newton's theoretical discovery that for every action there is an equal and opposite reaction,
or William Harvey's concept of circulation of the blood. Medical
and premedical education tends to ignore considerations of this
type while emphasizing "facts" almost exclusively.

Fortunately, now the situation has begun to change. As a science moves from pure empiricism to the insight that comes
from a sound theoretical foundation, it is no longer limited to
statistical analysis of "facts" for determining "truth" and no
longer limited to simply describing phenomena; it can begin to
explain phenomena in terms of fundamental laws. In basic research, we are beginning to focus not only on "parts," or molecules, but more and more on whole systems, such as living cells.
And with this more complete view, we are developing the begin-
nings of sound theory. With even a primitive theory, or working
model, we can make predictions, and these predictions can be
either confirmed or refuted. This gives us additional, more
powerful and reliable tests of scientific "truth."

Looking at More Than One Variable

Solving the problem of high blood pressure requires the application of theories in physiology and in biophysics to make
some predictions. In this model, we consider more than one
variable at a time. We hope we have made it clear that while
analyzing one thing at a time won't give us clear, consistent
answers, analyzing the *relation* between two or more variables
(such as expressed in the *K Factor*) does. This is a very simple
example of a systems approach (new paradigm) as opposed to a
reductionist approach (old paradigm).

Theoretical "Criteria" for Scientific "Proof"
To be accepted as true, a hypothesis, model, or theory of how
something in nature works must:

∘ Successfully predict results.
∘ Be consistent with all empirical (factual) tests.
∘ Be consistent with all established theories (conceptual frame-
  works).

In other words, although science cannot "prove" any idea, it
does provide tests (criteria for acceptance or rejection) that can
provide support for the idea. If we think all the tests have been
passed, the idea is supported. We then accept it as provisional
truth, and we go with it.

PREDICTABILITY. A critical test of whether a theory is "true" or
not is whether the theory correctly predicts real events: if x
happens, the probability is high that y will follow, as borne out
by repeated trials. The theory behind the *K Factor* approach did
predict accurately that potassium would lower blood pressure
in primary hypertension and also that people with diabetes
would have an increased chance of having high blood pressure.
Scientists often talk about the importance of repeatability;
that is, can something be repeated. Actually this is an example
of the requirement for predictability. If we can predict that
when we do certain things, a specific result will follow, then we
can repeatedly observe that result. And the elements of the
K Factor approach *are* repeatable—they have been tried successfully by several groups of investigators. So the *K Factor* approach has met the requirements for both predictability and
repeatability.

CONSISTENCY. Consistency is also an important consideration
in deciding if something is true. *All* lines of evidence, whether
empirical or theoretical, must be consistent with the hypothesis.
This is where statistics comes in. Statistical analysis is valu-
able—often essential—in determining the quality of the empirical data. Not only that, statistical analysis is required to

determine if the data match the predictions of the theory *beyond any reasonable doubt*. But by itself, statistical analysis can at best give us leads.

Scientific "Proof" and the K Factor?

What really should decide the outcome? What really determines whether a scientific idea is accepted? In the short term, authoritarianism and politics may carry the day in science. But in the long run, nature has the final say. Nature is the final authority. Remember, the proof of the pudding is in the eating.

Good science involves not only being open-minded but also having a healthy skepticism. Let's consider how this applies to hypertension.

First, the *K Factor* approach is consistent with current theories of how body cells are regulated. Remember at the end of Chapter 6, we gave six predictions of the model, each of which has received confirmation. And in Chapter 7, we point out that other known facts can, at least potentially, be understood in terms of the model.

To us, this consistency is very compelling—and it is an example of prediction. And the *K Factor* approach is consistent with the empirical evidence. As we discussed in Part II, there are five lines of evidence, four of them empirical, that support the conclusion that primary hypertension is not inevitable and beyond our control but instead is triggered by a nutritional imbalance, especially a low potassium-to-sodium ratio. Each of these widely different types of evidence points to the same conclusion. All the lines of evidence are consistent.

In fact, working on all these cell mechanisms and the concepts and model that we now have is what led us to expect that primary hypertension could be cured by both decreasing sodium and increasing potassium in the diet.

Since all the lines of evidence are consistent, the most probable conclusion is the one we adopt in this book. Although there are a lot of details yet to be clarified by research, the overwhelming weight of evidence points to the conclusion that primary hypertension is due to an imbalance within the living cell that involves the relation between potassium, sodium, calcium, and magnesium. Furthermore, although not all the i's have been dotted and not all the t's have been crossed, it is clear that drugs treat the blood pressure rather than the imbalance within the cell. Fortunately, we now know enough about the effect of both nutritional factors, such as the *K Factor*, and about exercise to restore normal cell function in people with primary hypertension and, as a result, allow their bodies to achieve normal blood pressure. If it makes sense, you should go along with it until proved otherwise.

Summary

The old scientific paradigm tended to focus thought away from a systems approach involving many variables and to discount concepts while emphasizing "facts" or data. Since it was reductionistic, it inevitably reinforced the tendency to focus upon molecules, including drugs, in the treatment of conditions such as hypertension.

The new scientific paradigm requires that we focus upon the whole system, realizes that understanding the parts doesn't enable us to understand the whole, and is consistent with the idea that human problems can only be "solved" by living with, rather than dominating, nature.

Intervention procedures, such as drugs, are to be used only when we can't do anything better. But in the case of hypertension, we can do something better. The theoretical criteria of consistency and predictability are already satisfied for the *K Factor* approach.

In addition, the empirical evidence (including a few double-blind studies using potassium pills) for the *K Factor* approach is abundant, although the very large "double-blind, random crossover" clinical trial required to convince the diehard empiricist has yet to be done and may never be. Thus far, however, the view that the dietary potassium-to-sodium ratio as well as the balance in the body among potassium, sodium, calcium, and magnesium is the key to primary hypertension has survived every known test.

Reliable prediction of events in unfamiliar circumstances can come only through theory and understanding. Understanding the main features of how nutritional changes can restore normal blood pressure allows you to be much more flexible and to design an eating plan that will fit your life-style. Understanding frees you from a purely rote approach, which would confine you to rigid recipes. And by making it possible for you to be more flexible, understanding makes it easier for you to stick to a diet that will help control your blood pressure.

The overall evidence leaves little doubt that the long-term answer to primary hypertension is nutrition and exercise, not drugs. The fact that we need further research to better understand the details and fine-tune the application does not mean we can't, or shouldn't, apply what we *do* know *now*.

Since this idea leads to recommended procedures that can do no harm, our approach should be presented to the public so that they and their physicians can have the opportunity to try it.

The Contrast to Drugs

The procedures we recommend involve restoring a natural balance within the body, as opposed to the introduction of drugs, which the human body has experienced only during the last few of its four-million-year existence on this planet. Drugs, such as are used in the therapy of hypertension, are often synthetic molecules that are primarily foreign to the body and as such often produce several unwanted side effects. Moreover, these drugs are usually designed to treat symptoms or signs, such as the elevated blood pressure per se, as opposed to correcting the basic imbalance that initially caused the high blood pressure.

It should seem obvious that a therapy that remedies the initial defect in cell function that led to a disease process is better than a therapy that treats merely the consequences of the basic defect. This should be especially evident when the treatment involves restoration of a balance in the diet in accord with that which supported the evolution of our ancestors.

This type of therapy—using substances natural to the body to restore normal balance, or homeostasis, in the body—is an example of what Nobel Prize–winner Linus Pauling has called orthomolecular medicine. The approach is a harmonious blend of concepts from advanced basic science on the one hand and a return to a more natural life-style on the other. In general, drugs treat signs, such as elevated blood pressure, and symptoms. Orthomolecular approaches, such as increasing the dietary potassium-to-sodium ratio, treat the primary biological defect and thus restore normal functioning of the body's cells.

Finally, in our experience thus far, when the procedure we recommend is really followed, *it works*.

CHAPTER 20

Additional Evidence: Low Dietary *K Factor*—A Main Cause of Primary Hypertension

If you're still skeptical—good! That means you're thinking for yourself. You're being scientific. But apply your skepticism equally to any view of hypertension. Don't swallow anything (drugs or bananas) without some thinking and consulting with your doctor.

In our cultural environment, primary hypertension acts as though it is inherited. A large percentage of people (about 25% to 30%, depending upon the population group) *appear* to inherit a genetic weakness in their ability to handle a diet overloaded with sodium chloride and deficient in potassium, magnesium, or calcium. Because of the imbalance of these minerals in the typical American diet, hypertension is almost inevitable in those with the genetic weakness. This apparent inevitability has helped reinforce dependency, as opposed to participation, between the patient and doctor, with a lifetime of drug-taking being the only option. But these people are *not* predestined to hypertension—provided they eat properly and maintain their weight through aerobic exercise. On a low-sodium high-potassium diet, only about 1 percent of people will develop hypertension (the rare cases seen in the cultures with diets low in sodium and high in potassium). Apparently this 1 percent has a very strong genetic tendency for hypertension, although some of them may have kidney disease.

A number of other studies also lead to this conclusion. For example, recall that Table 1 of Chapter 3 listed two groups from Tel Aviv, the only difference between them being diet. The vegetarian group (who ate a vegetarian diet that had a high *K Factor*) had a very low incidence of hypertension compared to the other group. So the evidence is clear that whether or not those people with a genetic tendency actually get hypertension depends upon their life-style, particularly their diet.

We have already summarized evidence that leads to the conclusion that in hypertension, the most important aspect of diet is the *K Factor*. This evidence included not only the population studies but also medical studies, animal studies, an understanding of the importance of the proper balance between potassium and sodium in the living cell, and the realization that obesity and lack of exercise can compromise the body's ability to balance potassium and sodium.

At this point, we want to emphasize that a central theme of this book is that when considering living systems, it is *never* enough to look at one thing at a time. We have emphasized this with respect to sodium. But although the balance between potassium and sodium seems to be a key factor, we pointed out in Chapter 8 that other substances, such as chloride, magnesium, and calcium, are also involved. Therefore, the *K Factor* is an approximation that will one day be replaced by something more complete, and more accurate. But at the present state of research, it appears to be not only the best we have, but adequate to the job.

Now we present additional evidence that supports the conclusion that the balance between potassium and sodium plays a key role in determining whether those with the genetic weakness will develop primary hypertension as they get older.

1. *The level of potassium in the blood plasma is correlated with hypertension.* As you will recall from Chapter 7, the sodium-

potassium pump requires an adequate amount of potassium in the fluid *outside* the cell in order to maintain the proper balance between potassium and sodium *inside* the cell. Since potassium in the fluid outside body cells is in equilibrium with plasma potassium, a decrease in the level of plasma potassium would be expected to decrease activity of the sodium-potassium pump in these cells. This in turn would increase the level of calcium *inside* the cell, causing contraction of the small resistance arteries and therefore raising blood pressure. Thus a low level of plasma potassium would be expected to contribute to high blood pressure.

In general, physicians have not noticed a difference in the level of potassium in the blood plasma of hypertensive individuals compared to the level of those with normal blood pressure. However, in a study of 1,462 middle-aged women in Sweden, serum potassium levels in hypertensive women, whether treated or untreated, were significantly lower than in women with normal blood pressure.[1] In another study of 91 patients with primary hypertension, a graph of both plasma potassium and total body potassium showed a significant tendency for both diastolic and systolic blood pressures to increase as the plasma potassium levels decreased.[2] These correlations were clearest in younger patients. This study also found that as the total amount of sodium in the body increased, blood pressure increased.

In a study in London of 3,578 men and women not taking antihypertensive drugs, it was observed that both systolic and diastolic blood pressures were significantly "negatively" associated with plasma potassium: that is, the lower the plasma potassium, the higher the blood pressure tended to be.[3]

Perhaps the most interesting study of serum potassium was of Japanese men in their forties. A total of 1,158 men from six different population groups, with different lifestyles, both urban and rural, were studied. When the average level of plasma potassium of each of the six groups was plotted against the incidence of high blood pressure, a clear tendency for the prevalence of hypertension to increase as plasma potassium decreased was seen.[4]

Data from that paper are summarized in Table 10 and show a steady increase (reported to be statistically significant) in the incidence of hypertension as the serum potassium level decreases; the apparent exception of line 3 is within the level of statistical error. The interpretation of this table is not clouded by possible effects of antihypertensive drugs, since none of the data in this table is from men taking these agents. As you can see, this study found that as the dietary *K Factor* (K/Na ratio) increases, hypertension decreases.

TABLE 10.

Region	Incidence of Hypertension (%)	Average Serum Potassium (meq/L)	Average Dietary Potassium/Sodium Ratio (gm K/gm Na)
A	10.3	4.26	0.197
B	12.0	4.24	0.192
C	13.3	4.29	0.213
D	19.9	4.11	0.187
E	24.9	4.02	0.168
F	33.3	3.85	0.141

In a government-sponsored nationwide study of a very large number of hypertensive patients it was found that when medication was not being used, serum potassium was lowest in groups with the highest blood pressure regardless of age, sex, or race (both blacks and whites were studied). The hypertensive patients taking medication tended to have even lower serum potassium levels—still another finding that raises questions about the use of drugs to treat high blood pressure.[5]

The "normal" values for plasma potassium may be too low. Until recently, most authorities did not recognize that serum potassium tends to be depressed in people with hypertension. Accordingly, the "normal" range of serum potassium is based upon large populations, about 20 percent of whom have high blood pressure. The four recent studies just quoted indicate that this 20 percent has lower levels of serum potassium than does the rest of the population. This suggests we reconsider the "normal" range of serum potassium. The lower limit of the "normal" level may well need to be revised upward.

2. *Total body potassium is decreased in untreated primary hypertension.* Since a decrease in plasma potassium slows the sodium-potassium pump, decreasing the amount of potassium inside body cells, a lower plasma potassium level indicates a decreased total body potassium. Therefore, we would expect that the total body potassium of people with primary hypertension would be decreased.

This prediction has been confirmed by a study in which total body potassium was measured in fifty-three patients with untreated primary hypertension and in sixty-two healthy people with normal blood pressure who were used as controls.[6] The total body potassium was an average of 13 percent lower in the people with untreated primary hypertension than in people with normal blood pressure (with the same amount of body fat). This decrease is statistically significant. The potassium content of small samples of muscle removed from these people confirmed that the decrease was not due to differences in amount of body fat. Analysis of these samples also revealed that the calcium content of the muscle tissue was greater in the subjects with primary hypertension. As we discussed in Chapter 6, if these changes in potassium and calcium occur in the smooth muscle cells surrounding the arterioles, the tension of these cells would increase, with a resulting constriction of the arterioles and consequent rise in blood pressure.

Another study showed that among ninety-one people with hypertension who were not taking drugs, there was a negative correlation between total body potassium and blood pressure.[7]

3. *Correlation of urinary K/Na ratio with hypertension.* The content of sodium and/or of potassium in a twenty-four-hour urine collection can be a fairly good reflection of the dietary intake. We would expect that as the urinary *K Factor* rises, the incidence of high blood pressure would fall.

IN JAPAN. This proved to be the case in a Japanese study in which Dr. Naosuke Sasaki of Hirosaki University studied blood pressure, urinary sodium and potassium, and apple consumption.[8] He noticed that in one apple-growing district of Japan, those who ate even one to three apples (which are high in potassium) each day had lower blood pressure than those who ate no apples. When examining middle-aged farmers from four different regions, Dr. Sasaki also found a definite correlation between their blood pressure and urinary K/Na ratio, which reflects the dietary *K Factor*. This is illustrated in Table 11 and shows that as the average urinary K/Na ratio decreases, both average diastolic and systolic blood pressure rise.

TABLE 11.

Region	Average Diastolic Blood Pressure (mm Hg)	Average Systolic Blood Pressure (mm Hg)	Average Urinary Ratio of Potassium/Sodium (gm K/gm Na)
A	78.6	131.4	0.293
B	80.9	139.3	0.252
C	85.9	149.7	0.229
D	86.6	152.5	0.223

IN THE UNITED STATES. In a 1979 study conducted by Dr. W. Gordon Walker and his colleagues[9] at Johns Hopkins School of Medicine, the average urinary K/Na ratio of the 274 volunteers with diastolic blood pressure less than 90 mm Hg was 0.88, while the ratio in urine of the 300 volunteers with hypertension (diastolic pressure greater than 90) was 0.71. There was no correlation with sodium excretion; the decrease in urinary K/Na ratio in the hypertensives was almost entirely due to a decrease in potassium in urine, and, therefore, presumably in the diet. This finding is especially important because none of the subjects was taking drugs of any kind, and therefore the difference in urinary K/Na ratio cannot be attributed to antihypertensive drugs, such as diuretics, which can cause the body to lose potassium.

IN AMERICAN BLACKS COMPARED TO WHITES. It is well known that blacks have a much higher incidence of hypertension than whites. What is not so widely appreciated is that the dietary K/Na ratio, as reflected by the urinary K/Na ratio, is also lower in blacks than in whites. In one study of women in their early twenties, the urinary K/Na ratio was 0.42 in blacks as compared to 0.62 to whites.[10]

One study, begun in 1961, was conducted in which both blacks and whites living in Evans County, Georgia, were selected randomly.[11] As in almost all American studies, the blacks had a significantly higher incidence of hypertension than did the whites. Surprisingly, black men actually had about 27 percent *less* sodium in their diet and about 20 percent less in their urine than the whites. However, the white men had over twice as much potassium in their diet and nearly that much more potassium in their urine. Thus in spite of a decrease in consumption of sodium as compared to whites, the dietary *K Factor* and the corresponding urinary K/Na ratio of blacks was less than that of the whites. Averaging the men and women together, the urinary K/Na ratio was 0.33 for blacks and 0.44 for whites.

In a study of 662 black and white female high school students in Jackson, Mississippi, there was only a weak correlation between urinary sodium excretion and blood pressure, but a highly significant relation between urinary K/Na ratio and blood pressure. Those young women with lower urinary K/Na ratio clearly had higher blood pressure.[12] (This study was also mentioned in Chapter 3.) In another study of hypertensive patients, the strong correlation between urinary K/Na ratio and hypertension was not observed, but Dr. Herbert Langford of Jackson, Mississippi, has suggested that the lack of correlation was probably due to the fact that most of the patients were taking antihypertensive medication, which had already lowered their blood pressure.[13]

IN AFRICAN BLACKS. In a study of an African tribe, those living in cities had a urinary K/Na ratio of 0.46 and significantly higher blood pressure than those living in villages, whose urinary K/Na ratio was 0.63. The difference was most striking in the men. The urban men had an average blood pressure of 140/88 mm Hg and a urinary K/Na ratio of 0.50, while the village men had an average blood pressure of 129/78 and a urinary K/Na ratio of 0.89.[14]

IN EUROPEANS. Finally, of 694 randomly selected people in a Belgian village, there was no significant relationship between blood pressure and urinary excretion of sodium.[15] However, there was a significant rise in blood pressure associated with decreased potassium excretion in the urine.

4. *The K Factor and hypertension in experimental animals.* In Nashville, Tennessee, a physician, Dr. George Meneely, and his colleague Con Ball had been studying the toxic action of table salt, NaCl, on laboratory rats. In 1958, they published the results of studies of the toxic effect of sodium chloride and the protective effect of potassium chloride on the life span of 825 rats.[16] It was probably this group that first suggested the use of the dietary *K Factor* as an indicator of the likelihood of having hypertension. They found some very surprising results. When rats were fed a diet with high levels of sodium chloride with a *K Factor* of only 0.11, the extra sodium resulted in a decrease in average life span from the normal of about twenty-four months to only sixteen months. When the dietary *K Factor* was increased to 0.8 by addition of potassium chloride while keeping the levels of sodium chloride in the food constant, the *average life span increased by 8 months*—back to the normal life span of rats without high blood pressure! (Into this technical scientific paper, the authors slipped the following comment: "There may, too, have been some potash (potassium) in the fountain of youth.")

Dr. Lewis K. Dahl and co-workers studied a strain of rats that became hypertensive on a high-sodium diet and confirmed that increasing the *K Factor* in the diet diminished the rise in blood pressure produced by giving salt. These salt-sensitive rats were divided into six different groups, and each group was placed on a different diet. Each diet contained the same high amount of sodium, but each had a different amount of potassium.[17] The results are summarized in Table 12.

The protective effect of adding potassium to increase the *K Factor* can be clearly seen. At twelve months (other data indicated that the mean blood pressure had reached nearly its highest level by then), the blood pressure of the different groups steadily decreases as the dietary *K Factor* increases. This effect is also evident at six months and begins to be evident at one month. Of even more significance, the authors also reported that the life span of the rats on the diets with higher *K Factor* was much longer than the others.

A second part of this study showed that not only is the *K Factor* important, but the *absolute* amounts of sodium and potassium also affect blood pressure. For example, when the *K Factor* was kept constant at either 0.57 or 1.7, increasing the amount of both sodium *and* potassium threefold resulted in a substantial (about 20 and 15 mm Hg respectively) rise in blood pressure. Therefore, not only must attention be given to the K/Na ratio of our diet but to the *amount* of sodium in the foods listed in the table in Chapter 13 as well.

TABLE 12. *Average Mean Blood Pressures of Rats on a Constant High Sodium Diet*

K/Na ratio → (gm K/gm Na)	0.17	0.34	0.42	0.57	0.85	1.7
Months on Diet	Mean Blood Pressure (in mm Hg)					
1	116	109	115	119	110	108
6	166	145	140	143	135	125
12	170	164	162	160	152	137

NOTE: Mean blood pressure = diastolic pressure plus 1/3 the difference between systolic and diastolic pressure.

In another animal study, rats were divided into three groups and given food that was identical except for a different *K Factor* for each group.[18] When the *K Factor* was lowered from the control value of 1.86 to 0.45 by the addition of sodium, the average systolic blood pressure rose significantly. When a small supplement of potassium was also added along with the sodium, thus raising the *K Factor* back up to 0.61, blood pressure did not rise nearly as much. This study also found that animals made hypertensive by a low K/Na ratio had a moderate increase in the amount of adrenaline (a hormone that raises blood pressure) excreted in their urine. When the *K Factor* was raised from 0.45 to 0.61, by addition of a small amount of potassium, the excretion of adrenaline decreased about 20 percent.

This effect of increased dietary *K Factor* on blood pressure has also been demonstrated in other animals with hypertension.[19]

How Increasing Dietary K Works

Increased potassium intake lowers blood pressure toward normal in persons with high blood pressure but has less effect on persons with normal blood pressure. This suggests that extra potassium in the diet does not change normal mechanisms of blood pressure regulation but instead restores "damaged" mechanisms toward normal.

A number of mechanisms have been suggested to account for the ability of potassium to lower blood pressure in people with hypertension. The effect of potassium to relax the smooth muscle surrounding the arterioles is probably both direct and indirect.

Direct Effect

A high-potassium diet has been shown to increase the potassium level in the blood serum by 10 to 15 percent, almost 0.6 meq/liter (see Table 10, p. 311, and the clinical trials of the high–*K Factor* diet described in Chapter 4). Since even a very in potassium in the fluid bathing the body cells will increase the activity of the sodium-potassium pumps, this should lower blood pressure by causing relaxation of the small arteries.

A direct effect of potassium has been demonstrated by Dr. F. J. Haddy, who showed that infusion of potassium directly into arteries causes them to relax, thus allowing increased blood flow.[20] In the presence of ouabain, a drug that specifically inhibits operation of the sodium-potassium pump, potassium did not produce this relaxing effect. When the sympathetic hormone adrenaline is used to cause contraction in strips of arteries taken from rats, potassium also causes relaxation. This relaxing effect is consistently greater in arteries taken from rats with the genetic tendency to have hypertension than from normal rats. Addition of ouabain blocks the ability of potassium to relax these strips of arteries.[21] These results indicate that potassium relaxes the smooth muscle cells by stimulating the sodium-potassium pump, as we described in Chapter 6.

At plasma concentrations that might be found with a high-potassium diet, potassium also has a direct relaxing effect upon arterioles, resulting in less resistance to blood flow.[22] Therefore, this relaxing effect of potassium is probably part of the explanation for the ability of extra dietary potassium to lower blood pressure toward normal.

The potassium level in the fluid bathing the body cells is very close to the same level found in the watery part (plasma) of the blood. Thus, it is significant that at least five studies have found that plasma potassium is decreased by 5 to 15 percent in patients suffering from untreated primary hypertension, as we described earlier in this chapter.

All these findings are consistent with a major working hypothesis, currently being tested in a number of research laboratories, that considers an increase in sodium inside the cell to be a main part of the cause of primary hypertension. We discussed this in Chapter 6. In fact, the authors of this book each became interested in this problem because of our own research upon regulation of the sodium-potassium pump and the known effect (mentioned in Chapter 6) of even small increases in potassium outside the cell to stimulate the sodium-potassium pump and thus keep sodium inside the cell at a low level.

Indirect Effects

Besides the probable direct effect of potassium on the sodium-potassium pump in the walls of the small arteries, there is strong evidence that potassium also exerts some of its effect on blood pressure by affecting the kidneys, by changing blood hormone levels, and by affecting nerve activity.

Extra potassium in the diet causes increased excretion of sodium by the kidney, which in turn leads to a decrease in the amount of sodium in the body and might decrease the release of natriuretic hormone from the brain (see Chapter 22). This would allow the sodium-potassium pump to reduce the level of sodium inside the cells and increase the voltage across their surface membrane. Both effects act to keep intracellular calcium at a low level, thus relaxing the smooth muscle cells.

Addition of potassium to the diet of people with primary hypertension not only significantly decreases blood pressure, but in at least one study, this decrease was shown to be correlated with a decrease in the level of noradrenaline in the blood.[23] In other words, with added dietary potassium, the sympathetic nervous system became less active, since noradrenaline is released from sympathetic nerve endings. Potassium may have an effect upon the sympathetic nerves that go directly to the arterioles and cause contraction and narrowing of these small resistance arteries.[24] This effect of potassium may be due to stimulation of the sodium-potassium pump in the sympathetic nerve cells, which would decrease their activity by increasing the voltage across their surface membrane, causing fewer impulses to be sent to the arterioles, allowing them to relax.

Hypertension in the Obese

It is widely recognized that being obese greatly increases your chances of developing primary hypertension. In all populations that have been studied, overweight people have an increased likelihood of high blood pressure.[25] In the HANES I study, the correlation of blood pressure with body weight was one of the strongest factors.

In clinical trials, loss of only a third to a half of excess body weight has been shown to reduce blood pressure significantly.[26] Moreover, very low calorie diets will decrease blood pressure in only three to four days in almost all obese people.[27] This is long before there is any sizable loss of weight. This clearly indicates that in the obese, high blood pressure is not due to the mechanical effects of body fat or, as was previously thought, to the increase in small blood vessels associated with excess fat. Rather, the increase in blood pressure must be due to a change in physiological *function* in obese people.

In Chapter 7, we outlined the fact that obesity results in increased levels of insulin (commonly known as a sugar hormone) and that insulin regulates the body's mechanism that exchanges potassium for sodium, the sodium-potassium pump.

In the late 1960s, the work from Dick's laboratory, which indicated that insulin increases the activity of the sodium-potassium pump, prompted Dr. Jean Crabbé, in Belgium, to study the effect of insulin upon the sodium-potassium pump in the kidney. The work of Dr. Crabbé's group[28] and then that of Dr. Ralph deFronzo[29] of Yale University Medical School has since conclusively demonstrated that elevation of blood insulin levels results in increased reabsorption of sodium by the kidney, causing the retention of more sodium in the body. For a review, see Sims[30] or Moore.[31]

The elevation of blood levels of insulin by obesity may be a form of compensation for the fact that in obese people, the enlarged fat cells have fewer receptors for the insulin molecule (for a given area of surface membrane). Dr. Ethan Sims,[32] of the University of Vermont, has pointed out that this elevation of blood insulin in obesity would be expected to cause the kidney to retain body sodium, producing essentially the same effect as having too much sodium in the diet. Drs. Berchtold and Sims quote the conclusion of an international meeting on hypertension and obesity held at Florence, Italy, in 1980: "Hyperinsulinemia and related disorders are common features of the syndromes of obesity. There is now much evidence that insulin promotes retention of sodium by the kidney, and this may be a major contributor to hypertension in the obese subgroup of patients."

Dr. Sims points out that modified fasting, which lowers blood insulin, rapidly "brings about an impressive decrease in blood pressure." In the experience of Dr. Wayne Gavryck, a physician friend of Dick's, when hypertensive patients who are obese are placed on a very low calorie diet (400 calories per day), the blood pressure almost always drops significantly within seven days. Exceptions are uncommon, and the blood pressure is usually down within three to four days.[33] This procedure also decreases blood pressure in many who are not obese, again demonstrating that it is not fat per se that causes the elevated blood pressure but altered physiology.

Also supporting the idea that insulin has an effect upon sodium excretion in obese hypertensives are the two studies quoted earlier in which high blood pressure was treated by weight reduction.[34] In both of these studies, about 75 percent of the people developed normal diastolic blood pressure without drug treatment when calories were restricted. And while caloric intake was restricted, sodium excretion in the urine was significantly increased in spite of the fact that there was no evident change in dietary sodium.

Insulin also affects blood pressure by acting on the hypothalamus, a part of the brain, causing it to step up the activity of the sympathetic nervous system,[35] which then elevates blood pressure by causing constriction of the arterioles, as discussed in chapters 7 and 22.

Noradrenaline, which is released by nerves in the sympathetic nervous system, not only plays a direct role in development of hypertension in the obese individual but also affects sodium and potassium balance.[36] Besides reducing plasma insulin levels, in obese people with high blood pressure, weight loss results in a fall in plasma levels of noradrenaline, renin, Angiotensin II, and aldosterone[37]—all hormones that tend to increase blood pressure.

Exercise and Hypertension

The effect of too little exercise, like obesity, probably relates to the body's regulation of potassium and sodium. Physical training of overweight middle-aged persons strikingly reduces the blood level of insulin even when there is no change in body fat while at the same time increasing the number of insulin receptors on skeletal muscle.[38] This drop in blood insulin level should allow the kidney to excrete more sodium, thus helping reduce elevated blood pressure. Physical training also has effects on other hormones, such as adrenaline, which affect blood pressure.

Diabetes and Hypertension

People who have Type II diabetes (the type that occurs in overweight adults) have a greatly increased chance of developing high blood pressure. Is there any evidence that the balance of sodium and potassium is involved in this? We know insulin stimulates the sodium-potassium pump that moves sodium out of and potassium into body cells. The muscle cells of Type II diabetics are resistant to insulin. Therefore they have a *relatively* low blood level of insulin (at least relative to what they need), so we would expect that the sodium-potassium pumps in their muscle cells might be slowed, with a resulting increase in the level of sodium inside the cell. This prediction has been verified in experiments with laboratory rats where the reduction of serum insulin due either to fasting or to diabetes results in an increase in the level of sodium inside skeletal muscle.[39] If this effect also occurs in the vascular smooth muscle that controls the diameter of the arterioles, the elevated level of intracellular sodium would be expected to result in an increase in intracellular free calcium, causing increased contraction of the arterioles, which would increase peripheral resistance and thus elevate blood pressure, as described before. Supporting this hypothesis is the observation that insulin has a direct effect that decreases arterial smooth muscle tension, causing the arteries to dilate.[40]

Both obese people, who have an excess of plasma insulin, and Type II diabetics, who act like they have a relative shortage of plasma insulin, are prone to high blood pressure. Therefore, one might question whether the proposed involvement of insulin and the sodium-potassium pump in diabetes on the one hand and in obesity on the other is consistent. Wouldn't the relative lack of insulin in diabetes lead to more excretion of sodium by the kidney? And in obesity, shouldn't the elevated blood level of insulin lead to *more* activity of the sodium-potassium pumps in their muscles? Not necessarily, because we have to keep in mind that the response of different tissues to insulin can change with respect to each other. For example, exercise training increases the sensitivity of muscle to insulin without much change in liver and adipose tissue.[41] More to the point, Type II diabetics actually have an *elevated* level of plasma insulin, their diabetes being due to a tissue resistance to the hormone. In fact, *all* groups that tend to have primary hypertension—Type II diabetics, obese people, and people who don't exercise—tend to have elevated levels of plasma insulin. Even more intriguing is the finding that *non*obese people who have primary hypertension *also* appear to have elevated levels of plasma insulin, compared to control groups with normal blood pressure.[42] It now appears that all groups with primary hypertension have elevated blood insulin levels. Type I diabetics, who have decreased levels of native insulin, are *not* prone to hypertension.

Although obese people have elevated levels of plasma insulin, they have a decrease in insulin receptors and insulin responsiveness of many of their body cells. The same relationship tends to hold for people who get little exercise. So in spite of the elevated plasma insulin, their body cells do not get enough *effect* of insulin. This is why obese people tend to become diabetic. But it is entirely possible that the response of their kidneys to insulin is not correspondingly decreased.

Until these details are worked out, we should not draw any final conclusions. The point is, however, that in contrast to a few years ago, there are several independent lines of research—insulin research, diabetes research, research into the natriuretic factor, research on the effects of obesity—each of which has independently come up with evidence, of varying degrees of development, that the altered activity of the sodium-potassium pump, and therefore the exchange of potassium for sodium, is a key factor in the development of primary hypertension.

Why Doesn't Potassium Always Lower Blood Pressure?

If potassium does relax the small arteries, whether directly or indirectly, and thus decreases the resistance of blood flow, why doesn't an increase in dietary potassium (and a decrease in dietary sodium) *always* produce a decrease in blood pressure within a few days? We don't know for sure, but we can make an educated guess. In fact, from what researchers have discovered about the structure of small arteries, we would expect that increasing potassium would result in a relatively rapid drop in blood pressure only in the early stages of hypertension. This should not be used as an argument against increasing the dietary K/Na ratio as a means of treating primary hypertension: experiments show that extra potassium extends the life of laboratory animals even when it doesn't lower blood pressure.

Thiazide diuretics produce a more rapid drop in blood pressure, but initially this is due to a decrease in cardiac output resulting from decreased blood volume, an effect that hardly seems desirable. Only after a considerable delay do these diuretics result in a reduction of resistance to blood flow and thus affect the primary problem.[43]

When the blood pressure is increased by mechanically constricting an artery in experimental animals, the result is an increased thickness of the wall of the artery upstream from the constriction. The mechanism for part of this is similar to the development of increased mass of other body muscles. The increased blood pressure causes increased strain, or tension, on the smooth muscles circling the artery.

We know that resistance exercises, either isometric or isotonic, increase the tension of the skeletal muscles and cause hypertrophy, or bulging, of the muscles. Similarly, we would expect the increased tension of the smooth muscles, caused by the high blood pressure, to cause hypertrophy. It does, and this causes part of the increased thickness of the artery wall seen in hypertensive people. The thickened arterial walls may remain even if the primary cellular imbalance in sodium, potassium, and calcium is corrected by stimulation of the sodium-potassium pump. Therefore, once hypertension has been present for a sufficient period of time, increasing dietary potassium would not be expected to decrease blood pressure, at least for some time.

However, with proper therapy over sufficient time, even this hypertrophy of the smooth muscles would be expected to decrease; when the stress on *any* muscle is decreased, the muscle gradually becomes smaller. For example, easier workouts allow the enlarged muscles of the weight lifter to decrease back toward normal size. Also, prolonged bed rest results in decrease in the size and strength of leg muscles. Therefore, the time required for elevated blood pressure to respond to an increase in the dietary K/Na ratio would be expected to be longer in those people whose high blood pressure has gone untreated for a longer time. The effect of the dietary change should be quickest—within several days to a few weeks—in those who have had hypertension only a very short time. In someone who has had untreated hypertension for a much longer period, it might take a few months for the blood pressure to drop.

Unfortunately, if the hypertension has been present for a sufficiently long period, increasing the dietary K/Na ratio, or even the use of drugs, may not decrease the blood pressure very much. We have a pretty good idea why this should be the case. In experimental animals, continued elevation of the blood pressure eventually leads to an increase in collagen in the wall of the artery after the smooth muscles of the arteries hypertrophy. Now collagen is a tough structural material; it is collagen that makes meat from an old cow tough to chew. Once the collagen has increased in the wall of the arteries, relaxation or even decrease in the size of the smooth muscles would not allow the artery to expand its interior so the blood can flow easier. The tough collagen would not allow it. At this point, it is improbable that dietary changes or even drugs would produce much lowering of the blood pressure. This is consistent with what is observed clinically.

The Whole Picture

Finally, it is important to emphasize again the need to realize that the reductionist view of looking at only one factor ignores the reality of the systems, or holistic functioning, of the human body. For example, a decrease of dietary sodium leads to a decreased loss of potassium through the kidneys, with a resulting increase in body potassium and in plasma potassium concentration, and also decreases the content of sodium in blood vessels.[44] These are precisely the same effects produced by increasing dietary potassium and are similar to the effects of reducing weight or increasing exercise.

Summary

Many lines of evidence point to the importance of increasing the amount of potassium and decreasing the amount of sodium in your diet (maintaining a high–*K Factor* diet) in order to prevent or reverse high blood pressure. People who do eat a high–*K Factor* diet have lower blood pressure, and tend to have a higher concentration of potassium in the blood plasma and less sodium inside body cells. High blood levels of insulin tend to increase the activity of the sodium-potassium pump in the kidneys, causing retention of sodium, but losing weight or exercising helps restore normal plasma insulin levels. This, and other evidence summarized earlier, suggests that decreasing dietary sodium and increasing dietary potassium, losing weight, and exercising more are in many ways *doing the same things* in the body. Changing only one component is doing only part of the job.

One might say that sodium and potassium balance each other. The push-pull effects, or the yin-yang aspect of increasing potassium while decreasing sodium is hard to ignore. One pushes while the other pulls. One is the yin and the other is the yang. To have an effect, *both* must be changed. Thus, it is important to keep an eye on the *K Factor* in the diet *and* to eliminate factors, such as obesity and lack of exercise, that prevent the body from maintaining a normal balance between potassium and sodium.

PART SIX

Salt, Blood Pressure Regulation, and Drug Action

CHAPTER 21

How Important Is Salt?

"Ye are the salt of the earth"—the well-known quote from the Bible (Matthew 5:13) not only has poetic and theological meaning, it is literally true.

We are what we eat. We eat plants and animals. The animals that we eat in turn eat plants. So, in effect, all the substances in our bodies ultimately come from plants. And the plants themselves get all their minerals—their salts—from the earth.

As we explained earlier, the most abundant mineral inside our body's cells is potassium, so it's not surprising that we need a fair amount of potassium in our food. Fortunately, because both plants and animals contain plenty of potassium, we can easily obtain enough in our food—as long as we don't boil it out.

Animals also need a certain amount of sodium in order for their muscles and nerves to work properly and to keep their "sodium battery" charged, as we discussed in Chapter 6. Carnivores—animals that eat other animals—obtain an adequate amount of sodium in their diet from the fluid surrounding the cells of their prey, as well as the prey's blood, both of which are rich in sodium.

Plants, unlike animals, contain very little sodium. Plants do not have the sodium requirement that animals have: they do not possess nerve or muscle cells; neither do they have a "sodium battery." The reason we humans, and many other animals, don't need nearly as much sodium as most of us get turns out to be because of our body's fantastic ability to conserve sodium.

The Body's Ability to Conserve Sodium

Our ancestors were plant eaters living on a low-sodium diet. In order for these prehumans to survive, they had to develop mechanisms to retain sodium in their bodies and still eliminate water. We have inherited these sodium-conserving mechanisms in our kidneys and in our sweat glands. We'll discuss how the kidneys work and their amazing ability to keep sodium in the body in the next chapter.

Sweat glands work like miniature kidneys. Although it is not widely recognized, our sweat glands are also capable of conserving sodium by secreting large amounts of sweat that is almost completely lacking in sodium.

In a 1949 study[1] at the University of Michigan Medical School, Dr. Jerome Conn found that when men were eating a low-salt (low sodium chloride) diet and working in a hot environment, their perspiration had only 0.1 grams of sodium chloride (about 40 mg of sodium) in a whole liter (more than a quart) of sweat. The men lost only an additional 0.05 grams of sodium chloride (about 20 mg of sodium) per day in their urine! In total, they lost only about 0.75 grams of sodium chloride (amounting to 300 mg of sodium) per day—which is about 7 percent of the amount the average American consumes. Thus these men were able to maintain a balance between the amount of salt they were eating and the amount they were losing in their sweat and urine, even though they were losing over seven quarts of sweat a day!

In contrast, when Dr. Conn put the men to work in the same hot environment and had them eat a typical American diet containing 11 grams of sodium chloride (amounting to 4,400 mg of sodium), they lost about 7 grams of sodium chloride in their sweat (1 gram per each of 7 liters). The other 4 grams were lost mostly in their urine; a small amount was lost in their feces. The sweat of the men eating the typical American high-salt diet contained ten times as much sodium as the sweat of the men when they were on the low-salt diet. Thus it appears that the reason we Americans put out a very salty sweat is that our bodies are trying to get rid of the excess salt we have eaten.

Both of us have noticed that when we exercise, our sweat has a very bland taste compared with the salty taste it used to have before we started our high–*K Factor* diet.

If you're sweating a lot, you don't need extra salt, but you *do* need to drink extra water. In *Eat to Win*, Dr. Robert Haas recommends the following drink for sweating athletes: To every 1 cup of water add 2 tablespoons of fresh orange juice and ⅓ teaspoon of table salt. This will have a *K Factor* of about 1. We believe it would be even better to cut the salt to ⅙ teaspoon or less, bringing the *K Factor* up to 2 or more.

Many Groups of People Do Quite Well Without Added Salt

In view of the fact that both our kidneys and our sweat glands can get rid of water without losing much sodium, it isn't surprising that people can live quite well without adding salt to their food, even in a very hot climate. In fact, the South American Indians and the Africans and Asians living near the Equator have been eating a low-sodium diet for thousands of years. As we pointed out in Chapter 3, the people who still eat a diet of unprocessed natural foods, with no added salt, have almost no hypertension: Less than 1 percent of these populations develop hypertension, and blood pressure does not increase with age. You will recall that these low-blood-pressure groups ranged from the Carajas Indians of Brazil to the Papuans of New Guinea.

Actually, the low-blood-pressure groups live in a variety of climates, and they eat a variety of diets. For example, the diet of the Yanomamo Indians is primarily vegetarian, a major component of their diet being plantain (a cooking banana). In contrast, the diet of the Greenland Eskimos—at least in the 1920s, when they were studied by Dr. William Thomas[2]—was completely carnivorous. It consisted of walrus, seal, polar bear, caribou, Arctic hare, fox, birds, and fish—all usually eaten raw and never with any added salt. (Unsalted meats have *K Factor*s of 4.5 or more.)

The Greenland Eskimos' diet was fairly low in fat, since this was carefully removed from the meat for use as fuel. Wild animals do not have fat "marbled" between the muscle cells, as do "fattened" beef cattle. (As we described in chapters 8 and 10, excess fat in our food can contribute to high blood pressure, atherosclerosis, heart attacks, and cancer.) Not only were the Greenland Eskimos free of high blood pressure, but they enjoyed general good health even into old age.

The Labrador Eskimos examined in the same study, however, were in very poor health. Their diet was augmented with dried and canned foods, which they purchased from the Hudson's Bay Company in exchange for furs. The latter foods contained added salt, and they were deficient in vitamin C.

How Much Sodium Do We Really Need?

The National Academy of Sciences has estimated that the "safe and adequate" daily dietary intake of sodium is 1,100 to 3,300 milligrams. However, there is considerable reason to believe that the amount of sodium we need is actually lower.

Some of the low-blood-pressure groups of people who eat primarily vegetarian diets have been getting along fine for thousands of years on sodium intakes ranging from 50 to 230 milligrams per day.[3] Some of Dr. Lewis Dahl's patients with hypertension lived on diets containing 50 to 300 milligrams of sodium per day for up to fifteen years with no ill effects.[4] Dr. Walter Kempner's rice-fruit diet has also been used for years by many patients, and this diet provides only 50 to 60 milligrams of sodium per day.[5] Thus there is considerable evidence that the required amount of sodium is well below the 1,100 milligrams figure, probably as low as 100 to 300 milligrams.

Our Appetite for Salt

So why do so many people think we need extra salt?

Some people say we need extra salt because they think animals do. This misconception probably arises from the well-known fact that cows like to lick salt blocks. However, this isn't so much that their vegetarian diet contains very little sodium as it is that they lose a lot of sodium in the very large amount of milk they produce. Holstein cows, for example, can produce as much as 30,000 pounds of milk per year, about 15 times the amount required to nurse a calf. This is about 10 gallons per day and up to 40 percent of the weight of the cow per week! Because a lactating cow loses so much sodium in her milk, she requires about 30 grams of supplemental salt per day.[6]

In contrast, dry cows (those not producing milk) or beef steers are equally healthy whether or not they are given supplemental salt,[7] and the same is true for other domestic animals.[8] And although wild herbivores such as deer have been reputed to travel great distances to go to natural salt licks, it is difficult to substantiate this belief. For example, Dr. A. R. Patton analyzed mud sent in by forest rangers from areas in the Montana Rockies where wild animals congregate to lick the soil. The rangers called these sites "salt licks," but Dr. Patton did not find sodium in any of the mud samples. What he did find, however, was iodine,[9] an element needed to make thyroid hormone.

Probably the biggest reason we have been conditioned to use so much salt is the history of our culture. About 4,000 years ago, trade routes were developed that made sea salt available even to people living far from the sea. Salt came into common use for seasoning and for preserving food. It was also an important item of commerce. In the Bible, it is written: "And every oblation of thy meat offering shalt thou season with salt" (Leviticus 2:13). This was written about 3,500 years ago. The word *salary* is derived from the Latin word *salarium* ("salt money"), which was used to pay the Roman soldiers. We still use the expression Is he worth his salt? But the 4,000 years during which there has been easy access to salt is only one-thousandth of the period of time that human life has existed on this planet.

Thus the "recent" abundance of salt has probably not had time to affect the evolution of humans significantly. This is especially true because the major harmful effect that excess salt produces in some people—high blood pressure—does not usually have lethal effects until after a person has passed breeding age.

The fact that we do not need much sodium in our diet is indicated by the low sodium content of human milk (37 to 39 mg per cup, with a *K Factor* of 3.2 to 3.5).[10] Many modern babies are nourished with cow's milk, however, which has over three times as much sodium as does human milk. Considering that the foods available to children after they are weaned typically have added salt, it is hardly surprising that our palates become habituated to the taste of salt. The result: any food without added salt doesn't taste right.

We believe that the major part of our craving for salt is acquired as a dietary habit. We have been taught, or conditioned, to like salt. In fact, one study reported that many people said that after they had been on a low-sodium diet for a few weeks, they actually began to prefer unsalted food.[11] We can testify to this from our own experience: We have even developed a taste preference for potassium salts, which most people dislike at first!

Summary

Since our kidneys and sweat glands are designed to hold on to sodium, we do not need to eat very much in our food. Our modern food habits, however, have caused us to develop a craving for salt. This craving has resulted in a major health problem— hypertension—in our modern society, where salted foods and foods with much of their natural potassium removed are readily available and extremely popular.

Fortunately, though, most of your craving for salt is a learned habit. And habits can be broken.

CHAPTER 22

How the Kidneys, Hormones, and Nervous System Work Together to Control Blood Pressure

Blood pressure depends on both the output from the heart (the volume of blood pumped per minute) and the peripheral resistance to the flow of blood. Blood pressure is regulated by three main systems: the kidneys, the endocrine system (hormones), and the nervous system. In other words, these three systems are able to control heart output and peripheral resistance.

The Kidneys and Blood Pressure

There are several ways the kidneys influence blood pressure. One is thought to be by regulating the volume of blood and other fluids in the body, which could affect both heart output and peripheral resistance. Another way the kidneys influence blood pressure is by controlling the amounts of sodium, potassium, and calcium in the body. We have already discussed how these minerals affect the degree of contraction of the smooth muscle cells in the arterioles.

It has long been known that some diseases of the kidney can

335

cause hypertension. When it is due to an identifiable disease, this type of hypertension is called secondary (see Chapter 9). One example of secondary hypertension involving the kidney occurs when there is an obstruction of the artery to a kidney. This causes an excessive secretion by cells in the kidney of the hormone renin, the effects of which we describe later in this chapter.

The Connection between the Kidneys, Sodium, and Blood Pressure

But blood pressure can be affected by the kidneys even when they are not obviously diseased. An example of this type of hypertension was discovered in laboratory rats by Dr. Lewis Dahl.[1] Through selective breeding, Dr. Dahl and his co-workers developed two strains of rats: salt-insensitive rats, which do not develop high blood pressure regardless of what they eat, and salt-sensitive rats, which do develop high blood pressure but only when they are raised on a high-salt (NaCl) diet.

In order to excrete the same amount of sodium, the kidneys of the salt-sensitive rats require a higher blood pressure than do those of the salt-insensitive rats. One way of looking at this is that the high blood pressure may be the salt-sensitive rat's way of getting rid of the extra sodium it gets when on a diet high in sodium. It is likely that something similar may be operating in some humans who inherit a tendency to high blood pressure.

The ability of the kidneys to affect blood pressure is dramatically demonstrated by kidney transplant experiments. When kidneys from salt-sensitive rats with high blood pressure are transplanted into rats with normal blood pressure, these recipient rats also develop high blood pressure.[2] On the other hand, when kidneys from rats with normal blood pressure are transplanted into hypertensive rats, the latter develop normal blood pressure.[3] Similar observations have been made in humans: when a good kidney is transplanted into a person with severe kidney disease and hypertension, the blood pressure often returns to normal.[4]

How the Kidneys Work

Now we'll review briefly how the kidneys work: by filtering a huge amount of fluid out of the blood and then reabsorbing most of it back into the blood. Only what the body doesn't need is left in the final urine.

Each of us has two kidneys inside the abdomen next to the back muscles. Each kidney consists of about one million tiny functional units that are called nephrons. The structure of a typical nephron is shown in Figure 21.

A very large volume of fluid enters the nephrons at the glomeruli, where the arterial blood pressure forces (filters) the fluid part of the blood through ultrafine pores. These pores are so small that they allow only salts and other small molecules, such as water and glucose, to pass through; they prevent the

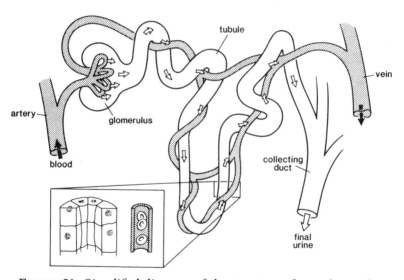

FIGURE 21. *Simplified diagram of the structure of a nephron, the unshaded tube; blood vessels are shaded.* The watery part of the blood is "filtered" into the glomerulus at the head end of the nephron. As this "preformed urine" passes along the nephron tubule, most of the water and dissolved substances are reabsorbed out of the tubule and back into the blood.

blood cells and proteins from entering the nephrons. The resulting ultrafiltrate of the blood ("preformed urine") contains about the same concentration of small molecules and of sodium and other ions as does the blood fluid.

In an average adult, about 50 gallons of this preformed urine are formed each day. Fortunately, the nephrons reabsorb most of this fluid back into the bloodstream; otherwise we would produce 50 gallons of urine per day! Normally all the glucose and amino acids are reabsorbed back into the blood, and more than 99 percent of the sodium is reabsorbed.

Most of the energy for the reabsorption of sodium comes from the sodium-potassium pump we described in Chapter 6. Water follows the reabsorbed substances passively by the process of osmosis. A simplified diagram of how most of the sodium and potassium are reabsorbed from one portion of the nephron tubule is shown in Figure 22.

The inner and outer membranes of the tubule cells are different. The net effect of the ion movements is the movement of sodium, potassium, and chloride (along with water) from the nephron passageway back into the blood. The "Na-K-Cl pump" (the "triangle" in Figure 22) is a recently discovered "piggyback" membrane pump that moves one potassium ion, one sodium ion, and two chloride ions simultaneously across the cell membrane into the nephron cell from the nephron passageway, using energy from the sodium battery we described in Chapter 6.

Because the membrane of the tubule cell that faces outward pumps sodium out and potassium into the cell, and because of membrane leakiness, the net effect of all of the membrane transport systems is primarily to move sodium and chloride from the inside of the nephron (that is, from the preformed urine) to the blood.

In the piggyback pump system just described, sodium must be transported back into the body together with chloride; therefore the amount of sodium that can be reabsorbed back into the body from the ultrafiltrate in the tubule is partly limited by the amount of chloride present. For this reason, *a low-chloride diet helps the body get rid of sodium* in the urine, while a high-chloride diet helps keep sodium in the body. Thus table salt (in

NEPHRON   BLOOD VESSEL

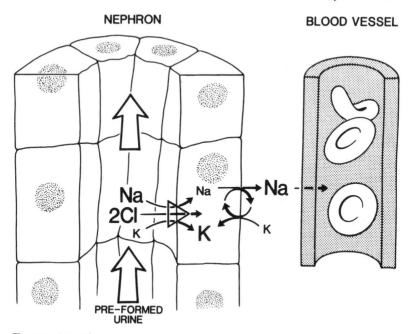

FIGURE 22. *The movement of Na, K, and Cl (chloride) through the wall of the nephron.* (Only some of the most important pathways for these ions are shown.) The circle on the outer nephron membrane represents the metabolically driven sodium potassium pump described in Chapter 6. The triangle represents a "piggyback" pump that carries Na, K, and Cl together into the nephrone cell. Electrical voltages across the cell membranes are not shown.

which *all* the sodium comes packaged with chloride) is generally the *worst* form of sodium to have in your diet.

The sodium in natural food isn't quite so bad. In meat, for example, about 15 percent of the sodium is combined with organic anions rather than chloride. In unprocessed foods, relatively little potassium is complexed with chloride (for example, about 20% in potatoes). In both plant and animal cells, potassium is associated primarily with a variety of organic negative ions rather than with chloride (Cl^-). So you can see that the best way to get potassium is in natural foods. Mother Nature has it prepared just right for us. If you take supplemental potassium, such as in pills or a salt substitute, it may be better not to take it as the chloride salt.

In summary, the kidneys are good at conserving sodium for the body and at the same time excreting large amounts of potassium into the urine. So it's understandable why we don't need much sodium (only about 100 or 200 mg) but do need a lot of potassium in our diet. Since the kidneys can excrete so much potassium into the urine, the amounts in natural foods certainly are not dangerous unless severe kidney disease is present.

Regulation of the Kidneys by Hormones

ANTIDIURETIC HORMONE. The volume of urine output is regulated by several factors. One of these is *antidiuretic hormone* (ADH), which is secreted by the pituitary gland at the base of the brain. The rate of secretion of ADH depends on blood volume and especially the concentration of salts in the blood. The hormone is carried by the bloodstream to the kidneys, where it causes a reduction in the volume of urine production.

Deficient ADH secretion is known as diabetes insipidus. The people who have this relatively rare condition produce up to 20 liters of urine each day. Because it is so dilute, physicians in the old days noticed that the urine of these patients has an insipid taste, hence the name of the condition. (The more common diabetes is called diabetes mellitus because of the sugar in the urine; *mellitus* means "sweet.")

The volume of urine output is also tied to the rate at which the kidneys excrete sodium, which is largely under the control of the hormones *aldosterone, natriuretic factors*, and *insulin*.

INSULIN. Insulin is best known for its ability to regulate blood sugar levels and for its role in diabetes mellitus. Although the finding is not yet in the textbooks, insulin is also one of the most potent sodium-retaining hormones.

After Dick's laboratory discovered that insulin stimulates the sodium-potassium pump,[5] a colleague, Dr. Jean Crabbé from the University of Louvain Medical School in Belgium, visited his laboratory and discussed this. Back in Belgium, Dr. Crabbé and his co-workers demonstrated that insulin stimulates the sodium-potassium pump in the kidney so much that at about twice the normal blood level, insulin can cause almost total reabsorption of sodium from the preformed urine back into the blood.[6]

This effect of insulin partly explains why obese people tend to retain sodium in their body and thus frequently develop high blood pressure. It also explains why people who have been on a very low calorie diet or on a total fast (which lowers blood insulin) develop retention of fluid after taking a lot of carbohydrate in their first full meal. The carbohydrate sharply raises their blood sugar, which, in turn, causes the pancreas to release lots of insulin into the blood. This increase in blood insulin then stimulates the sodium-potassium pumps in the kidneys to cause retention of sodium ions (Na^+). Since water always follows Na^+, their kidneys also retain fluid, causing a temporary weight gain of several pounds.

ALDOSTERONE. *Aldosterone* is sometimes considered the primary salt-retaining hormone. Aldosterone is secreted into the blood by the adrenal glands that sit on top of each kidney. At high levels of aldosterone secretion, almost no sodium is lost in the urine or sweat. In Addison's disease, there is a deficiency in the secretion of aldosterone. This results in the excessive loss of sodium from the body, a hunger for salt, decreased blood volume, and *low* blood pressure.

The opposite symptoms occur in Conn's syndrome, which can be caused by an adrenal-gland tumor that secretes excess aldosterone. The resulting retention of sodium and water causes high blood pressure. High blood pressure due to this type of Conn's disease cannot be cured either by drugs or raising the *K Factor* but must be corrected by surgical removal of the tumor.

Aldosterone also causes the kidneys to excrete more potassium. The fact that a high blood level of aldosterone leads not only to retention of sodium in the body and to loss of potassium but also to elevated blood pressure presents one more piece of evidence that excess sodium or too little potassium in the body can cause hypertension.

ANGIOTENSIN AND RENIN. The rate of secretion of aldosterone is controlled partly by the blood level of another hormone called angiotensin, which is in turn controlled by an enzyme called renin, which is secreted into the blood by specialized cells in the kidney.

Renin secretion by the kidney is increased by sympathetic nerve activity and/or by low arterial blood pressure in the kidneys. In addition to causing increased secretion of aldosterone, angiotensin also acts directly on the smooth muscle cells of the arterioles, causing them to contract and raising blood pressure. We mentioned earlier in this chapter that a few cases of human hypertension result from the increased renin secretion (and thus higher levels of angiotensin) caused by an obstruction of the artery leading to a kidney.

The action of renin is summarized in the following diagram:

Decreased Kidney Blood Pressure or
Increased Sympathetic Nerve Activity

Increased Release of Renin from the Kidneys

Increased Level of Angiotensin in the Blood

Constriction of Arterioles   Secretion of Aldosterone

Kidneys Retain Sodium

High Blood Pressure

NATRIURETIC FACTORS. Natriuretic factors are recently discovered substances that increase the rate of sodium excretion by the kidneys. The word *natriuretic* comes from *natrium*, for "sodium," and *uresis*, meaning "excretion in the urine." Increased consumption of sodium or an increase in the blood volume stimulates the secretion of these factors into the blood.

One natriuretic hormone, or factor, is secreted by cells at the base of the brain. This natriuretic factor acts partly by inhibiting the sodium-potassium pumps in the kidney tubules. This slows sodium reabsorption, allowing more sodium to be lost in the urine. Researchers have suggested that if the blood level of this natriuretic factor rises sufficiently (for example, as it does when you eat a lot of sodium), it may inhibit the sodium-potassium pumps located in the smooth muscle cells in the arterioles throughout the body. This would cause the "sodium batteries" of these cells to run down. Some scientists believe that this is what causes many cases of primary hypertension, since the discharged sodium batteries would result in constriction of the arterioles.[7] As you already know, this would result in increased peripheral resistance, causing the blood pressure to rise.

The other natriuretic factor is a peptide, or small protein, manufactured and released from a small "ear," or auricle, which sticks out from the atrium of the heart. Accordingly it is called the atrial natriuretic factor, or ANF. It does not inhibit the sodium-potassium pump but instead increases sodium excretion by another means.

Until recently, it was thought odd that the heart would have this part, which apparently served no useful function in the body. Now it has been shown that stretching out the auricle of the heart by increased blood volume causes it to secrete atrial natriuretic factor. The atrial natriuretic factor then causes the arterioles in the kidney to enlarge, allowing more preformed urine to be filtered and thus more sodium and water to be lost in the urine. ANF also dilates other blood vessels. ANF is the only hormone known to effectively lower blood pressure and has been proposed as a new drug for that purpose.

OTHER HORMONES. Other hormones, whose functions are still poorly understood, are secreted by the kidneys and are probably very important. Only recently has it been recognized that a class of hormones called prostaglandins are secreted by cells in the kidneys. Prostaglandins appear to help the kidneys excrete sodium. This may account for the reduction in blood pressure that occurs when safflower oil is added to the diet (see Chapter 8), since linoleic acid (the major component of safflower oil) is necessary for the synthesis of prostaglandins.

Regulation of Blood Pressure by the Nervous System

Our blood pressure is regulated from minute to minute by nerves. At specific locations in the walls of the large arteries, special sensors "measure" blood pressure by responding to the amount of stretch in the walls of the arteries. An important location of these sensors is called the *carotid sinus*, which is in the arteries that run up the neck to supply the head with blood.

When blood pressure increases for any reason, these sensors send nerve signals to the blood-pressure-regulating center located in the lower portion of the brain. In response to the nerve signals, the blood-pressure-regulating center sends out nerve signals that slow the heart and dilate the arterioles. The lower output of blood by the heart and the lower peripheral resistance to blood flow both result in lowering the arterial blood pressure back toward normal.

By rubbing the carotid sinus area on the side of your neck near your voice box, you can stimulate these receptors and cause a quick (but temporary) reduction of your blood pressure.

Another example of this reflex occurs when you suddenly sit or stand after lying down. Gravity pulls the blood downward, lowering the blood pressure in the carotid sinus in your neck. If the carotid sinus reflex didn't act promptly, sending out nerve impulses (over sympathetic nerves) to increase heart output and constrict the arterioles, you would faint from the decreased flow of blood to your head. In fact, fainting when standing up is one of the side effects of some of the blood pressure medicines that act by inhibiting the sympathetic (adrenergic) nervous system, as we will describe in the next chapter.

The sympathetic nervous system is the portion of the autonomic (involuntary) nervous system that has as its main function the preparation of our bodies for emergency situations. The sympathetic (adrenergic) nervous system sends nerve signals to the blood-pressure-regulating center, which tell it to raise the blood pressure, which the center accomplishes by sending signals over sympathetic nerves that go to the heart and blood vessels. This system becomes active when we are frightened, preparing us to run away or to fight by increasing our heart rate and reducing the blood flow to the stomach, intestines, and skin. Some cases of primary hypertension appear to be associated with increased sympathetic nervous system activity. This could be partly the result of a decrease in the voltage across the surface membrane of the sympathetic nerve cells caused by accumulation of sodium and depletion of potassium inside the cell, which could be helped by dietary changes. The decreased membrane voltage of the sympathetic nerve cells would cause them to fire off nerve signals more often, thus raising blood pressure. Increased sympathetic nervous system activity can also result from the psychological stress caused by our reaction to unpleasant situations.

Summary

The kidneys, the endocrine system (hormones), and the nervous system all play important roles in regulating blood pressure. Since our lives depend on maintaining our blood pressure, it is not surprising that so many systems have evolved to take care of this important function. We have suggested how our dietary sodium and potassium intake might affect these systems. In different individuals, one particular system might be more susceptible to the deleterious effects of a low K/Na ratio than another. In Chapter 6, we showed how dietary potassium and sodium can affect the final determiners of peripheral resistance: the arteriolar smooth muscle cells.

CHAPTER 23
Antihypertensive Drugs

In this chapter, we will briefly describe how antihypertensive drugs reduce your blood pressure. The types of drugs most often used for treating high blood pressure are listed in Table 13.

TABLE 13. *Antihypertensive Drugs*

Type	Generic Name	Trade Names	Common Side Effects*
Step 1: Diuretics			
Thiazide diuretics	Chlorothiazide	Diuril Aldoclor† Diupress	Low blood plasma potassium due to urinary loss of potassium, muscle weakness or cramping, faintness upon standing, sexual dysfunction
	Chlorthalidone	Hygroton Regroton Novothalidon Tenoretic Uridon	

Type	Generic Name	Trade Names	Common Side Effects*
	Hydro-chlorothiazide	Maxzide† Aldoril† Dyazide†	
Potassium-sparing diuretics	Spirono-lactone	Aldactone Aldactazide	Lethargy, enlargement of male breasts, breast pain, menstrual irregularities, intestinal problems
	Triamterene	Dyremium Maxzide† Dyazide†	Nausea, weakness, leg cramps
Other diuretics	Furosemide	Lasix	Potassium loss, nausea, vomiting, diarrhea, headache, weakness

Step 2: Adrenergic (Sympathetic) Inhibiting Drugs

Central-acting adrenergic inhibitors	Clonidine	Catapres Combipres	Drowsiness, fatigue, dry mouth, constipation, dizziness, sexual dysfunction
	Methyldopa	Aldoclor† Aldomet Aldoril†	Headache, weakness, nausea, dry mouth, drowsiness, fatigue, constipation, dizziness, sexual dysfunction
Sympathetic nerve ending blockers	Guanethidine (STEP 4)	Ismelin Esimil	Faintness upon standing up, diarrhea, weakness, stuffy nose, failure to ejaculate, slow heart rate
	Rauwolfia alkaloids	Harmonyl Raudixin	Sexual dysfunction, stuffy nose, depression, lethargy
	Reserpine	Diupress† Serpasil	Faintness upon standing up, diarrhea, weakness, stuffy nose, failure to ejaculate, slow heart rate, depression, lethargy

Type	Generic Name	Trade Names	Common Side Effects*
Alpha adrenergic blockers	Phenoxy-benzamine	Dibenzyline	Dizziness on standing, stuffy nose, fast heart beat, failure of ejaculation
	Phentolamine	Regitine	Dizziness on standing, weakness, failure of ejaculation, stuffy nose, fast heart beat, nausea, vomiting, diarrhea
	Prazosin	Minipress	Dizziness on standing, weakness, drowsiness, headache, failure of ejaculation, stuffy nose, fast heart beat, nausea, vomiting, diarrhea
Beta adrenergic blockers (ALSO USED FOR STEP 1)	Metoprolol	Lopressor	Slow heart beat, nausea, loss of appetite, insomnia, fatigue, sexual dysfunction
	Nadolol	Corgard	
	Propanolol	Inderal Inderide	

Step 3: Vasodilators

Vasodilators	Hydrazaline	Apresoline Dralzine Unipres	Headache, fast heart beat, nausea
	Minoxidil	Loniten	Fast heart beat, fluid retention, excess hair growth, breast pain

Newer Drugs (not yet included in the stepped care recommendations)

Angiotensin inhibitors	Captopril	Capoten Lopirin	Rash
	Saralasin	Sarenin	
Calcium entry blockers	Diltiazem	Anginyl Cardizem	Headache, dizziness, nausea
	Nifedipine	Adalat Nifedin	

Type	Generic Name	Trade Names	Common Side Effects*
	Verapamil	Calan Cordilox Isoptin Vasolan	Flushing, fluid retention, constipation

*All these drugs also have many other less common side effects that are not listed here.

The sources for this table are given under reference 1.[1]

†Many of the trade-name drugs combine two or more generic drugs in one pill; thus these trade names appear twice.

Warning: If you are currently taking one of the adrenergic inhibiting drugs, do not suddenly stop taking it, as this could cause a heart attack or sudden death. In fact, any change in your current medication should only be done in consultation with your physician.

Diuretics

Thiazide Diuretics

Diuretics are drugs that stimulate the kidneys to produce a larger volume of urine. Thiazide diuretics accomplish this by causing the kidneys to reabsorb less sodium back into the blood and thus to excrete extra sodium. Water accompanies this extra sodium in the urine, leading to the increased urine volume.

Thiazide diuretics decrease blood pressure in two ways: First, the loss of sodium and water leads to a decrease in blood volume, which in turn reduces blood pressure by decreasing output of blood from the heart. Later the heart output returns to normal, but the blood pressure stays down because the loss of sodium from the body results in a decrease in the peripheral resistance to blood flow (by mechanisms we described in Chapter 6).

In people whose kidneys are no longer functioning—patients on artificial kidney machines—thiazide diuretics have no effect on blood pressure.[2] Since diuretics do not affect the amount of sodium removed by the artificial kidney machine, this suggests that the decreased peripheral resistance induced by the thiazide diuretics is due to the loss of sodium. As Dr. Louis Tobian has repeatedly pointed out, every physician who uses a thiazide diuretic for treating hypertension is casting a vote for the idea that too much sodium is a key factor in causing essential hypertension.

Unfortunately, the thiazide diuretics also cause the excretion of extra potassium. This can lead to a deficiency of potassium in skeletal muscles,[3] which can cause mild weakness, a fairly common side effect of these drugs. The extra loss of potassium through the kidney can also result in a decrease in the level of plasma potassium.[4] If you are also taking a digitalis compound for your heart, this drop in plasma potassium can be very dangerous, leading to an irregular rhythm of your heart (cardiac arrhythmia).

Of course, the irony of the thiazide diuretics is that a deficiency in potassium is part of the problem in your developing high blood pressure in the first place. Although we don't yet know all the effects of a deficiency in body potassium, it is established that they include abnormal carbohydrate metabolism, glycosuria, disturbed acid base balance, and kidney disease.[5]

A frequent complication of the thiazide diuretics is an elevation of the blood uric acid level. This can precipitate an attack of gout. Thiazide diuretics also elevate blood levels of cholesterol and other fats, which are known to increase your chances of having a heart attack. Recall from Chapter 2 that treatment of borderline hypertension with thiazide diuretics apparently doubles the death rate, with most of the deaths resulting from heart attacks.[6]

Prolonged use of thiazide diuretics results in a decrease not only in blood potassium but also in body magnesium content,[7] which can, in turn, make it difficult for the body to restore its potassium.

Potassium-sparing Diuretics

The potassium-sparing diuretic spironolactone is thought to block the action of the hormone aldosterone.[8] Remember from

Chapter 22 that aldosterone causes the kidneys to conserve sodium by causing more of it to be reabsorbed out of the preformed urine in the nephrons, thus putting it back into the blood. Therefore, when spironolactone is given, this action of aldosterone is blocked and more sodium (and water) is lost in the urine.

Aldosterone also stimulates secretion of potassium from the blood into the forming urine in the kidney nephrons. Therefore, spironolactone causes the kidneys to conserve potassium, keeping it in the body instead of excreting it in the urine along with the excreted sodium. For this reason, spironolactone lacks one of the undesirable side effects of the thiazide diuretics—loss of body potassium. You can see that spironolactone will have some of the same beneficial effects on blood pressure as a diet with a high *K Factor*. The high–*K Factor* diet, however, does not have any undesirable side effects, whereas spironolactone use can result in lethargy, enlargement of male breasts, breast pain, menstrual irregularities, or intestinal problems.[9]

The other potassium-sparing diuretic listed in the table is triamterene. Triamterene directly inhibits the transport of sodium out of and the secretion of potassium into the preformed urine in the kidney tubules.[10] Thus, like spironolactone, triamterene promotes the loss of sodium through urination while conserving potassium. Both these effects will reduce the blood pressure by the mechanisms we described in Chapter 6. However, triamterene can cause nausea, leg cramps, or weakness.

Other Diuretics

Furosemide is sometimes used for treating hypertension as well as for treating congestive heart failure and other conditions that cause fluid accumulation. It acts on the kidney tubules to inhibit the reabsorption of sodium and chloride and, to some degree, potassium. Thus more salts and water remain in the final urine. Getting rid of extra sodium is beneficial for reducing the blood pressure, but the extra loss of potassium may be a harmful side effect, as we discussed in the thiazide diuretic section.

Adrenergic Inhibitors

There are four types of antihypertensive drugs that inhibit the sympathetic nervous system. The major function of the sympathetic nervous system is to prepare the body for "fight or flight." In order to fight or take flight, more blood must be delivered to the arm and leg muscles. To accomplish this, the sympathetic nervous system causes the heart to pump out more blood by increasing the heart's rate of beating and the strength of its contractions. In addition, the sympathetic nervous system tightens the blood vessels going to the stomach, intestines, skin, and other regions, since it's more important to run away from a tiger than to digest your hamburger or stay cool. Both the increased cardiac output and the increased peripheral blood vessel resistance caused by sympathetic nerve activity will lead to increased blood pressure.

Even when a person is sitting or standing at rest and not frightened, there is a basal level of sympathetic nervous system activity. Thus there is a constant stream of nerve impulses arriving at the arteriolar smooth muscles, causing them to have a "resting" tone or tension. Therefore, a drug that inhibits the sympathetic nervous system will tend to lower the blood pressure by decreasing the basal smooth muscle tone, allowing the arterioles to widen.

Centrally Acting Adrenergic Inhibitors

Adrenergic inhibitors can be centrally acting or peripherally acting. The centrally acting adrenergic inhibitors block the sympathetic nervous system in the brain or spinal cord. Both types have a variety of undesirable side effects (see Table 13).

METHYLDOPA. Methyldopa inhibits the outflow of nerve signals from the sympathetic nervous system.[11] Since sympathetic nerve signals generally tell smooth muscle cells in the blood vessels to contract, the inhibition of these signals allows the arteriolar smooth muscle cells to relax, thus lowering peripheral resistance and blood pressure.

CLONIDINE. Clonidine's major hypotensive effect stems from its action on the blood-pressure-regulating center in the medulla of the brain stem.[12] It inhibits sympathetic nerve output and stimulates parasympathetic nerve outflow; both these central effects result in a lowering of the blood pressure. *Caution: sudden withdrawal of clonidine can cause a life-threatening hypertensive crisis.*

Peripheral-Acting Adrenergic Inhibitors

The rest of the adrenergic inhibiting drugs act primarily at the endings of the sympathetic nerves, where they make functional contact with smooth muscle cells. By *functional contact*, we mean that this is where the nerve signals are transmitted to the muscle cells, causing them to increase their level of contraction. The nerve endings do not actually physically touch the smooth muscle cells; instead they are separated by a narrow *synaptic* gap. Thus the electrical nerve signals cannot be directly conducted from the nerve cell endings to the smooth (or heart) muscle cells. To get the signal across the synaptic gap, the electric nerve signal causes the sympathetic nerve endings to release the chemical *norepinephrine* (we will call it by the common name, *noradrenaline*), which is stored in the nerve terminal. The noradrenaline then diffuses across the synaptic gap and attaches to *receptor* protein molecules on the surface of the smooth muscle cells. This attachment causes a pore in the muscle cell membrane to open, allowing calcium to enter the cell, where it activates the contractile machinery. This is illustrated in Figure 23.

RESERPINE AND THE RAUWOLFIA ALKALOIDS. Several chemicals called alkaloids may be extracted from the root of the plant *Rauwolfia serpentina*, a climbing shrublike plant that is native to India. The ancient Hindus used these alkaloids for treating snake bites and hypertension.[13] One of these alkaloids has been named reserpine and has been widely used for treating high blood pressure since the rediscovery of the rauwolfia alkaloids in the 1950s.

Reserpine and the other rauwolfia alkaloids act by depleting

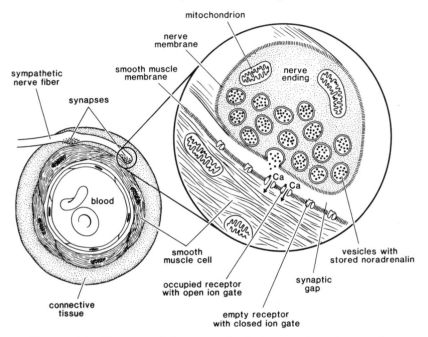

FIGURE 23. *Diagram of the sympathetic innervation of arteriolar smooth muscle. Left*: cross section of an arteriole; *right*: an enlargement (circled portion).

the stores of noradrenaline in the nerve endings. This affects the brain as well as the peripheral nerve endings, but the peripheral effects are considered to be the most important. Because of the depletion of stored noradrenaline, the nerve signals do not release as much noradrenaline, and fewer calcium channels open in the smooth muscle membrane, resulting in less tension in the muscle cells. This dilates the arterioles and lowers blood pressure. The effect of reserpine lasts for about a week, so the physician must be aware of the cumulative effect of daily doses.

GUANETHIDINE. Guanethidine, like reserpine, also inhibits the *presynaptic* release of noradrenaline. It does this both by directly inhibiting the release mechanism and by depleting the amount of stored noradrenaline.

Adrenergic Blockers

In contrast to reserpine and guanethidine, which act on the nerve endings, the drugs we will discuss next act by inhibiting the postsynaptic receptors on the smooth muscle membrane—that is, they block the membrane from receiving noradrenaline. The postsynaptic receptors normally respond to the noradrenaline released by the nerve endings. There are two major types of noradrenaline receptors: *alpha* receptors and *beta* receptors—and there are "blocker" drugs for each.

ALPHA BLOCKERS. Alpha receptors are found on the smooth muscle cells in almost all the body's arterioles. Thus the alpha blocking drugs—phenoxybenzamine, phentolamine, and prazosin—reduce blood pressure by blocking the transmission of sympathetic nerve signals to the arterioles, allowing the arteriolar smooth muscle to relax and widening the passageway for blood flow. This effect is greatest when you are standing and is minimal when lying down (very few sympathetic nerve signals are sent out when you are lying at rest). The side effects of the alpha blocking drugs result from the fact that alpha receptors are found not only in arteriolar muscle but also in heart muscle, intestinal muscle, and sexual tract muscle. As listed in Table 13, these side effects include fast heartbeat, diarrhea, and failure of ejaculation.

BETA BLOCKERS. Beta receptors are found on smooth muscle cells in the arterioles of the heart, liver, and skeletal muscles. These receptors are activated by adrenaline. Adrenaline hormone is released from the inner cells of the adrenal glands when they are stimulated by sympathetic nerve signals. It then circulates in the blood.

In contrast to the alpha receptors just discussed, activation of the beta receptors by the circulating adrenaline causes a *dilation*, not a constriction, of the arterioles that have beta receptors. Thus one would think that a beta blocker such as propranolol, which blocks these "dilation" receptors, might constrict the arterioles of the heart, intestines, and arm and leg muscles, and thus cause an increase in blood pressure. But because the blood level of adrenaline is normally fairly low and because the drugs have other effects, beta blockers do reduce blood pressure.

The exact mechanisms by which the beta blockers reduce blood pressure are not known for certain, but one mechanism appears to be by inhibiting the kidneys' secretion of renin into the blood. Ordinarily the secretion of renin is stimulated by activation of beta receptors on the secretory cells in the kidneys. As we described in the previous chapter, renin causes an increased production of angiotensin in the blood. Angiotensin has two actions that raise the blood pressure: It causes arteriolar smooth muscle to contract, and it acts on the adrenal gland, causing the outer cells to secrete more aldosterone into the blood. Aldosterone in turn acts on the kidneys to cause sodium and water to be retained by the body and potassium to be lost in the urine. Thus beta blockers, by inhibiting this process, actually help improve the body's *K Factor.*

Another mechanism by which beta blockers may reduce blood pressure is by reducing the amount of noradrenaline that is released from sympathetic nerve terminals. This can occur because there are beta receptors on the nerve terminal membrane that, when activated, cause more noradrenaline to be released. Propranolol and the other beta blockers block this noradrenaline release.

Vasodilators

Hydrazaline and minoxidil both reduce blood pressure by acting directly on the arteriolar smooth muscle cells and causing them to relax. An interesting side effect of minoxidil is that it stimulates hair growth. A solution of the drug is now being applied to the heads of younger bald men to stimulate the regrowth of hair, but as of this writing it has not been approved for this purpose by the FDA.

Newer Drugs

Angiotensin Inhibitors

We have described how propranolol, a beta blocker, can reduce blood pressure by inhibiting renin secretion. This renin inhibition in turn reduces the amount of angiotensin in the blood. There are also drugs that specifically inhibit angiotensin. Captopril reduces the level of angiotensin in the blood by inhibiting the renin-stimulated angiotensin production. Saralasin inhibits the actions of angiotensin on the kidneys and on arteriolar smooth muscle. These angiotensin inhibitors are especially effective in reducing the blood pressure of hypertensive people who have higher than normal blood levels of renin.

Calcium Entry Blockers

As we pointed out in Chapter 6, the amount of tension in smooth muscle cells is controlled by the intracellular concentration of calcium. Much of this calcium enters the cells through "slow" calcium channels in the cell membrane, which can be opened by a decrease in the membrane voltage, such as occurs in sympathetically stimulated cells. The calcium entry blockers block these channels so that they cannot open, thus reducing the tension in the smooth muscle cells. These drugs are currently being used in Europe to treat high blood pressure, but at this writing they have not yet been approved for this purpose by the FDA.

Summary

The drugs used for treating hypertension work by a wide variety of mechanisms. Usually these mechanisms merely treat the symptom (high blood pressure) without curing the basic cause. All these drugs have undesirable side effects because they act at several locations and tend to upset the body's normal balance. In contrast, our eating and exercise program corrects the basic imbalance that causes hypertension in the first place. And instead of the drug side effects, which make you feel worse, our program makes you feel better!

PART SEVEN
For The Physician

CHAPTER 24

Recommendations for the Physician

Some of you physicians have had reservations about drugs for some time. But until 1984, the official medical position of the Joint National Committee[1] was that all hypertensives be treated with drugs. Even as recently as 1983, Dr. Norman Kaplan pointed out that treating borderline and mild hypertensives without drugs would "fly in the face of current dogma and practice."[2]

But the movement away from drugs has begun. More and more specialists are treating some of their patients with dietary programs. Interest in low-sodium diets has revived, and the importance of potassium and calcium is discussed more and more. By 1982, Dr. Edward Freis[3] of the Veterans Administration Medical Center in Washington, D.C., had expressed reservations about the routine use of drugs for the treatment of people with mild hypertension. Some physicians, such as Kaplan, have been recommending that people with diastolic pressure below 100 mm Hg not be treated with drugs unless they have risk factors.

And now, since its 1984 Special Report, even the prestigious

Joint National Committee has begun to recommend that patients with diastolic pressure of less than 95 mm Hg no longer be started on drug therapy unless they have risk factors. In its Special Report the committee recommends: "For those with diastolic blood pressure in the 90- to 94-mm Hg range who are otherwise at low risk, nonpharmacologic therapy should be pursued aggressively while blood pressures are carefully monitored."

This recommendation was based in part on the surprising results of the MRFIT study,[4] which demonstrated a dissociation between the effect of drugs upon blood pressure and upon mortality: when stepped-care drug therapy, as opposed to "usual care," was used to lower blood pressure, mortality was unchanged in the group with diastolic pressure between 95 and 100 mm Hg, and it was actually *increased* in the group with diastolic pressure between 90 and 94 mm Hg.

Up to 75 percent of those U.S. citizens suffering from hypertension have diastolic blood pressure between 90 and 104 mm Hg.[5] Thus perhaps half of the people with hypertension have diastolic blood pressures in the range from 90 to 100 mm Hg and fall into the category of those not benefited by drug therapy, according to the MRFIT study.

Not only is a lifetime of drug therapy expensive, but unpleasant side effects are frequent. Many of these side effects are well known, but as Drs. Berchtold, Sims, Horton, and Berger[6] of the University of Vermont School of Medicine have pointed out, there is as yet no way "of knowing or of evaluating possible long-term effects in a population that may be taking drugs for a matter of decades." If primary hypertension* is due to a genetic predisposition that only becomes manifest due to mistakes of life-style (especially improper food preparation and obesity), the only long-term answer is a return to proper nutrition and normal weight, as we have outlined in this book.

We think that as time goes by, the majority of patients with

---

*Instead of the term *essential hypertension*, we use the older term, *primary hypertension*. We found that some readers got confused by the term *essential* because they felt it implied that if something is "essential" it must be necessary or good.

primary hypertension will eventually be treated without drugs. With uncommon exceptions, even those people being treated with drugs should also change their approach to nutrition and, if possible, to exercise. In fact, we look forward to the day when our entire society corrects its habits of food preparation, and primary hypertension becomes an uncommon problem.

The Goal of Hypertension Treatment

The goal is not merely to get blood pressure down. What we really want to do is correct the imbalances that caused the high blood pressure.

As the Joint National Committee states in its 1984 Special Report: "The goal of treating patients with hypertension is to prevent the morbidity and mortality attributed to high blood pressure."

Restoring the Balance

In this book, we have summarized the evidence that primary hypertension is most often a consequence of an imbalance between the amounts of sodium, potassium, calcium, and magnesium in the body. Direct evidence of this imbalance is provided by the observation that *untreated* hypertensives have a significant deficiency in total body potassium. This imbalance causes abnormal functioning of body cells, with high blood pressure being just *one* consequence. (Defects in blood vessel integrity, including thickening, are probably another.)

The importance of the experiments with hypertensive rats demonstrating that increasing dietary potassium—that is, increasing the *K Factor*—protects against strokes cannot be overemphasized. There isn't much doubt about this in rats; the original study by Dr. George Meneely and Con Ball has been confirmed by Dr. Lou Tobian (see Chapter 5). Although it will take ten to twenty years to confirm this statistically in humans, there is no reason to believe the same effect won't hold.

In fact, from what we understand about the basic physiology and biophysics involved, this protective effect of potassium, independent of blood pressure, might have been predicted if we had thought about it earlier. The effect of potassium upon blood pressure *was* predicted from our knowledge of basic biophysics and physiology (that's what got one of us thinking along these lines in the first place).

(We now know that the balance of such ions as potassium, sodium, and calcium, as well as pH, play an important role in regulating several fundamental cell processes, including cell division. Thus it is not out of the question that the dietary stress that causes hypertension in those so disposed genetically may produce other problems. As one possible example, there is some evidence that a high-sodium diet can increase the probability of getting cancer of the digestive tract.)

The fact that potassium can extend life regardless of changes in blood pressure emphasizes that the goal should be much more than just lowering blood pressure. This not only indicates the importance of adequate dietary potassium but underscores the fact that blood pressure is a sign of an underlying problem and not the primary problem, as we used to think.

The obvious way to achieve our goal is to restore a normal balance within body cells. Although drugs may assist in ridding the body of excess sodium, they seldom if ever restore the normal *balance* between sodium, potassium, calcium, and magnesium in body cells. The way to restore the proper cellular balance is to eat a diet with that balance while eliminating such factors as obesity and lack of exercise, which prevent the body from maintaining the normal ionic balance. In other words, people should keep themselves physically fit and eat the foods their physiological systems were designed to handle over a million years of human evolution.

The "Dangers" of Potassium

Isn't a program that significantly increases potassium intake dangerous? Not if the change is made gradually, as outlined in Chapter 10, and kidney function is normal. It has yet to be sufficiently recognized that the gradual change, over a few days, allows *extrarenal* mechanisms (which take potassium up into body cells) as well as *renal* mechanisms[7] (which excrete part of an excess potassium load) to become more effective in "buffering" plasma potassium against elevations.

Physicians tend to be wary of giving anything orally that contains a potassium salt. A typical illustration of this reservation is the statement in a book published in 1978 on the management of essential hypertension: "The indiscriminate use of salt substitutes is to be condemned as a dangerous practice. Indeed, severe toxicity with near-fatal hyperkalemia (high blood potassium) has been reported in a small child who ingested approximately 1 to 1.5 teaspoonsful of a salt substitute from his father's 'medicines.' "[8]

To put things in perspective, we would like to point out that even table salt (NaCl) can also be poisonous, especially to small children. For example, in an Associated Press release in U.S. newspapers in March 1984, it was reported that an infant died as a result of drinking a milk formula that was accidentally contaminated with NaCl.

Potassium is Not to Be Feared—Just Respected

Why are many physicians so afraid of potassium? Dick has given this a lot of thought. Although it's just a speculation, perhaps the following may make sense to you: Our first exposure to the use of potassium is in a hospital setting, where potassium is often given intravenously. As we all know, if the flow of potassium-containing fluid directly into the blood speeds up too much, it is possible to raise the concentration of potassium in the blood to levels that can trigger a cardiac arrhythmia. Accordingly, it must be drilled into medical students and nurses that (in the hospital setting) potassium can be *very* dangerous. This wariness with regard to potassium may be reinforced by the fact that potassium-containing pills can cause a stomach ulcer.* Every time we physicians have heard about potassium,

*The tendency of potassium pills to cause ulcers is due to the high local concentration of potassium salt in the intestine when the pill dissolves. "Slow-release" pills have greatly reduced this problem. For slow-release potassium pills, the incidence is one small bowel ulcer out of 100,000 patient-years. The ulcer problem can be essentially eliminated by using liquid or effervescent potassium preparations.

it's been with a warning—and, for these particular situations, a warning well heeded.

However, we are talking about a *health*, not a *disease* (or hospital) setting. In a health setting, such as the home, where potassium is taken only orally, additional potassium is a different matter, especially when it is taken in natural foods, such as fruits and vegetables. Potassium in natural foods is partly complexed to organic material and therefore is absorbed more slowly into the blood. There is no doubt that normal kidneys can handle the amounts of potassium we recommend if it is taken in as food.

In fact, the high-potassium diet required to prevent or cure high blood pressure is eaten today by precisely those groups of native people where hypertension is rare. And our ancestors evolved over millions of years on a high-potassium diet; during that time our kidneys and extrarenal mechanisms developed the means to cope with rather large amounts of potassium compared with what most of us eat now. If potassium were dangerous, the human race would have died out long ago. And if the large amount of potassium in many natural foods (a potato or banana, for example) were dangerous to people, vegetarianism would be a dying fad (pun intended).

Provided the guidelines we outline are followed, and the patient does not have kidney or endocrine disease, all the evidence indicates that in contrast to drugs, *this procedure can do no conceivable harm.*

The Importance of Extrarenal Potassium Regulation

Many physicians are afraid of oral potassium because of the possibility of hyperkalemia. It's widely recognized that this can result from kidney disease, which can involve a decreased ability to excrete potassium. This is an important consideration, but a large part of an acute potassium load is handled by *extrarenal mechanisms*.

Dr. Ralph DeFronzo of Yale University Medical School has

studied this.[9] When 50 meq of potassium is given intravenously over a four-hour period, the rise in blood plasma K⁺ is only 1 meq/L, rather than the 3 meq/L expected if all had remained in the extracellular fluid. Nevertheless, during this time, only 40 percent of the potassium load is excreted by the kidneys. The remaining potassium is removed from the blood into body cells by extrarenal mechanisms.

The most important of these extrarenal mechanisms involves the elevation of blood insulin by plasma potassium. The elevated insulin level then acts through the mechanism Dick documented, namely insulin stimulation of the sodium-potassium pump. Dr. DeFronzo has called insulin the "most potent hormone for extrarenal potassium regulation."[10] This has practical implications, as evidenced by the fact that in dogs, diabetes results in a doubling of the elevation of plasma potassium level in response to potassium loads.

When body potassium is replenished, the ability to handle a potassium load without spiking plasma potassium is greatly improved. This is known as potassium tolerance. Conversely, if a person is deficient in body potassium, the ability to handle a potassium load is compromised. So potassium deficiency presents a catch-22. The potassium needs to be restored, but not too fast.

Diminished ability to handle potassium may possibly be explained at least in part by the finding by Dr. Torben Clausen,[11] in Aarhus, Denmark, that in rats, potassium deprivation leads to an 80 percent decrease in the number of sodium-potassium pumps in muscle. Since insulin affects only the rate of each pump, this would blunt the ability of insulin to remove potassium from the plasma during a potassium load.

There are at least two clinical lessons to be drawn from this:

1. In people suspected of having a decreased amount of total body potassium, restoration of potassium through diet and especially if intravenously should be done *gradually*. One or two weeks should be enough time, and we have taken this into account in our nutritional suggestions about getting started on the program as well as in the menu plan in Chap-

ter 10. The evidence clearly indicates that the majority of untreated hypertensives have diminished amounts of total body potassium. If they have been on thiazide diuretics, this condition may have been exacerbated.

2. Because of a relative hypoinsulinemia, most diabetics may have their extrarenal potassium regulatory mechanism compromised. Until further research is done, it is especially important that dietary potassium in diabetics should be increased gradually. In addition, in these patients, the plasma potassium should probably be checked—perhaps as often as every other day—for a couple of weeks until a new steady state is obtained. Of course, insulin dosage should be maintained at adequate levels to normalize not only blood glucose, but also plasma potassium.

What About Kidney Disease?

As you know, potassium supplements in pill or liquid form can be hazardous to persons with decreased kidney function. This also applies to potassium-containing salt substitutes, which patients may take even if you don't advise it. So a urinalysis and serum creatinine for evaluation of kidney function in the initial physical examination is especially important.

If the patient has a kidney problem, a thorough evaluation of kidney function (including GFR, clearance tests, etc.) should be made. Your approach must be tailored for that patient. Of course, if the patient's serum creatinine *and* serum potassium are elevated, you have some definite indications that the patient's kidneys are having trouble handling potassium. Of course, if the kidney disease is so extreme as to indicate need of a dialysis machine, you should be wary even of high-potassium foods.

But remember, we're not really talking about large amounts of potassium in an absolute sense—just about amounts that are large relative to the deficient levels in our present diet. The amounts required are those found naturally in food before it is processed or prepared in the kitchen. Virtually any patient who can handle lots of vegetables and fruits can be on a high–*K Factor* diet! If there is a suspicion of a kidney problem, in spite of the protection of extrarenal mechanisms, we suggest you advise the patient to avoid potassium-containing salt substitutes. This is probably overconservative, but the proper *K Factor* can be obtained by food (natural dietary means) alone if it is properly selected and prepared.

Recommendations for Treating Primary Hypertension

With the appearance of the 1984 Special Report, there is now a consensus that those with diastolic blood pressure below 95 mm Hg should be treated by a nondrug approach. The 1984 Special Report also points out that such nondrug approaches as weight reduction have value even in people with more severe hypertension who *do* receive drug treatment.

The MRFIT study failed to demonstrate that those with diastolic pressures between 95 and 100 were noticeably benefited by stepped-care drug therapy. In view of this fact, as well as consideration of the side effects common to these drugs, our uncertainty as to their long-term safety, and the fact that they treat only the symptom, we suggest you consider the guidelines advanced in 1983 by Dr. Norman Kaplan[12] of Dallas, that unless the diastolic pressure is above 100 mm Hg or risk factors are present, drugs not be used initially.

"1. All patients with elevated blood pressure should be kept under surveillance by a physician.
2. Those persons at relatively high cardiovascular risk can be identified by using the Framingham data in the Coronary Risk Handbook provided by the American Heart Association or slide rule calculators provided by pharmaceutical companies. They may benefit enough to justify antihypertensive drug therapy even if their diastolic blood pressures are only in the 90-to-100 mm Hg range.
3. Persons at relatively low risk will likely not suffer from and

may be protected by the deferral of drug therapy.

4. All patients, regardless of risk status, should be offered and strongly encouraged to follow nondrug therapies that are likely to help—weight reduction for the obese, moderate sodium restriction for all, or one or another relaxation technique for those willing to use them. Moderate sodium restriction, to 75 to 100 millimoles (4.4 to 5.8 grams NaCl, table salt, or 1,745 to 2,300 mg sodium) per day from the usual 150 to 200 millimoles (8.7 to 11.6 grams NaCl or 3,450 to 4,600 mg sodium) per day, should be feasible for all patients and can be easily monitored. The evidence for benefit from such moderate dietary sodium restriction has been strengthened by the positive results of two controlled trials. Since such moderate sodium restriction can do no harm, it should be attempted by all hypertensives.

5. Persons whose diastolic blood pressure is above 100 mm Hg should be given drug therapy."

The recommendation that excess dietary sodium chloride be decreased does not go far enough, since it overlooks the importance of correcting dietary *imbalances* due to deficiencies of potassium, calcium, and magnesium. Compared with drugs, the relatively innocuous procedure of adjusting the ratio of potassium to sodium in the food we eat to a more "natural" balance, correcting dietary deficiencies in calcium and magnesium, decreasing excess body fat, and exercising regularly would seem the safer approach.

You may decide to continue to use drug therapy for all patients with diastolic blood pressure of 95 mm Hg or higher. This would be in keeping with the 1984 Special Report. And of course, this judgment should in the final analysis be left to the physician-patient team.

At the present time, the purely statistical evidence is insufficient to recommend a nondrug approach for those with diastolic pressure above 100 mm Hg. So until further evidence is in, we believe that the treatment of those with diastolic blood pressure greater than 100 mm Hg should be begun with judicious use of antihypertensive drugs in addition to a nutritional approach, such as the *K Factor*. Frankly, this view is based more on medical-legal considerations than upon sound principles of biophysics and physiology.

But remember that Kempner, Priddle, and other pioneers found evidence that blood pressure could be lowered by dietary change even when the diastolic pressure was well over 100 mm Hg. And if you agree with the anthropologists, as we do, that hypertension is a cultural disease, then it should be clear that drugs are only a stopgap.

For those of you not ready to accept this, the information in this book will still help you motivate your patients and educate them concerning the dietary changes that will provide the greatest chances of success for those with diastolic pressure between 90 and 94 mm Hg. And we believe that even when drugs are used, the *K Factor* approach should still be employed (unless the drugs are potassium-sparing diuretics or beta blockers—see following warning), since the aim should include correcting the primary problem, not just lowering blood pressure. Not only should this approach increase the effectiveness of the treatment, it very likely may enable a lower drug dose to be used, thus minimizing side effects.

The clear advantage of drugs remains in situations in which you want to get the blood pressure down fast; if a patient walks in the door with severe hypertension, we would all probably agree to use drugs to get the pressure down out of the high danger zone, and worry about nutrition and exercise later.

What Is a Desirable K Factor?

You will recall from evidence summarized in chapters 3 and 7 that any person with a dietary *K Factor* of less than about 2 and a genetic predisposition is a candidate for primary hypertension. As the potassium-to-sodium ratio drops below about 0.8, the probability of getting hypertension—and that it will be severe—rapidly increases. As we pointed out in Chapter 3, the dietary *K Factor* of the average American adult male is only 0.38, right in the high danger zone!

In Chapter 3, we pointed out that hypertension is rare in populations in which the *K Factor* was increased to values closer to 2 or more. In clinical trials, only when the *K Factor* is raised above about 3 (the same value found in human milk) is blood pressure consistently restored toward normal. So we recommend that the dietary *K Factor* be kept well above 3. But remember from Chapter 20 that increasing the *total* amount of sodium and potassium too much can be bad even if the *K Factor* is well above 3. Therefore, not only should the level of potassium be increased; be certain that the level of sodium is *decreased*. Keep in mind that in our country, people consume several times the required amount of sodium. Remember that although the minimum safe daily sodium requirement has been set at 1,100 mg per day, more likely it is only about 200 to 300 mg per day (500 to 800 mg of NaCl) (see evidence in Chapter 20). When food is processed and prepared the way the average American gets it, it contains several *grams* of sodium per day. In the United States, it's almost impossible to get too little sodium. Remember that most Americans have a long way to go: from an average dietary *K Factor* of 0.38 to a recommended value about ten times that.

Getting Started

Because of the reduced ability to handle potassium in potassium deficiency, restoring body potassium should be started slowly. As stated in Chapter 10, we recommend eliminating the use of table salt for one week before starting the first, or transition, week of the menu program. During the transition week, the *K Factor* is increased to about 4. If there is any question about kidney function, insulin deficiency, or if the patient is elderly, you might make some dietary substitutions to increase the *K Factor* more slowly.

Potassium-containing Salt Substitutes

Moderate use of potassium-containing salt substitutes is not unduly dangerous. If a person has normal kidney function, up to 175 meq per day (6.8 g/day) of potassium[13] has been reported as not being dangerous for an adult. It is extremely unlikely that an adult will take more than this amount of potassium salts to add taste to his or her food, since 6.8 g would be 2¼ teaspoonsful! The greatest danger is probably to young children, who might ingest these salts in excess, as indicated by the quote earlier in this chapter. Therefore, although we do recommend the use of salt substitutes, like many other things, *they should be kept out of the reach of young children.*

Potassium Supplements in Pill or Liquid Form

Only in cases in which the patient will not adopt the appropriate dietary changes—and especially if thiazide diuretics are also used—a physician might, after evaluation of kidney function and serum potassium level, also want to prescribe potassium in liquid or slow-release form.

If the patient must be on a thiazide diuretic (which may be a dubious choice; see Chapter 23), we're not sure if the *K Factor* diet is able to provide adequate potassium. If while on thiazide diuretics, the patient's serum potassium level remains low after a month on the *K Factor* approach, potassium supplements in pill or liquid may then be indicated. When present, hypokalemia is probably part of the pathophysiological mechanism of primary hypertension. Therefore, it is *especially* important to evaluate periodically the serum potassium level of patients taking thiazide diuretics.

Advantages of Increasing the Dietary K Factor When Drug Therapy Is Used

Even when drugs are used, especially if they are thiazide diuretics, increasing the dietary *K Factor* will not only oppose diuretic-induced depletion of body potassium, it may potentiate the action of these drugs, allowing smaller doses to be used.[14]

Drugs That May Make the K Factor Dangerous

A note of caution about potassium-sparing diuretics: These are uncharted waters. You will need to use your own judgment. If the patient is on these when dietary potassium is increased, we recommend you follow their plasma potassium carefully. It may be best to decrease the potassium-sparing diuretics somewhat before, or during, the dietary changes. Another option would be to replace them with another drug during the transition to a high–*K Factor* diet.

A note of caution about beta blockers: Beta blockers diminish the regulation of plasma K during potassium loading. In the presence of beta blockers, plasma potassium can spike during a potassium load.

A note of caution about thiazide diuretics: You already know that thiazide diuretics tend to cause loss of body potassium. This is precisely what should *not* happen in the hypertensive patient. From what we know of the role of potassium in the body, we would expect the thiazides to make the patient more prone to sequelae of decreased body potassium, including cardiac arrhythmias, sudden death, and perhaps weakened arterial system. Unfortunately, this expectation is borne out by evidence that indicates that treatment with thiazides is especially dangerous in patients with EKG abnormalities.[15] Based upon these considerations, it seems that there is a very good chance that in the near future, thiazides will rarely be used for hypertension. Indeed, the trend in that direction seems already evident in the most recent version of stepped care.

A note about the importance of serum potassium: Knowing basic physiology as we do, it's difficult for us to understand the resistance some clinicians seem to have for careful monitoring of serum potassium levels even if the patient is on a thiazide diuretic. Remember, people with primary hypertension have deficient body potassium stores even before they are given drugs such as thiazides. Four different studies show they also tend to have, as expected on physiological considerations, lowered serum potassium levels. Not enough attention has been paid to these facts.

The level of serum potassium is often, but not always, an

indicator of total body potassium. A decrease in serum potassium is correlated in a fairly linear fashion with a decrease in total body potassium; as a rough guide, a drop of 0.25 meq/L in serum potassium represents roughly a 100 meq (the total is roughly 3000 meq) decrease in total body potassium.[16] Because of this, and the key importance of potassium, we recommend that every untreated hypertensive have a serum potassium determination before starting treatment, whether the treatment is drugs, diet, or both. If the patient is already on drugs, especially if those drugs are thiazide diuretics, a serum potassium should be obtained as a benchmark before starting the *K Factor* approach.

Based upon evidence that indicates that a low serum potassium level can be part of the pathological mechanism of primary hypertension *and* the fact that the "normal" serum potassium range is probably skewed too low by inclusion of hypertensives in the data, we suggest the following guidelines. Though not cast in concrete, they are based upon the presently available information and should be of use.

If the serum potassium is:

○ Between 4.0 and 5.0 meq/liter, it is probably still a good idea to recheck it twice, say at monthly intervals.
○ 4.0 or less (*especially* if it is below the "accepted" lower limit of 3.5), it should be rechecked every 2 or 3 weeks until at least two successive readings are between 4.0 and 5.0.

If a patient is on thiazide diuretics, the serum potassium level should be monitored closely—probably at least once a month—even if the level is between 4.0 and 5.0 meq/liter. We realize this is not the usual practice but believe that it will become so as the importance of potassium is better appreciated (at least until thiazide diuretics are no longer widely used for primary hypertension).

Hypokalemia

Physicians realize the danger of *hyper*kalemia, but what about *hypo*kalemia? In the context of primary hypertension, debates about hypokalemia usually fail to take into account the evidence (summarized in chapters 6 and 20) indicating that hypokalemia is also prevalent in untreated hypertensives. Moreover, it is probably part of the pathophysiological mechanism *contributing* to the elevation of blood pressure.

Causes

Hypokalemia is often associated with hypertension (see Chapter 20). In addition, hypokalemia can be caused by thiazide diuretics, loop diuretics, osmotic diuretics, carbonic anhydrase inhibitors, magnesium deficiency, Cushing's disease, licorice intoxication, primary aldosteronism, and some high renin hypertension (especially malignant hypertension).

Consequences

Besides making hypertension worse, hypokalemia can decrease glomerular filtration rate, decrease renal concentrating ability, increase sodium reabsorption, increase ammoniagenesis, and cause glucose intolerance. Although the extent of the danger is debated,[17] there is considerable evidence that hypokalemia can cause arrhythmias. An increased risk for cardiac irregularities has been correlated with decreases in serum potassium levels of greater than 0.6 mEq/L.[18] Some specialists suspect that some of the sudden deaths observed in the MRFIT study may have been due to hypokalemia. In patients with myocardial infarction, a higher frequency of ventricular fibrillation occurs among those with hypokalemia.[19] Patients with diuretic-induced hypokalemia have an increased incidence of serious ventricular ectopic activity.

Because the activity of the membrane sodium-potassium pump depends upon potassium, hypokalemia is especially dangerous under conditions in which this pump has already been slowed, as in digitalis therapy[20] or hypoinsulinemia.[21]

Treating Obese Hypertensives

As you are well aware, obesity is a major contributor to hypertension. In clinical trials, loss of only a third to half of excess body weight has reduced blood pressure significantly. We discussed the effect of obesity on cellular regulation of potassium and sodium in Chapter 6.

Because of the increased risk of diabetes and heart attack associated with any degree of obesity, it is better if body weight (actually body fat) is reduced to a normal level. So it is essential that those who are overweight and have hypertension reduce excess weight by at least half and preferably to a normal level.

Evaluating the Patient for Aerobic Exercise

It's not a bad idea to put the patient on a reduced fat diet before beginning exercise, and you should screen for evidence of cardiovascular disease. Although nothing is foolproof, the two best indicators are probably the serum cholesterol and an exercise EKG, although family history of heart disease, history of smoking, and excess dietary fat should also be noted.

As an example of the value of proper medical evaluation, at Dr. Kenneth Cooper's Aerobics Center in Dallas, over five thousand participants have been followed. They have collectively run more than six million miles (an average of over 1,000 miles per person) with only two cardiac-related events and *no* fatalities. These people had all been screened with an exercise tolerance stress test to maximum heart rate as well as a complete physical and history.

Withdrawing Drugs

Even if drugs should be discontinued in a given patient, the actual change can be dangerous. NEVER WITHDRAW ANY DRUG SUDDENLY. This should be emphasized to the patient. *Any* sudden change in the physiological state of a person can be dangerous. For example, sudden withdrawal of Clonidine can precipitate a rebound hypertension. If a patient has angina, a sudden withdrawal of beta blockers can precipitate anginal attacks. So drug withdrawal should always be done under your supervision and it should be gradual, in a series of steps.

Since there is relatively little experience in taking hypertensive patients completely off drugs, we offer these thoughts for your consideration: Even when you think a patient should eventually be taken off drugs, unless the patient is taking potassium-sparing diuretics or beta blockers, it is probably best to establish the patient on our recommended dietary procedures for a few weeks and then reevaluate before starting to taper the drug dosage. During this time, the patient should be monitored carefully. Then, if the blood pressure is normal, or at least the diastolic pressure is less than 100 mm Hg, the dose of drugs could be adjusted in small decrements. Based upon the biological half-life of drugs and the adaptive processes within the body, the dose should be changed probably no more than perhaps every two to four weeks. By monitoring blood pressure, serum potassium, and other appropriate signs (depending upon the drugs and upon the presence of other conditions, such as diabetes, obesity, and so on), you can use your judgment as to whether and when to make the next reduction in drug dosage.

Summary

There are many things a person can do to lower his or her blood pressure and to protect against the consequences of hypertension, such as stroke. A holistic approach is needed. Before taking drugs to reduce blood pressure, we and a growing number of physicians recommend trying a nondrug approach unless the hypertension is severe.

The key steps to protecting your patients from hypertension include reducing dietary sodium, increasing potassium, magnesium, and calcium, starting regular moderate aerobic exercise, and losing excess body weight. Provided that your patient has normal kidney function, there are no known harmful effects of increasing the dietary *K Factor* above 3, exercising, and losing excess weight.

If this program doesn't decrease blood pressure, don't let the patient get discouraged; motivate him or her to stay with it. It may take weeks or months for blood pressure to respond to the program, especially if the hypertension has been present for several years. Remember that increased blood pressure is a sign of an abnormal balance in the body's cells. Increasing the dietary *K Factor*, magnesium, and calcium level to normal will act to correct this imbalance in these cells.

Correcting this imbalance by a proper dietary *K Factor*, exercise, and weight loss can improve health and increase life span, even if blood pressure doesn't return to normal levels. You can't say that about drugs.

REFERENCES

The following notes are numbered sequentially by superscripts within each chapter. *Ibid* means "same as the reference above." "*See* xx" means "same as reference number xx in this chapter."

Introduction to Part I. The Problem

1. The Joint National Committee on Detection, Evaluation, and Treatment of High Blood Pressure. The 1984 report of the Joint National Committee on Detection, Evaluation, and Treatment of High Blood Pressure. *Arch. Intern. Med.* 144:1045–57 (1984).
2. Subcommittee on Definition and Prevalence of the 1984 Joint National Committee. Hypertension Prevalence and the Status of Awareness, Treatment, and Control in the United States. *Hypertension* 7:457–68 (1985).
3. Kempner, W. Treatment of hypertensive vascular disease with rice diet. *Amer. J. Med.* 4:545–577 (1948).
4. Dahl, L. K. Salt and hypertension. *Amer. J. Clin. Nutr.* 25:231–44 (1972).
5. Page, L. B., A. Damon, and R. C. Moellering, Jr. Antecedents of cardiovascular disease in six Solomon Islands societies. *Circulation* 49:1132–46 (1974).

6. Multiple Risk Factor Intervention Trial Research Group. Multiple risk factor intervention trial. Risk factor changes and mortality results. *J. Amer. Med. Assoc.* 248:1465–77 (1982).
7. American Heart Association, Vermont Affiliate. Hypertension: One Major Risk Factor for Your Heart. *Heartline* 5:2 (1985).

Chapter 1. What Is High Blood Pressure?
1. Subcommittee on Definition and Prevalence of the 1984 Joint National Committee. Hypertension Prevalence and the Status of Awareness, Treatment, and Control in the United States. *Hypertension* 7:457–68 (1985).
2. The Joint National Committee on Detection, Evaluation, and Treatment of High Blood Pressure. The 1984 report of the Joint National Committee on Detection, Evaluation, and Treatment of High Blood Pressure. *Arch. Intern. Med.* 144:1045–57 (1984).
3. Soc. of Actuaries & Assoc. of Life Insurance Med. Directors of America, *Blood Pressure Study 1979*, published by Soc. of Actuaries & Assoc. of Life Insurance Med. Directors of America (1980).
4. *See 2.*
5. *See 3.*

Chapter 2. Drugs—The Usual Treatment
1. Kempner, W. Treatment of hypertensive vascular disease with rice diet. *Amer. J. Med.* 4:545–77 (1948).
2. Cade , R., D. Mars, H. Wagemaker, C. Zauner, D. Packer, M. Privette, M. Cade, J. Peterson, and D. Hood-Lewis. Effect of Aerobic Exercise Training on Patients with Systemic Arterial Hypertension. *Amer. J. Med.* 77:785–90 (1984); and McCarron, D. A., L. E. Hare, and B. R. Walker. Therapeutic and economic controversies in antihypertensive therapy. *J. Cardiovasc. Pharmacol.* 6:837–40 (1984).
   The estimate of the amount Americans spend on antihypertensive drugs is based on the average drug cost per year per patient being $500. This is a compromise between the average of $1,350 spent by the patients in the Cade et al. study above, most of whom were probably taking more than one drug, and the average cost for only one drug of $125 per year reported by McCarron et al. From reference number 2 of Chapter 1, we know that 18 million Americans are taking antihypertensive drugs. This calculates out to an estimate of *$9 billion* spent each year by Americans for drugs to treat high blood pressure.
3. U.S. Public Health Service. The 1980 report of the Joint National

Committee on Detection, Evaluation, and Treatment of High Blood Pressure. NIH Publication No. 81–1088 (1980).

4. The Joint National Committee on Detection, Evaluation, and Treatment of High Blood Pressure. The 1984 report of the Joint National Committee on Detection, Evaluation, and Treatment of High Blood Pressure. *Arch. Intern. Med.* 144:1045–57 (1984).

5. *See* 4.

6. Baker, C. E. Jr., *Physicians' Desk Reference (PDR 34th Ed.)*. Medical Economics, Oradell, NJ (1980).

7. Curb, J. D., N. O. Borhani, T. P. Blaszkowski, N. Zimbaldi, S. Fotin, and W. Williams. Long-term surveillance for adverse effects of antihypertensive drugs. *J. Amer. Med. Assoc.* 253:3263–68 (1985).

8. Veterans Administration Cooperative Study Group on Antihypertensive Agents. Comparison of propranalol and hydrochlorothiazide for the initial treatment of hypertension. II. Results of long-term therapy. *J. Amer. Med. Assoc.* 248:2004–11 (1982); and Flamenbaum, W. Metabolic consequences of antihypertensive therapy. *Ann. Intern. Med.* 98:875–80 (1983); and Leren, P., P. O. Foss, A. Helgeland, I. Hjermann, I. Holme, and P. G. Lund-Larsen. Effect of propranolol and prazosin on blood lipids. The Oslo study. *Lancet* II:4–6 (1980).

9. Smith, W. M. Treatment of mild hypertension. Results of a ten-year intervention trial. *Circulation* 40 (Suppl. 1):I98–I-105 (1977).

10. Veterans Administration Cooperative Study Group on Antihypertensive Agents. Effects of treatment on morbidity in hypertension. II. Results in patients with diastolic blood pressures averaging 90 through 114 mm Hg. *J. Amer. Med. Assoc.* 213:1143–52 (1970).

11. Hypertension Detection and Follow-up Program Cooperative Group. Five-year findings of the hypertension detection and follow-up program. I. Reduction in mortality of persons with high blood pressure, including mild hypertension. *J. Amer. Med. Assoc.* 242:2562–71 (1979).

12. Management Committee: The Australian therapeutic trial in mild hypertension. *Lancet* 1:1261–67 (1980).

13. Oliver, M. P. Risks of correcting the risks of coronary disease and stroke with drugs. *New Eng. J. Med.* 306:297–98 (1982).

14. *See* 4.

15. Multiple Risk Factor Intervention Trial Research Group. Multiple risk factor intervention trial. Risk factor changes and mortality results. *J. Amer. Med. Assoc.* 248:1465–77 (1982).

16. Morgan, T. O., W. R. Adam, M. Hodgson, and R. W. Gibberd. Failure of therapy to improve prognosis in elderly males with hypertension. *Med. J. Austral.* 2:27–31 (1980).

17. Lundberg, G. D. Editorial: MRFIT and the goals of the Journal. *J. Amer. Med. Assoc.* 248:1501 (1982).
18. *See* 4.
19. *See* 9.
20. Kaplan, Norman M. Hypertension: prevalence, risks, and effect of therapy. *Ann. Intern. Med.* 98:705–709 (1983).

Introduction to Part II. The Answer

1. Vieth, I. *The Yellow Emperor's Classic in Internal Medicine.* (Translated from Huang ti Nei thing Su Wen, 2600 B.C.) Berkeley University Press, CA (1966).

Chapter 3. High Blood Pressure Is Not Inevitable

1. Trowell, H., and D. P. Burkitt. *Western Diseases: Their Emergence and Prevention.* Edward Arnold, Publisher, London (1981).
2. Acsadi, Gy, and J. Nemeskeri. *History of Human Lifespan and Mortality.* Akademai Kiado, Budapest (1970).
3. *See* 1; and Truswell, A. S., and J. D. L. Hansen. Medical research among the !Kung, in *Kalahari Hunter-Gatherers*, R. B. Lee and I. DeVore, eds. Harvard University Press, Cambridge (1976).
4. Page, L. B., A. Damon, and R. C. Moellering, Jr. Antecedents of cardiovascular disease in six Solomon Islands societies. *Circulation* 49:1132–46 (1974).
5. Hicks, C. S., and R. F. Matters. The standard metabolism of the Australian aborigines. *Austral. J. Exper. Biol. Med. Sci.* 11:177–83 (1933); and Nye, L. J., and L. J. Jarvis. Blood pressure in Australian aboriginal, with consideration of possible aetiological factors in hyperplesia and its relation to civilization. *Med. J. Austral.* 2:1000–1001 (1937).
6. Truswell, A. S., B. M. Kennelly, J. D. Hansen, and R. B. Lee. Blood pressure of !Kung bushmen in northern Botswana. *Amer. Heart J.* 84:5–12 (1972); and Truswell, A. S., and J. D. L. Hansen. Medical research among the !Kung, in *Kalahari Hunter-Gatherers*, R. B. Lee and I. DeVore, eds. Harvard University Press, Cambridge (1976).
7. Lowenstein, F. W. Blood-pressure in relation to age and sex in the tropics and subtropics. *Lancet* 1:389–92 (1961).
8. Kean, B. H. The blood pressure of the Cuna Indians. *Amer. J. Trop. Med.* 24:341–43 (1944).
9. Thomas, W. A. Health of a carnivorous race. A study of the Eskimo. *J. Amer. Med. Assoc.* 88:1559–60 (1927).
10. Donnison, C. P. Blood pressure in the African native. *Lancet* 1:6–7 (1929).

11. Murphy, W. Some observations on blood pressures in humid tropics. *New Z. Med. J.* 54:64–73 (1955).
12. Whyte, H. M. Body fat and blood pressure of natives in New Guinea: reflections on essential hypertension. *Austral. Ann. Med.* 7:36–46 (1958).
13. Kaminer, B., and W. P. W. Lutz. Blood pressure in bushmen of the Kalahari desert. *Circulation* 22:289–95 (1960).
14. Connor, W. E., M. T. Cerqueira, R. W. Connor, R. B. Wallace, M. R. Malinow, and H. R. Casdorph. The plasma lipids, lipoproteins, and the diet of the Tarahumara Indians of Mexico. *Amer. J. Clin. Nutr.* 31:1131–42 (1978); and Cerqueria, M. T., M. McMurry Fry, and W. E. Connor. The food and nutrient intakes of the Tarahumara Indians of Mexico. *Amer. J. Clin. Nutr.* 32:905–15 (1979).
15. Williams, A. W. Blood pressure of Africans. *E. Africa Med. J.* 18:109–17 (1941).
16. Morse, W. R., and Y. T. Beh. Blood pressure amongst aboriginal ethnic groups of Szechwan province, west China. *Lancet* 1:966–67 (1937).
17. Oliver, W. J., E. L. Cohen, and J. V. Neel. Blood pressure, sodium intake, and sodium related hormones in the Yanomamo Indians, a "no-salt" culture. *Circulation* 52:146–51 (1975).
18. *See* 14.
19. *See* 14 (2nd ref.).
20. *See* 1; and Tobian, L. Salt and hypertension. *J. Med. Assoc. Georgia.* 69:827–34 (1980).
21. *See* 1.
22. Personal communication with Dr. Mark Cohen, Professor of Anthropology, SUNY, Plattsburg, NY; presently on sabbatical at University of Cambridge, U.K.
23. *See* 22.
24. *See* 8.
25. Page, Lot B., David Vandevert, Karim Nader, Nancy Lubin, and Jesse R. Page. Blood pressure, diet, and body form in traditional nomads of the Qash'qai tribe, southern Iran. *Acta Cardiol.* 33:102–103 (1978).
26. *See* 22.
27. *See* 17; and Chagnon, N. A. *Yanomamo, the Fierce People.* Holt, Reinhart and Winston, New York (1968).
28. Eaton, S. B., and M. Konner. Paleolithic nutrition. *New Eng. J. Med.* 312:283–89 (1985).
29. *See* 17.
30. *See* 6.

31. Ophir, O., G. Peer (Peresecenschi), J. Gilad, M. Blum, and A. Aviram. Low blood pressure in vegetarians: the possible role of potassium. *Amer. J. Clin. Nutr.* 37:755–62 (1983).

32. Grim, C. E., F. C. Luft, J. Z. Miller, G. R. Meneely, H. D. Battarbee, C. G. Hames, and L. K. Dahl. Racial differences in blood pressure in Evans County, Georgia: relationship to sodium and potassium intake and plasma renin activity. *J. Chron. Dis.* 33:87–94 (1980).

33. Ueshima, H., M. Tanigaki, M. Iida, T. Shimamoto, M. Konishi, and Y. Komachi. Hypertension, salt, and potassium. *Lancet* 1:504 (1981).

34. See 32.

35. Zinner, S. H., H. S. Margolius, B. Rosner, H. R. Keiser, and E. H. Kass. Familial aggregation of urinary kallikrein concentration in childhood: relation to blood pressure, race and urinary electrolytes. *Amer. J. Epidemiol.* 104:124–32 (1976); and Luft, F. C., C. E. Grim, N. Fineberg, and M. C. Weinberger. Effects of volume expansion and contraction in normotensive whites, blacks, and subjects of different ages. *Circulation* 59:643–50 (1979); and Watson, R. L., H. G. Langford, J. Abernethy, T. Y. Barnes, and M. J. Watson. Urinary electrolytes, body weight, and blood pressure. Pooled cross-sectional results among four groups of adolescent females. *Hypertension* 2 (Suppl. I):193–98 (1980).

36. Tobian, L., D. MacNeill, M. A. Johnson, M. C. Ganguli, and J. Iwai. Potassium protection against lesions of the renal tubules, arteries, and glomeruli and nephron loss in salt-loaded hypertensive Dahl S rats. *Hypertension* 6 (Suppl. I):170–76 (1984).

37. Sasaki, N., T. Mitsuhashi, and S. Fukushi. Effects of the ingestion of large amounts of apples on blood pressure in farmers in Akita prefecture. *Igaku Seibutsugaku* 51:103–105 (1959); and Sasaki, N. High blood pressure and the salt intake of the Japanese. *Jap. Heart J.* 3:313–24 (1962).

38. Reed, D., D. McGee, K. Yano, and J. Hankin. Diet, blood pressure, and multicollinearity. *Hypertension* 7:405–10 (1985).

39. See 31; and Armstrong, B., A. J. van Merwyk, and H. Coates. Blood pressure in seventh-day adventist vegetarians. *Amer. J. Epidemiol.* 105: 444–49 (1977); and Rouse, I. L., L. J. Beilin, B. K. Armstrong, and R. Vandongen. Blood-pressure-lowering effect of a vegetarian diet: controlled trial in normotensive subjects. *Lancet* 1:5–9 (1983).

40. See 31.

41. Altman, P. L., and D. S. Dittmer (ed.) *Biological Handbooks. Blood and Other Body Fluids.* Fed. Amer. Soc. for Exper. Biol., Washington, D.C. (1961), pp. 455–58.

Chapter 4. Human Studies

1. Kramer S. N., and M. Levry. The oldest medical text in man's recorded history: a Sumerian physician's prescription book of 4000 years ago. In *Illustrated London News* 226:370. Ingram House, Strand (1955).
2. Ambard, L., and Beaujard. Causes de l'hypertension arterielle. *Arch. Gen. Med.* (Paris) 81:520–33 (1904).
3. Addison, W. L. T. The use of sodium chloride, potassium chloride, sodium bromide and potassium bromide in cases of arterial hypertension which are amenable to potassium chloride. *Can. Med. Assoc. J.* 18:281–85 (1928).
4. Addison, W. L. T. The use of calcium chloride in arterial hypertension. *Can. Med. Assoc. J.* 14:1059–61 (1924).
5. Resnick, L. Calcium effective for low-renin hypertension. *Cardiology Observer* 1(3):4 (1984); and Resnick, L. M., J. P. Nicholson, and J. H. Laragh. Calcium metabolism and the renin-aldosterone system in essential hypertension. *J. Cardiovasc. Pharmacol.* 7 (Suppl. 6):5187–93 (1985).
6. McCarron, D. A., and C. D. Morris. Blood pressure response to oral calcium in persons with mild to moderate hypertension. *Ann. Intern. Med.* 103:825–31 (1985).
7. See 3.
8. Addison, W. L. T., and H. G. Clark. Calcium and potassium chlorides in the treatment of arterial hypertension. *Can. Med. Assoc. J.* 15:913–15 (1925).
9. Priddle, W. W. Observations on the management of hypertension. *Can. Med. Assoc. J.* 25:5–8 (1931).
10. McQuarrie, I., W. H. Thompson, and J. A. Anderson. Effects of excessive ingestion of sodium and potassium salts on carbohydrate metabolism and blood pressure in diabetic children. *J. Nutr.* 11:77–101 (1936).
11. Kempner, W. Treatment of hypertensive vascular disease with rice diet. *Amer. J. Med.* 4:545–77 (1948).
12. See 11; and Dole, V. P., L. K. Dahl, G. C. Cotzias, H. A. Eder, and M. E. Krebs. Dietary treatment of hypertension: clinical and metabolic studies of patients on rice-fruit diet. *J. Clin. Invest.* 29:1189–1206 (1950).
13. Dahl, L. K. Salt and hypertension. *Amer. J. Clin. Nutr.* 25:231–44 (1972).
14. Pritikin, N. Optimal dietary recommendations: a public health responsibility. *Preventive Med.* 11:733–39 (1982).
15. Beard, T. C., W. R. Gray, H. M. Cooke, and R. Barge. Randomized

controlled trial of a no added sodium diet for mild hypertension. *Lancet* 11:455–58 (1982).

16. MacGregor, G. A., N. D. Markandu, F. E. Best, D. M. Elder, J. M. Cam, G. A. Sagnella, and M. Squires. Double-blind randomized crossover trial of moderate sodium restriction in essential hypertension. *Lancet* 1:351–55 (1982); and MacGregor, G. A., S. J. Smith, N. D. Markandu, R. A. Banks, and G. A. Sagnella. Moderate potassium supplementation in essential hypertension. *Lancet* 11:567–70 (1982).

17. *See* 15 (1st ref.).

18. *See* 15 (2nd ref.).

19. Iimura, O., T. Kijima, K. Kikuchi, A. Miyama, T. Ando, T. Nakao, and Y. Takigami. Studies on the hypotensive effect of high potassium intake in patients with essential hypertension. *Clin. Sci.* 61:77–80 (1981).

20. McCarron, D. A., C. D. Morris, H. J. Henry, and J. L. Stanton. Blood pressure and nutrient intake in the United States. *Science* 224:1392–98 (1984).

21. Gruchow, H. W., K. A. Sobocinski, and J. J. Barboriak. Alcohol, nutrient intake, and hypertension in U.S. adults. *J. Amer. Med. Assoc.* 253:1567–70 (1985).

22. Richards, A. M., M. G. Nicholls, E. A. Espiner, H. Ikram, A. H. Maslowski, E. J. Hamilton, and J. E. Wells. Blood-pressure response to moderate sodium restriction and to potassium supplementation in mild essential hypertension. *Lancet* 1:757 (1984).

23. Priddle, W. W. Hypertension—sodium and potassium studies. *J. Assoc. Med. Can.* 86:1–9 (1962).

Chapter 5. Animal Studies

1. Gordon, D. B., and D. R. Drury. The effect of potassium on the occurrence of petechial hemorrhages in renal hypertensive rabbits. *Circulation Res.* 4:167–72 (1956).

2. Meneely, George R., and Con O. T. Ball. Experimental epidemiology of chronic sodium chloride toxicity and the protective effect of potassium chloride. *Amer. J. Med.* 25:713–25 (1958).

3. Dahl, L. K., G. Leitl, and M. Heine. Influence of dietary potassium and sodium/potassium molar ratios on the development of salt hypertension. *J. Exper. Med.* 136:318–30 (1972).

4. Tobian, L. The protective effects of dietary K against the lesions of NaCl-induced hypertension. *Abstracts of Papers of the 149th National Meeting of the American Association for the Advancement of Science* 64 (1983).

5. Tobian, Louis. Potassium protection against lesions of the renal tubules, arteries, and glomeruli and nephron loss in salt-loaded hypertensive Dahl S rats. *Hypertension* 6 (Suppl. I):170–I-176 (1984).

6. Emanuel, D. A., J. B. Scott, and F. J. Haddy. Effect of potassium on small and large blood vessels of the dog forelimb. *Amer. J. Physiol.* 197:637–42 (1959).

7. Chen, W. T., R. A. Brace, J. B. Scott, D. K. Anderson, and F. J. Haddy. The mechanism of the vasodilator action of potassium. *Proc. Soc. Exper. Biol. Med.* 140:820–24 (1972).

8. Overbeck, H. W. Vascular responses to cations, osmolality, and angiotensin in renal hypertensive dogs. *Amer. J. Physiol.* 223:1358–64 (1972).

9. Dahl, L. K., K. D. Knudsen, and J. Iwai. Humoral transmission of hypertension: evidence from parabiosis. *Circulation Res.* (Suppl. 1) 16:I-21–I-33 (1969).

10. Moore, R. D. Effect of insulin upon sodium pump in frog skeletal muscle. *J. Physiol.* 232:23–45 (1973); and Gavryck, W. A., R. D. Moore, and R. C. Thompson. Effect of insulin upon membrane-bound ($Na^+ = K^+$) = ATPase extracted from frog skeletal muscle. *J. Physiol.* 252:43–58 (1975).

11. Clausen, T., and P. G. Kohn. Effect of insulin on transport of sodium and potassium in rat soleus muscle. *J. Physiol.* 265:19–42 (1977).

12. Kitasato, H., S. Sato, K. Murayama, and K. Nishio. Interaction between the effects of insulin and ouabain on the activity of Na-transport system in frog skeletal muscle. *Jap. J. Physiol.* 30:115–30 (1980).

13. Haddy, F. J., and H. W. Overbeck. The role of humoral agents in volume expanded hypertension. *Life Sci.* 19:935–48 (1976).

14. Hamlyn, J. M., P. D. Levinson, R. Ringel, P. A. Levin, B. P. Hamilton, M. P. Blaustein, and A. A. Kowarski. Relationships among endogenous digitalis-like factors in essential hypertension. *Fed. Proc.* 44:2782–88 (1985); and Haddy, F. J., and M. B. Pamnani. Evidence for a circulating endogenous $Na^+ = K^+$ pump inhibitor in low-renin hypertension. *Fed. Proc.* 44:2789–94 (1985); and Gruber, K. A., C. H. Metzler, T. E. J. Robinson, J. Buggy, B. C. Bullock, and J. R. Lymangrover. Cardiovascular investigations of an endogenous digoxin-like factor. *Fed. Proc.* 44:2795–99 (1985).

15. Valdes, R., Jr. Endogenous digoxin-immunoactive factor in human subjects. *Fed. Proc.* 44:2800–2805 (1985).

16. *See* 14.

17. *See* 14 (2nd ref.).

18. *See* 14 (3rd ref.).
19. *See* 14 (2nd ref.).
20. *See* 13; and Blaustein, M. P. Sodium ions, calcium ions, blood pressure regulation, and hypertension: a reassessment and a hypothesis. *Amer. J. Physiol.* 232:C165–73 (1977).

Chapter 6. The Action at the Cell Membrane

1. Smith, T. J., and I. S. Edelman. The role of sodium transport in thyroid thermogenesis. *Fed. Proc.* 38:2150–53 (1979).
2. Moore, R. D. Effect of insulin upon sodium pump in frog skeletal muscle. *J. Physiol.* 232:23–45 (1973).
3. Moore, R. D., J. W. Munford, and T. J. Pillsworth, Jr. Effects of streptozotocin diabetes and fasting on intracellular sodium and adenosine triphosphate in rat soleus muscle. *J. Physiol.* 338:277–94 (1983).
4. *See* 3.
5. Webb, G. D. Increased passive sodium flux associated with human essential hypertension. *Biophys. J.* 45:203a (1984).
6. Daniel, E. E., A. K. Grover, and C. Y. Kwan. Isolation and properties of plasma membrane from smooth muscle. *Fed. Proc.* 41:2898–904 (1982).
7. Cone, C. D., Jr. Control of cell division by the electrical voltage of the surface membrane. Presentation to the Twelfth Annual Science Writers Seminar, American Cancer Society, San Antonio, TX, March (1970).
8. Tuyns, A. J. Sodium chloride and cancer of the digestive tract. *Nutr. and Cancer* 4:198–205 (1983).
9. Glassman, J. *The Cancer Survivors.* The Dial Press, New York (1983).
10. Glynn, I. M. Sodium and potassium movements in human red cells. *J. Physiol.* (London) 124:278–310 (1956); and Sjodin, R. A. The kinetics of sodium extrusion in striated muscle as functions of the external sodium and potassium ion concentrations. *J. Gen. Physiol.* 57:164–87 (1971).
11. Chen, W. T., R. A. Brace, J. B. Scott, D. K. Anderson, and F. J. Haddy. The mechanism of the vasodilator action of potassium. *Proc. Soc. Exper. Biol. Med.* 140:820–24 (1972).
12. Blaustein, M. P. Sodium ions, calcium ions, blood pressure regulation, and hypertension: a reassessment and a hypothesis. *Amer. J. Physiol.* 232:C165–73 (1977).
13. *Ibid.*
14. Winkler, M. M. Regulation of protein synthesis in sea urchin eggs by intracellular pH. *Intracellular pH: Its measurement, regula-*

tion, and utilization in cellular functions. Ed. by R. Nuccitelli & D. Deamer. 325–40. Alan R. Liss, New York (1982).
15. *Ibid.*
16. Avolio, A. P., K. M. Clyde, T. C. Beard, H. M. Cooke, and M. O'Rourke. Low-salt diet and improvement of arterial distensibility in normotensive subjects. *Circulation* 72 (Suppl. III):39 (Abst.) (1985).
17. Ericsson, F. Intracellular potassium in man. *Scand. J. Clin. Lab. Invest.* 42 (Suppl. 163):1–58 (1982).
18. Parker, J. C., and L. R. Berkowitz. Physiologically instructive genetic variants involving the human red cell membrane. *Physiol. Rev.* 63:261–313 (1983).
19. *See* 10.
20. *See* 10.
21. Christlieb, A. R. Diabetes and hypertensive vascular disease: mechanisms and treatment. *Amer. J. Cardiol.* 32:592–606 (1973).

Chapter 7. Where Does Being Fit Fit In?

1. Reisin, E., R. Abel, M. Modan, D. S. Silverberg, H. E. Eliahou, and B. Modan. Effect of weight loss without salt restriction on the reduction of blood pressure in overweight patients. *New Eng. J. Med.* 298:1–6 (1978); and Eliahou, H. E., A. Iaina, T. Gaon, J. Shochat, and M. Modan. Body weight reduction necessary to attain normotension in the overweight hypertensive patient. *Inter. J. Obes.* 5 (Suppl. 1):157–63 (1981).
2. Stamler, J., E. Farinaro, L. M. Mojonnier, Y. Hall, D. Moss, and R. Stamler. Prevention and control of hypertension by nutritional-hygienic means. *J. Amer. Med. Assoc.* 243:1819–23 (1980).
3. Krotkiewski, M., K. Mandroukas, L. Sjostrom, L. Sullivan, H. Wetterqvist, and P. Bjorntorp. Effects of long-term physical training on body fat, metabolism, and blood pressure in obesity. *Metabolism* 28:650–58 (1979); and Cade, R., D. Mars, H. Wagemaker, C. Zauner, D. Packer, M. Privette, M. Cade, J. Peterson, and D. Hood-Lewis. Effect of aerobic exercise training on patients with systemic arterial hypertension. *Amer. J. Med.* 77:785–90 (1984).
4. *See* 3 (1st ref.).
5. Martin, J. E., and P. M. Dubbert, and W. C. Cushman. Controlled trial of aerobic exercise in hypertension. *Circulation* 72 (Suppl. III): 111–13 (Abst.) (1985).
6. *See* 3 (2nd ref.).
7. *See* 5.

8. Moore, R. D. Effects of insulin upon ion transport. *Biochem. Biophys. Acta* 737:1–49 (1983).
9. *See* 3 (1st ref.); and Bjorntorp, P., K. de Jounge, L. Sjostrom, and L. Sullivan. The effect of physical training on insulin production in obesity. *Metabolism* 19:631–38 (1970).
10. Welborn, T. A., A. Breckenridge, A. H. Rubinstein, C. T. Dollery, and T. Russell Frazer. Serum-insulin in essential hypertension and in peripheral vascular disease. *Lancet* 1:1336–37 (1966).
11. Modan, M., H. Halkin, S. Almog, A. Lusky, A. Eshkol, M. Shefi, A. Shitrit, and Z. Fuchs. Hyperinsulinemia. A link between hypertension obesity and glucose intolerance. *J. Clin. Invest.* 75:809–17 (1985).
12. Nizet, A., P. Lefebvre, and J. Crabbé. Control by insulin of sodium-potassium and water excretion by isolated dog kidneys. *Pflug. Arch.* 323:11–20 (1971).
13. Rowe, J. W., J. B. Young, K. L. Minaker, A. L. Stevens, J. Pallotta, and L. Landsberg. Effect of insulin and glucose infusions on sympathetic nervous system activity in normal man. *Diabetes* 30:219–25 (1981).
14. *See* 13, and 12.
15. *See* 9.
16. Landsberg, L., and J. B. Young. Diet and the sympathetic nervous system: relationship to hypertension. *Int. J. Obes.* 5 (Suppl. 1): 79–90 (1981).
17. *See* 13.
18. Mineur, P., and J. Kolanowski. Changes in blood pressure and cardiovascular indices of adrenergic activity in obese subjects undergoing total starvation. *J. Obes. Weight Regul.* 2:69–79 (1983).
19. Kolanowski, J. Pathophysiology of hypertension in overweight subjects. *Medicographia* 7:29–31 (1985).

Chapter 8. Other Factors That Influence Blood Pressure

1. Dawson, E. B., M. J. Frey, T. D. Moore, and W. J. McGanity. Relationship of metal metabolism to vascular disease mortality rates in Texas. *Amer. J. Clin. Nutr.* 31:1188–97 (1978).
2. Altura, B. M., B. T. Altura, A. Gebrewold, H. Ising, and T. Gunther. Magnesium deficiency and hypertension: correlation between magnesium-deficient diets and microcirculatory changes *in situ*. *Science* 223:1315–17 (1984).
3. Haddy, F. J. Local effects of sodium, calcium, and magnesium upon small and large blood vessels of the dog forelimb. *Circulation Res.* VIII:57–70 (1960).

4. Altura, B. M., B. T. Altura, and A. Carella. Magnesium deficiency-induced spasms of umbilical vessels: relation to preeclampsia, hypertension, growth retardation. *Science* 221:376–78 (1983).

5. Albert, D. G., M. Yoshikazu, and L. T. Iseri. Serum magnesium and plasma sodium levels in essential hypertension. *Circulation* XVII:761–64 (1958).

6. Resnick, L. M., J. H. Laragh, J. E. Sealey, and M. H. Alderman. Divalent cations in essential hypertension. *New Eng. J. of Med.* 309:888–91 (1983).

7. Resnick, L. M., R. K. Gupta, and J. H. Laragh. Intracellular free magnesium in red blood cells of essential hypertension: relation to blood pressure and serum divalent cations. *Proc. Nat. Acad. Sci.* 81:6511–15 (1984).

8. Whang, R., and J. K. Aikawa. Magnesium deficiency and refractoriness to potassium repletion. *J. Chron. Dis.* 30:65–68 (1977); and Dyckner, T., and P. O. Wester. Intracellular potassium after magnesium infusion. *Brit. Med. J.* April 1:822–23 (1978).

9. Berthelot, A., and J. Esposito. Effects of dietary magnesium on the development of hypertension in the spontaneously hypertensive rat. *J. Amer. College of Nutr.* 4:343–53 (1983).

10. Lim, P., and E. Jacob. Magnesium deficiency in patients on long-term diuretic therapy for heart failure. *Brit. Med. J.* Sept. 9:620–622 (1972).

11. Blackfan, K. D., and B. Hamilton. Uremia in acute glomerular nephritis. *Boston Med. Surg. J.* 193:617–628 (1925).

12. Conradt, A. H. Weidinger, and H. Algayer. Evidence that magnesium deficiency could be a causal factor of (essential) gestosis. In *Recent Advances in Pathophysiological Conditions in Pregnancy* ed. by J. G. Schenker, E. T. Rippmann, and D. Weinstein. Elsevier Science Publishers B. V., pp. 36–39 (1984).

13. Dyckner, T., and P. O. Wester. Effect of magnesium on blood pressure. *Brit. Med. J.* 286:1847–49 (1983).

14. Addison, W. L. T. The use of calcium chloride in arterial hypertension. *Can. Med. Assoc. J.* 14:1059–61 (1924).

15. Johnson, N. E., E .L. Smith, and J. L. Freudenheim. Effects on blood pressure of calcium supplementation of women. *Amer. J. Clin. Nutr.* 42:12–17 (1985).

16. Resnick, L., as reported in: Calcium effective for low-renin hypertension. *Cardiol. Observ.* 1(3):4 (1984).

17. Belizan, J. M., J. Villar. A. Zalazar, L. Rohas, D. Chan, and G. F. Bryce. Preliminary evidence of the effect of calcium supplementa-

tion on blood pressure in normal pregnant women. *Amer. J. Obstet. & Gyn.* 146:175–180 (1983).

18. McCarron, D. A., C. D. Morris, H. J. Henry, and J. L. Stanton. Blood pressure and nutrient intake in the United States. *Science* 224:1392–98 (1984); and Harlan, W. R., A. L. Hull, R. L. Schoulder, J. R. Landis, F. E. Thompson, and F. A. Larkin. Blood pressure and nutrition in adults. The national Health and Nutrition Examination Survey. *Amer. J. Epidemiol.* 120:17–28 (1984).

19. Strazzullo, P., V. Nunziata, M. Cirillo, R. Giannattasio, L. A. Ferrara, P. L. Mattioli, and M. Mancini. Abnormalities of calcium metabolism in essential hypertension. *Clin. Sci.* 65:137–41 (1983).

20. Kesteloot, H., J. Geboers, and R. Van Hoof. Epidemiological study of the relationship between calcium and blood pressure. *Hypertension* 5(Suppl. II):52–56 (1983).

21. See 20.

22. McCarron, D. A. Calcium, Magnesium, and phosphorus balance in human and experimental hypertension. *Hypertension* 4(Suppl. III):27–33 (1982).

23. Kotchen, T. A., R. G. Luke, C. E. Ott, J. H. Galla, and B. G. S. Whitescarver. Effect of chloride on renin and blood pressure response to sodium chloride. *Ann. Int. Med.* 98(Part 2):817–22 (1983); and Kurtz, T. W., and R. C. Morris. Dietary Chloride as a determinant of "sodium-dependent" hypertension. *Science* 222:1139–41 (1983).

24. Addison, W. L. T. The use of sodium chloride, potassium chloride, sodium bromide and potassium bromide in cases of arterial hypertension which are amenable to potassium chloride. *Can. Med. Assoc. J.* 18:281–85 (1928).

25. Iacono, J. M., R. M. Dougherty, and P. Puska. Reduction of blood pressure associated with dietary polyunsaturated fat. *Hypertension* 4(Suppl. III):34–42 (1982); and Puska, P., J. M. Iacono, A. Nissinen, H. J. Korhonen, E. Vartiainen, P. Pientinen, R. Dougherty, U. Leino, M. Mutanen, S. Moisio, J. Huttunen. Controlled, randomized trial of the effect of dietary fat on blood pressure. *Lancet* 1:1–5 (1983).

26. Fleischman, A. I., M. L. Bierenbaum, A. Stier, S. H. Somol, P. Watson, and A. M. Naso. Hypotensive effect of increased dietary linoleic acid in mildly hypertensive humans. *J. Med. Soc. New Jersey* 76:181–83 (1979).

27. Tobian, L., M. Ganguli, M. A. Johnson, and J. Iwai. Influence of renal prostaglandins and dietary linoleate on hypertension in Dahl S. rats. *Hypertension* 4:(Suppl. II):149–53 (1982).

28. Iacono, J. M., P. Puska, R. M. Dougherty, P. Pietinen, E. Vartiainen, U. Leino, M. Mutanen, and S. Moisio. Effect of dietary fat on blood pressure in a rural Finnish population. *Amer. J. Clin. Nutr.* 38:860–69 (1983).

29. Cooke, K. M., G. W. Frost, I. R. Thornell, and G. S. Stokes. Alcohol consumption and blood pressure survey of the relationship at a health-screening clinic. *Med. J. Austral.* 1:65–69 (1982); and Kromhout, D., E. D. Bosschieter, and C. de L. Coulander. Potassium, calcium, alcohol intake and blood pressure: the Zutphen study. *Amer. J. Clin. Nutr.* 41:1299–1304 (1985).

30. Klatsky, A. L., G. D. Friedman, A. B. Siegelaub, and M. J. Gerard. Alcohol consumption and blood pressure. *New Eng. J. Med.* 296:1194–1200 (1977).

31. Knutsson, E., and S. Katz. The effect of ethanol on the membrane permeability to sodium and potassium ions in frog muscle fibres. *Acta Pharmacol. Toxicol.* 25:54–64 (1967).

32. Seelig, M. S. *Magnesium Deficiency in the Pathogenesis of Disease.* Plenum Medical Book Co., New York (1980).

33. Stanton, J. L., L. E. Braitman, A. M. Riley Jr., C. S. Khoo, and J. L. Smith. Demographic, dietary, life style, and anthropometric correlates of blood pressure. *Hypertension* 4(Suppl. III):136–42 (1982).

34. Skrabal, F., J. Aubock, H. Hortnagl, H. Braunsteiner. Effect of moderate salt restriction and high potassium intake on pressor hormones, response to noradrenaline and baroreceptor function in man. *Clin. Sci.* 59:157–60 (1980).

35. Seer, P. Psychological control of essential hypertension: review of the literature and methodical critique. *Psychol. Bull.* 86:1015–43 (1979).

36. Aoki, K, K. Sato, S. Kondo, C. B. Pyon, and M. Yamamoto. Increased response of blood pressure to rest and handgrip in subjects with essential hypertension. *Jap. Circ. J.* 47:802–809 (1983).

37. See 35.

38. Brennan, P. J., G. Greenberg, W. E. Miall, and S. G. Thompson. Seasonal variation in arterial blood pressure. *Brit. Med. J.* 285:919–23 (1982).

Chapter 10. Eat Right

1. Eaton, S. B., and M. Konner. Paleolithic nutrition. *New Eng. J. Med.* 312:283–289 (1985).

2. Jacobson, M., B. F. Liebman, and G. Moyer. *Salt: The Brand Name Guide to Sodium Content.* Workman, New York (1983).

3. Ledger, H. P. Body composition as a basis for a comparative study of some east African mammals. *Symp. Zool. Soc. Lond.* 21:289–310 (1968).
4. Phillipson, B. E., D. W. Rothrock, W. E. Conner, W. S. Harris, and D. R. Illingworth. Reduction of plasma lipids, lipoproteins, and apoproteins by dietary fish oils in patients with hypertriglyceridemia. *New Eng. J. Med.* 312:1210–16 (1985); and Kromhout, D., E. B. Bosschieter, and C. de L. Coulander. The inverse relation between fish consumption and 20-year mortality from coronary heart disease. *New Eng. J. Med.* 312:1205–1209 (1985).
5. Johnson, N. E., E. L. Smith, and J. L. Freudenheim. Effects on blood pressure of calcium supplementation of women. *Amer. J. Clin. Nutr.* 42:12–17 (1985).
6. Conradt, A., H. Weidinger, and H. Algayer. On the role of magnesium in fetal hypotrophy, pregnancy induced hypertension, and pre-eclampsia. *Magn. Bull.* 2:68–76 (1984).
7. Lipid Research Clinics Program. The lipid research clinics coronary primary prevention trial results. *J. Amer. Med. Assoc.* 251:351–374 (1984).
8. Singer, P., W. Jaeger, M. Wirth, S. Voight, E. Naumann, S. Zimontkowski, I. Hajdu, and W. Goedicke. Lipid and blood pressure-lowering effect of mackerel diet in man. *Atherosclerosis* 49:99–108 (1983).
9. *See* 4. (1st ref.).
10. *See* 4. (2nd ref.).
11. Henningsen, N. C., L. Larson, and D. Nelson. Hypertension, potassium, and the kitchen. *Lancet* 1:133 (1983).
12. Silva, P., J. F. Hayslett, and F. H. Epstein. The role of Na-K–activated adenosine triphosphate in potassium adaptation. *J. Clin. Invest.* 52:2665–71 (1973).
13. *See* 12.

Chapter 11. Exercise

1. Cade, R., D. Mars, H. Wagemaker, C. Zauner, D. Packer, M. Privette, M. Cade, J. Peterson, D. Hood-Lewis. Effect of aerobic exercise training on patients with systemic arterial hypertension. *Amer. J. Med.* 77:785–90 (1984).
2. Yeater, R. A., and I. H. Ullrich. The role of physical activity in disease prevention and treatment. *W. Virg. Med. J.* 81:35–39 (1985).
3. Blair, S. N., N. N. Goodyear, L. W. Gibbons, and K. H. Cooper. Physical Fitness and incidence of hypertension in healthy nor-

motensive men and women. *J. Amer. Med. Assoc.* 252:487–90 (1984).
4. Hanson, P., and R. Kochan. Exercise and diabetes. *Prim. Care* 10:653–62 (1982).
5. *See 4.*
6. Billman, G. E., P. J. Schwartz, and H. L. Stone. The effects of daily exercise on susceptibility to sudden cardiac death. *Circulation* 69:1182–89 (1984).
7. Cooper, K. H., M. D., M. P. H. *Running With Fear: How to Reduce the Risk of Heart Attack and Sudden Death During Aerobic Exercise.* M. Evans and Co., New York (1985).
8. *See 7.*
9. Thompson, P. D., E. J. Funk, R. A. Carleton, and W. Q. Sturner. Incidence of death during jogging in Rhode Island from 1975 through 1980. *J. Amer. Med. Assoc.* 247:2535–38 (1980).
10. Siscovick, D. S., N. S. Weiss, R. H. Fletcher, and T. Lasky. The incidence of primary cardiac arrest during vigorous exercise. *New Eng. J. Med.* 311:874–77 (1984).
11. Ragosta, M. Death during recreational exercise in the state of Rhode Island. *Med. Sci. Sports Exer.* 16:339–342 (1984).
12. Vuori, I., M. Makarainen, and A. Jaaskelainen. Sudden death and physical activity. *Cardiology* 63:287–304 (1978).
13. *See 7.*
14. Sheenan, G. Live to win. The Keynote Address at the Wellness Strategies Conference, Trenton, N.J., June 1985.
15. Pritikin, N. In *The Pritikin Promise: 28 days to a longer Healthier Life.* Simon & Schuster, New York (1983).
16. Lamb, L. E. *Health Letter* 13:1–4 (1979).
17. Paffenbarger, R. S., Jr., A. L. Wing, and R. T. Hyde. Physical activity as an index of heart attack risk in college alumni. *Amer. J. Epidemiol.* 108:161–75 (1978).
18. Paffenbarger, R. S., Jr., R. T. Hyde, A. L. Wing, and C. H. Steinmetz. A natural history of athleticism and cardiovascular health. *J. Amer. Med. Assoc.* 252:491–95 (1984).
19. *See 10.*
20. Nabokov, P. *Indian Running.* Capra Press, Santa Barbara (1981).
21. Yeater, R. A., and R. B. Martin. Senile osteoporosis: the effects of exercise. *Postgrad. Med.* 75:147–59 (1984).
22. MacDougall, J. D. Tuxen, D. G. Sale, J. R. Moroz, and J. R. Sutton. Arterial blood pressure responses to heavy resistance exercise. *J. Appl. Physiol.* 58:785–90 (1985).
23. Freedson, P. More on hypertension and lifting. *Physic. Sportsmed.* 12(#10):21 (1984).

24. Dr. Rachel A. Yeater, Univ. of W. Virg., personal communication.
25. Shephard, R. J. *Endurance Fitness*. Univ of Toronto Press, Toronto (1977).
26. White, M. K., R. A. Yeater, R. B. Martin, *et al.* The effects of aerobic dancing and walking on the cardiovascular and muscular systems of post-menopausal females. *J. Sports Med. Phys. Fit.* 24:159–66 (1984); and Milburn, S., and N. K. Butts. A comparison of the training responses to aerobic dance and jogging in college females. *Med. Sci. Sports and Exer.* 15:510–13 (1984).
27. *See* 12.
28. Allen, C. J., M. A. Craven, D. Rosenbloom, and J. R. Sutton. Beta-blockade and exercise in normal subjects and patients with coronary artery disease. *Physic. Sportsmed.* 12:51–63 (1984).
29. American College of Sports Medicine. Position statement on the recommended quantity of exercise for developing and maintaining fitness in healthy adults. *Amer. Coll. Sportsmed.* 10:1–4 (1978).
30. *See* 29.
31. Seals, D. R., and J. M. Hagberg. The effect of exercise training on human hypertension: a review. *Med. Sci. Sports Exer.* 16:207–215 (1984).
32. *See* 7.
33. *See* 29.
34. *See* 29.
35. Krotkiewski, M., K. Mandroukas, L. Sjostrom, L. Sullivan, H. Wetterqvist, and P. Bjorntorp. Effects of long-term physical training on body fat, metabolism, and blood pressure in obesity. *Metab.* 28:650–658 (1979).
36. *See* 1.
37. *See* 14.
38. Sheehan G. A. *Running and Being. The Total Experience*. Simon & Schuster, New York, (1978).
39. *See* 7.

Chapter 12. *Help Your Body Find Its Proper Weight*

1. Sims, E. A. H. Diabesity and obitension: common mechanisms and common management. In *Controversies in Obesity*, ed. by B. C. Hansen. Praeger, New York (1983); and Kolanowski, J. Pathophysiology of hypertension in overweight subjects. *Medicographia* 7:29–31, 51 (1985).
2. Reisin, E., R. Abel, M. Modan, D. S. Silverberg, H. E. Eliahou, and B. Modan. Effect of weight loss without salt restriction on the re-

duction of blood pressure in overweight patients. *New Eng. J. Med.* 298:1–6 (1978); and Eliahou, H. E., A. Iaina, T. Gaon, J. Shochat, and M. Modan. Body weight reduction necessary to attain normotension in the overweight hypertensive patient. *Int. J. Obes.* 5(Suppl. 1):157–63 (1981).

3. Presta, E., J. Wang, G. G. Harrison, P. Bjorntorp, W. H. Harker, and T. B. van Itallie. Measurement of total body electrical conductivity: a new method for estimation of body composition. *Amer. J. Clin. Nutr.:* 37:735–39 (1983).

4. Ismail-Beigi, F., and I. S. Edelman. Mechanism of thyroid calorigenesis: role of active sodium transport. *Proc. Natl. Acad. Sci.* 67:1071–78 (1970).

5. Remington, D. W., A. G. Fisher, and E. A. Parent. *How to Lower your Fat Thermostat.* Vitality House, Provo, UT (1983).

6. Clausen, T., O. Hansen, K. Kjeldsen, and A. Norgaard. Effect of age, potassium depletion and denervation on specific displaceable [^{3}H]ouabain binding in rat skeletal muscle *in vivo. J. Physiol.* 333:367–81 (1982); and Kjeldsen, K., A. Norgaard, and T. Clausen. Effect of K-depletion on ^{3}H-ouabain binding and Na-K contents in mammalian skeletal muscle. *Acta Physiol. Scand.* 122:103–17 (1984).

7. Kolata, G. Why do people get fat? *Science* 227:1327–28 (1985).

8. Oscai, L. B., M. M. Brown, and W. C. Miller. Effect of dietary fat of food intake, growth and body composition. *Growth* 48:415–24 (1984).

9. Flatt, J. P. The biochemistry of energy expenditure. *Recent Adv. Obes. Res.* II:211–18. Ed. by G. S. Bray. Newmann Pub. Co., London, (1978); and Flatt, J. P. Energetics of intermediary metabolism in substrate and energy metabolism in man. *Int. J. Obes.* 9(Suppl. 2):58–69. Ed. by J. S. Garrow and J. Halliday. John Libby, London (1985).

10. Danforth, E., Jr. Diet and obesity. *Amer. J. Clin. Nutr.* 41:1132–45 (1985).

11. Hanson, P., and R. Kochan. Exercise and diabetes. *Prim. Care* 10:653–62 (1983).

12. Rowe, J. W., J. B. Young, K. L. Minaker, A. L. Stevens, J. Palotta, and L. Landsbert. Effect of insulin and glucose infusions on sympathetic nervous system activity in normal man. *Diabetes* 30:219–25 (1981).

13. Fagerberg, B., O. Andersson, U. Nilsson, T. Hedner, B. Isaksson, and P. Bjorntorp. Weight-reducing diets: role of carbohydrates on sym-

pathetic nervous activity and hypotensive response. *Int. J. Obes.* 8:237–43 (1984).
14. *See* 5.

Chapter 18. The Emphasis on Drugs

1. Toffler, A. Science and Change. Forward to *Order out of Chaos* by I. Prigogine and I. Stengers. Bantam Books, Toronto (1984).
2. Guttmacher, S., M. Teitelman, G. Chapin, G. Garbowski, and P. Schnall. Ethics and preventive medicine: the case of borderline hypertension. *Hastings Center Report* 12–20 (Feb. 1981).
3. Dahl, L. K. Salt and hypertension. *Amer. J. Clin. Nutr.* 25:231–44 (1972).

Chapter 19. Scientific Paradigm and Scientific "Proof"

1. D. O. Edge, personal communication.
2. Wheeler, J. The universe as home for man. *The Nature of Scientific Discovery*, ed. by G. Owen. Smithsonian Institution Press, Washington, D.C. (1975).
3. Wheeler, John. In a talk delivered to the National Academy of Sciences (1975).
4. Jung, C. G. *The Interpretation of Nature and the Psyche. Synchronicity: an Acausal Connecting Principle*; and Pauli, W. *The Influence of Archetypal Ideals on the Scientific Theories of Kepler.* Pantheon Books, New York (1955).
5. Capra, F. *The Tao of Physics.* Shambhala Publications, Boulder, CO (1975); Herbert, N. *Quantum Reality.* Anchor Press/Doubleday, Garden City, NY (1985); Pagels, H. R. *The Cosmic Code.* Simon & Schuster, New York (1982); Wolf, F. A. *Taking the Quantum Leap.* Harper & Row, San Francisco (1981); and Zukav, G. *The Dancing Wu Li Masters.* William Morrow, New York (1979).
6. Gliedman, J. Turning Einstein upside down. In The quantum universe of John Archibald Wheeler nothing exists until it is observed. *Sci. Digest*:34–97 (October, 1984).
7. Teilhard de Chardin, P. *The Future of Man.* Harper & Row, New York (1964); and Teilhard de Chardin, P. *The Phenomenon of Man.* Harper & Bro., New York (1959).
8. Naisbitt, J. *Megatrends. Ten New Directions Transforming Our Lives.* Warner Books, New York (1982).
9. Ferguson, M. *the Aquarian Conspiracy: Personal and Social Transformation in the 1980's.* Houghton Mifflin, Boston (1980).

10. Warren, J. V., D. N. Plumb, and G. L. Trzebiatowski. A crisis in medical education. Thoughts on listening to a conference on medical education for the 21st century. *J. Amer. Med. Assoc.* 253:2404–2407 (1985).

11. Flexner, A. *Medical Education in the United States and Canada. A Report to the Carnegie Foundation for the Advancement of Teaching.* Merrymount Press, Boston (1910).

12. Becker, R. O., and A. A. Marino. *Electromagnetism and Life.* State University of New York Press, Albany (1982).

13. See 12.

14. See 2.

15. Harlan, W. R., A. L. Hull, R. L. Schoulder, J. R. Landis, F. E. Thompson, and F. A. Larkin. Blood pressure and nutrition in adults. The national Health and Nutrition Examination Survey. *Amer. J. Epidemiol.* 120:17–28 (1984).

16. Stanton, J. L., L. E. Braitman, A. M. Riley, Jr., C. S. Khoo, and J. L. Smith. Demographic, dietary, life style, and anthropometric correlates of blood pressure. *Hypertension* 4(Suppl. III):136–42. (1982).

17. McCarron, D. A., C. D. Morris, H. J. Henry, and J. L. Stanton. Blood pressure and nutrient intake in the United States. *Science* 244:1392–98 (1984).

18. Gruchow, H. W., K. A. Sobocinski, and J. J. Barboriak. Alcohol, nutrient intake, and hypertension in U.S. adults. *J. Amer. Med. Assoc.* 253:1567–70 (1985).

19. Multiple Risk Factor Intervention Trial Research Group. Multiple risk factor intervention trial. Risk factor changes and mortality results. *J. Amer. Med. Assoc.* 248:1465–77 (1982).

20. Morgan, T. O., W. R. Adam, M. Hodgson, and R. W. Gibberd. Failure of therapy to improve prognosis in elderly males with hypertension. *Med. J. Austral.* 2:27–31 (1980).

21. Hypertension Detection and Follow-up Program Cooperative Group. Five-year findings of the hypertension detection and follow-up program. I. Reduction in mortality of persons with high blood pressure, including mild hypertension. *J. Amer. Med. Assoc.* 242:2562–71 (1979).

22. Veterans Administration Cooperative Study Group on Antihypertensive Agents. Effects of treatment on morbidity in hypertension. II. Results in patients with diastolic blood pressures averaging 90 through 114 mm Hg. *J. Amer. Med. Assoc.* 213:1143–52 (1970).

23. Management Committee: The Australian therapeutic trail in mild hypertension. *Lancet* 1:1261–67 (1980).

24. Cade, R., D. Mars, H. Wagemaker, C. Zauner, D. Packer, M. Privette,

M. Cade, J. Peterson, and D. Hood-Lewis. Effect of aerobic exercise training on patients with systemic arterial hypertension. *Amer. J. Med.* 77:785–90 (1984).

25. Gould, Steven J. *Ever Since Darwin.* Norton, New York (1977).

Chapter 20. *Additional Evidence*

1. Sigurdsson, J. A., and C. Bengtsson. Urinary findings and renal function in hypertensive and normotensive women. (from the Korpilampi Hypertension Meeting, 1980). *Acta Med. Scand.* (Suppl. 646):51–53 (1981).
2. Lever, A. F., C. Beretta-Piccoli, J. J. Brown, D. L. Davies, R. Fraser, and J.I.S. Robertson. Sodium and potassium in essential hypertension. *Brit. Med. J.* 283:463–68 (1981).
3. Bulpitt, C. J., M. J. Shipley, and A. Semmence. Blood pressure and plasma sodium and potassium. *Clin. Sci.* 61:85–87 (1981).
4. Usehima, H., M. Tanigaki, M. Ida, T. Shimamoto, M. Konishi, and Y. Komachi. Hypertension, salt, and potassium. *Lancet* I:504 (1981).
5. Maxwell, M. H., E. Fitzsimmons, R. Harrist, J. Hotchkiss, H. G. Langford, G. H. Payne, K. A. Schneider, and P. Varaday. Baseline laboratory examination characteristics of the hypertensive participants. *Hypertension* 5(Part 2):133–59 (1983).
6. Ericsson, F. Intracellular potassium in man. *Scand. J. Clin. Lab. Invest.* 42(Suppl. 163):1–58 (1982).
7. *See* 2.
8. Sasaki, N. High blood pressure and the salt intake of the Japanese. *Jap. Heart J.* 3:313–24 (1962).
9. Walker, W. G., P. K. Whelton, H. Saito, R. P. Russell, and J. Hermann. Relation between blood pressure and renin, renin substrate, angiotensin II, aldosterone and urinary sodium and potassium in 574 ambulatory subjects. *Hypertension* 1:287–91 (1979).
10. Watson, R. L., H. G. Langford, J. Abernethy, T. Y. Barnes, and M. J. Watson. Urinary electrolytes, body weight, and blood pressure: pooled cross-sectional results among four groups of adolescent females. *Hypertension* 2:93–98 (1980).
11. Grim, C. E., F. C. Luft, J. Z. Miller, G. R. Meneely, H. D. Battarbee, C. G. Hames, and L. K. Dahl. Racial differences in blood pressure in Evans County, Georgia: relationship to sodium and potassium intake and plasma renin activity. *J. Chron. Dis.* 33:87–94 (1980).
12. *See* 10.
13. Langford, H. G. Dietary potassium and hypertension: epidemiologic data. *Ann. Intern. Med.* 98(Part 2):770–72 (1983).

14. Sever, P. S., D. Gordon, W. S. Peart, and P. Beighton. Blood-pressure and its correlates in urban and tribal Africa. *Lancet* 2:60–64. (1980).

15. Stressen, J., K. Jagard, P. Lynsn, A. Amery, C. Bulpitt, and J. V. Joossens. Salt and blood pressure in Belgium. *J. Epidem. Commun. Health* 35:256–61 (1981).

16. Meneely, George R., and Con O. T. Ball. Experimental epidemiology of chronic sodium chloride toxicity and the protective effect of potassium chloride. *Amer. J. Med.* 25:713–25 (1958).

17. Dahl, L. K., G. Leitl, and M. Heine. Influence of dietary potassium and sodium/potassium molar ratios on the development of salt hypertension. *J. Exp. Med.* 136:318–30 (1972).

18. Battarbee, H. D., D. P. Funch, and J. W. Dailey. The effect of dietary sodium and potassium upon blood pressure and catecholamine excretion in the rat. *Proc. Soc. Exp. Biol. Med.* 161:32–37 (1979).

19. Treasure, J., and D. Ploth. Role of dietary potassium in the treatment of hypertension. *Hypertension* 5:864–72 (1983).

20. Haddy, F. J. Minireview. Potassium and blood vessels. *Life Sci.* 16:1489–98 (1975).

21. Webb, R. C., and D. F. Bohr. Potassium relaxation of vascular smooth muscle from spontaneously hypertensive rats. *Blood Vessels* 16:71–79 (1979).

22. Tannen, R. L. Effects of potassium on blood pressure control. *Ann. Intern. Med.* 98(Part 2):773–80 (1983).

23. Fujita, T., Y. Sato, and K. Ando. Role of sympathetic nerve activity and natriuresis in the antihypertensive actions of potassium in NaCl hypertension. *Jap. Circ. J.* 47:1227–31 (1983).

24. See 22.

25. Dustin, H. P. Mechanisms of hypertension associated with obesity. *Ann. Int. Med.* 98(Part 2):860–64 (1983); and Havlik, R. J., H. B. Hubert, R. R. Fabsitz, and M. Feinleib. Weight and hypertension. *Ann. Intern. Med.* 98(Part 2):855–59 (1983).

26. Eliahou, H. E., A. Iaina, T. Gaon, J. Shochat, and M. Modan. Body weight reduction necessary to attain normotension in the overweight hypertensive patient. *Int. J. Obes.* 5(Suppl. 1):157–163 (1981).

27. Mineur, P., and J. Kolanowski. Changes in blood pressure and cardiovascular indices of adrenergic activity in obese subjects undergoing total starvation. *J. Obes. Weight Regul.* 2:69–79 (1983).

28. Nizet, A., P. Lefebvre, and J. Crabbé. Control by insulin of sodium-potassium and water excretion by isolated dog kidneys. *Pflug. Arch.* 323:11–20 (1971).

29. Defronzo, R. A., R. Sherwin, M. Dillingham, R. Hendeler, W. Tamborlane, and P. Felig. Influence of basil insulin and glucagon secretion on potassium and on sodium metabolism studies with somatostatin in normal dogs and in normal and diabetic human beings. *J. Clin. Invest.* 61:472–479 (1978).

30. Sims, E.A.H. Diabesity and obitension: common mechanisms and common management. In *Controversies in Obesity*, B. C. Hansen, ed. Praeger, New York (1983).

31. Moore, R. D. Effect of insulin on ion transport. *Biochem. Biophys. Acta* 737:1–49 (1983).

32. Berchtold, P., and E.A.H. Sims. Obesity and hypertension: conclusions and recommendations. *Int. J. Obes.* 5(Suppl. 1):183–184 (1981).

33. Wayne Gavryck, personal communication.

34. See 26, and 27.

35. Rowe, J. W., J. B. Young, K. L. Minaker, A. L. Stevens, J. Palotta, and L. Landsberg. Effect of insulin and glucose infusions on sympathetic nervous system activity in normal man. *Diabetes* 30:219–25 (1981).

36. Besarab, A., P. Silva, and L. Landsberg. Effect of catecholamines on tubular function in the isolated perfused rat kidney. *Amer. J. Physiol.* 233:39–45 (1977); and Gullner, H. G. The role of the adrenergic nervous system in sodium and water excretion. *Klin. Wochenschr.* 61:1063–66 (1983).

37. Marks, P., B. Wilson, and A. Delassalle. Aldosterone studies in obese patients with hypertension. *Amer. J. Med. Sci.* 289:224–28 (1985).

38. Krotkiewski, M., P. Bjorntorp, G. Holm, V. Marks, L. Morgan, U. Smith, and G. E. Feurle. Effects of physical training on insulin, connecting peptide (C-peptide) gastric inhibitory polypeptide (GIP) and pancreatic polypeptide (PP) levels in obese subjects. *Int. J. Obes.* 8:193–99 (1984); and Bjorntorp, P., K. De Jounge, L. Sjostrom, and L. Sullivan. The effect of physical training on insulin production in obesity. *Metabolism* 19:631–38 (1970).

39. Moore, R. D., J. W. Munford, and T. J. Pillsworth. Effects of streptozotocin diabetes and fasting on intracellular sodium and adenosine triphosphate in rat soleus muscle. *J. Physiol.* 338:277–94 (1983).

40. Page, M. McB., R.B.W. Smith, and P. J. Watkins. Postural hypotension and tachycardia induced by insulin. *Austral. New Z. J. Med.* 6:169 (1976).

41. Koivisto, V. A., and L. Groop. Physical training in juvenile diabetes.

Ann. Clin. Res. 14(Suppl. 34):74–79 (1982).

42. Welborn, T. A., A. Breckenridge, A. H. Rubinstein, C. T. Dollery, and T. Russell Frazer. Serum-insulin in essential hypertension and in peripheral vascular disease. *Lancet* 1:1336–37 (1966).

43. Haddy, F. J. Mechanism, prevention and therapy of sodium-dependent hypertension. *Amer. J. Med.* 69:746–58 (1980).

44. *See* 43.

Chapter 21. How Important Is Salt?

1. Conn, J. W. The mechanism of acclimatization to heat. *Adv. Intern. Med.* 3:373–93 (1949).

2. Thomas, W. A. Health of a carnivorous race. A study of the Eskimo. *J. Amer. Med. Assoc.* 88:1559–60 (1927).

3. Dahl, L. K. Salt and hypertension. *Amer. J. Clin. Nutr.* 25:231–44 (1972).

4. *Ibid. See* 3.

5. Dole, V. P., L. K. Dahl, G. C. Cotzias, H. A. Eder, and M. E. Krebs. Dietary treatment of hypertension: clinical and metabolic studies of patients on rice-fruit diet. *J. Clin. Invest.* 29:1189–1206 (1950).

6. Smith, S. E., and P. D. Aines. Salt requirements of dairy cows. *N.Y. Agr. Exp. Sta. Ithaca Bull.* 938:1–26 (1959).

7. Babcock, S. M. The addition of salt to the ration of dairy cows. *Wisc. Agr. Exper. Sta. Ann. Rpt.*, 129 (1905); and Cox, R. F., and E. F. Smith. Salt for beef cattle and sheep. Salt Institute, Chicago (1957).

8. Tobe, J. H. *Salt and Your Health*, 37. Hearthside Press, New York (1965).

9. Patton, A. R. A letter in *Nutr. Rev.* 11:159 (1953).

10. Watt, B. K., and A. L. Merrill. *Composition of Foods.* Agriculture Handbook No. 8, U.S. Dept. of Agriculture, U.S. Government Printing Office, Washington, D.C. (1975); and Altman, P. L., and D. S. Dittmer, ed. *Biological Handbooks. Blood and Other Body Fluids.* Fed. Amer. Soc. for Exptl. Biol., Washington, D.C. (1961), 455–58.

11. Beauchamp, G. K., M. Bertino, and K. Engelman. Modification of salt taste. *Ann. Intern. Med.* 98(Part 2):763–69 (1983).

Chapter 22. Kidneys, Hormones, and Nervous System

1. Dahl, L. K., M. Heine, and K. Thompson. Genetic influence of the kidneys on blood pressure. Evidence from chronic renal homografts in rats with opposite predispositions to hypertension. *Circulation Res.* 34:94–100 (1974).

2. *See* 1; and Bianchi, G., U. Fox, G. F. Di Francesco, A. M. Giovanetti,

and D. Pagetti, Blood pressure changes produced by kidney cross-transplantation between spontaneously hypertensive rats and normotensive rats. *Clin. Sci. & Molec. Med.* 47:435–48 (1974).
3. *Ibid. See 2.*
4. Tobian, L. Salt and Hypertension. In *Hypertension, Physiopathology and Treatment*, J. Genest, O. Kuchel, P. Hamet, and M. Cantin, eds., McGraw-Hill Book Company, New York (1983), 73–83.
5. Moore, R. D. Effect of insulin upon sodium pump in frog skeletal muscle. *J. Physiol.* 232:23–45 (1973).
6. Nizet, A., P. Lefebvre, and J. Crabbé. Control by insulin of sodium potassium and water excretion by the isolated dog kidney. *Pflug. Arch.* 323:11–20 (1971).
7. Hamlyn, J. M., P. D. Levinson, R. Ringel, P. A. Levin, B. P. Hamilton, M. P. Blaustein, and A. A. Kowarski. Relationships among endogenous digitalis-like factors in essential hypertension. *Fed. Proc.* 44:2782–88 (1985); and de Wardener, H. E., and G. A. MacGregor. The relation of a circulating sodium transport inhibitor (the natriuretic hormone?) to hypertension. *Medicine* 62:310–26 (1983).

Chapter 23. Antihypertensive Drugs

1. The Joint National Committee of Detection, Evaluation, and Treatment of High Blood Pressure. The 1984 report of the Joint National Committee of Detection, Evaluation, and Treatment of High Blood Pressure. *Arch. Intern. Med.* 144:1045–57 (1984).
Baker, C. E., Jr. *Physicians' Desk Reference (PDR 34th Ed.)*. Medical Economics, Oradell, N.J. (1980).
2. Bennett, W. M., W. J. McDonald, E. Kuehnel, M. N. Hartnett, and G. A. Porter. Do diuretics have antihypertensive properties independent of natriuresis? *Clin. Pharmacol. Ther.* 22:499–504 (1977).
3. Edmonds, C. J., and B. Jasani. Total-body potassium in hypertensive patients during prolonged diuretic therapy. *Lancet* 2:8–12 (1972).
4. *See 3*; and Wilkinson, P. R., H. Issler, R. Hesp, and E. B. Raftery. Total body and serum potassium during prolonged thiazide therapy for essential hypertension. *Lancet* 1:759–62 (1975).
5. Schwartz, W. B. Potassium and the kidney. *New Eng. J. Med.* 253:601–608 (1955).
6. Morgan, T. O., W. R. Adam, M. Hodgson, and R. W. Gibberd. Failure of therapy to improve prognosis in elderly males with hypertension. *Med. J. Aust.* 2:27–31 (1980).
7. Lim, P., and E. Jacob. Magnesium deficiency in patients on long-term diuretic therapy for heart failure. *Brit. Med. J.* 3:620–22 (1972).

8. Gilman, A. G., L. S. Goodman, and A. Gilman, eds. *The Pharmacological Basis of Therapeutics* (6th edition). MacMillan, New York (1980).
9. *See* 1.
10. *See* 8.
11. *See* 8.
12. *See* 8.
13. *See* 8.

Chapter 24. *Recommendations for the Physician*

1. The Joint National Committee of Detection, Evaluation, and Treatment of High Blood Pressure. The 1984 report of the Joint National Committee of Detection, Evaluation, and Treatment of High Blood Pressure. *Arch. Intern. Med.* 144:1045–57 (1984).
2. Kaplan, Norman M. Hypertension: prevalance, risks, and effect of therapy. *Ann. Intern. Med.* 98:705–709 (1983).
3. Freis E. D. Should mild hypertension be treated? *New Eng. J. Med.* 307:306–309 (1982).
4. Multiple Risk Factor Intervention Trial Research Group. Multiple risk factor intervention trial. Risk factor changes and mortality results. *J. Amer. Med. Assoc.* 248:1465–77 (1982).
5. *See* 2.
6. Sims, E. A. H., and P. Berchtold. Obesity and hypertension. Mechanisms and implications for management. *J. Amer. Med. Assoc.* 247:49–52 (1982).
7. Silva, P., J. F. Hayslett, and F. H. Eptstein. The role of Na-K–activated adenosine triphosphate in potassium adaptation. *J. Clin. Invest.* 52:2665–71 (1973); and DeFronzo, R. Extrarenal K+ regulation. A talk at the Eleventh Yale Symposium on Membrane Transport Processes, New Haven, April, 1985.
8. McMahon, F. G. The role of diet in the management of essential hypertension. *Management of Essential Hypertension*. Futura Publ., Mt. Kisco, NY (1978).
9. *See* 7 (2nd ref.)
10. *See* 7 (2nd ref.)
11. Clausen, T., O. Hansen, K. Kjeldsen, and A. Norgaard. Effect of age, potassium depletion and denervation of specific displaceable [^{3}H]ouabain binding in rat skeletal muscle *in vivo*. *J. Physiol.* 333:367–81 (1982).
12. Kaplan, N. M. Therapy for mild hypertension: toward a more balanced view. *J. Amer. Med. Assoc.* 249:365–67 (1983).

13. Iimura, O., T. Kijima, K. Kikuchi, A. Miyama, T. Ando, T. Nakao, and Y. Takigami. Studies on the hypotensive effects of high potassium intake in patients with essential hypertension. *Clin. Sci.* 61:77–80 (1981).
14. Hunt, J. C. Sodium intake and hypertension: a cause for concern. *Ann. Intern. Med.* 98:724–28 (1983).
15. Kuller, L. H., P. H. Stephen, B. Hulley, J. D. Cohen, and J. Neaton. Unexpected effects of treating hypertension in men with electrocardiographic abnormalities: a critical analysis. *Circulation* 73:114–23 (1986).
16. Sterns, R. H., M. Cox, P. U. Feig, and I. Singer. Internal potassium balance and the control of the plasma potassium concentration. *Medicine* 60:339–54 (1981).
17. Struthers A. D., R. Whitesmith, and J. L. Reid. Prior thiazide diuretic treatment increases adrenaline-induced hypokalaemia. *Lancet* 1:1358–60 (1983); and Kaplan, N. M. Our appropriate concern about hypokalemia. *Amer. J. Med.* 77:1–4 (1984).
18. Holland, O. B., J. V. Nixon, and L. Kuhnert. Diuretic-induced ventricular ectopic activity. *Amer. J. Med.* 70:762–68 (1981).
19. Nordrehaug, J. E., and G. von der Lippe. Hypokalaemia and ventricular fibrillation in acute myocardial infarction. *Brit. Heart J.* 50:525–29 (1983).
20. See 18.
21. See 17 (2nd ref.)
22. Moore, R. D., J. W. Munford, and T. J. Pillsworth, Jr. Effects of streptozotocin diabetes and fasting on intracellular sodium and adenosine triphosphate in rat soleus muscle. *J. Physiol.* 338:277–94 (1983).
23. Cooper, K. H. *Running Without Fear* M. Evans and Co., New York (1985).

Progress Chart

Age_____   Initial weight_____   Height_____   Sex_____

Week	1	2	3	4	5	6	7	8	9	10	11	12
Blood Pressure Systolic												
Diastolic												
Pulse upon awakening												
Weight (lbs.)												
Number of workouts (aerobic exercise)												
less than 20 minutes												
20 to 30 minutes												
greater than 30 minutes												
K Factor (K/Na ratio)												
Serum K (mEq./liter)												
Drugs												

Week	13	14	15	16	17	18	19	20	21	22	23	24
Blood Pressure Systolic												
Diastolic												
Pulse upon awakening												
Weight (lbs.)												
Number of workouts (aerobic exercise)												
less than 20 minutes												
20 to 30 minutes												
greater than 30 minutes												
K Factor (K/Na ratio)												
Serum K (mEq./liter)												
Drugs												

Index

Rodale Press, Inc., publishes PREVENTION®, the better health magazine.
For information on how to order your subscription,
write to PREVENTION®, Emmaus, PA 18049.

AD Biography
Roosevelt Fra 2017

Dallek, Robert, author. Franklin D. Roosevelt : a
political life   9001136995

DISCARDED BY
MEAD PUBLIC LIBRARY